Regulation
in
Metabolism

Regulation in Metabolism

E. A. Newsholme

Department of Biochemistry
University of Oxford

and

C. Start

A Wiley–Interscience Publication

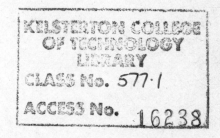
JOHN WILEY & SONS

London · New York · Sydney · Toronto

Library of Congress catalog card number 72-5721

ISBN 0 471 63530 8   Cloth bound

ISBN 0 471 63531 6   Paper bound

Reprinted December 1974

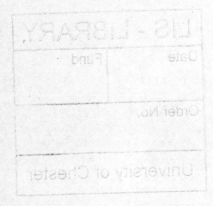

Printed in England by J. W. Arrowsmith Ltd. Bristol

PREFACE

The elucidation of the chemical reactions that constitute the major metabolic pathways during the last 30 to 40 years has provided a vast amount of information about metabolism. This information has been used to construct metabolic maps, which tend to suggest that metabolism is now fully understood. This is certainly not the case. The information contained in such maps merely provides a factual basis from which new and exciting fields of research are being developed. This research will no doubt lead to a fuller understanding of biological phenomena at a biochemical level. The new fields of research include metabolic regulation and the interrelationships of metabolism. Knowledge of metabolic regulation and pathway-interrelationships has become available at a remarkable rate during the past decade and has made it possible, now, to construct a reasonably coherent account of the regulation of some of the more universally important pathways, particularly those involved in energy release and utilization. We hope that in this book we have provided such an account.

Since most of the research in the field of metabolic regulation has been carried out relatively recently, and since certain of the theories presented are still controversial, we have discussed the available experimental evidence and its various, sometimes opposing, interpretations in some detail and we have provided a comprehensive bibliography. In some cases we have laid emphasis upon a particular theory at the expense of other plausible theories. This bias obviously reflects our personal opinions, although often these are strongly influenced by the consensus of opinion amongst research workers in the particular field. Despite the fact that certain of these theories will be modified with the acquisition of new data, the experimental basis on which the original theories were constructed should not change; it is only the interpretation of the evidence that will change. Consequently, this book should help not only in the understanding of current theories but also in following the logical developments of new theories of metabolic regulation.

The basic approach to the study of metabolic regulation, to which we have adhered throughout this book, is presented in the first chapter, along with a brief outline of the theoretical aspects of energy transfer in living organisms. Chapter 2 consists of a discussion of the regulation of enzyme activity at a molecular level and describes the various ways in which amplification of a small metabolic signal may be achieved, in particular via sigmoid response curves, whether these be of allosteric or purely kinetic origin. In particular, the sequential model of Koshland and the symmetry model of Monod, Wyman and Changeux have been discussed at length. It has been our intention to provide mathematical derivations that are entirely comprehensible to a non-mathematician and, for this reason, certain derivations (such as of heterotropic effects in the Monod–Wyman–Changeux model) are placed in an appendix so that they do not interrupt the flow of the text.

In the remaining chapters the theoretical principles and experimental techniques outlined in the first two chapters are actually applied to specific pathways in specific tissues. In some cases there is adequate knowledge available only in the case of mammalian tissues, but wherever possible other classes of animals have been included. The pathways under discussion include glycolysis, glycogen synthesis and degradation, the tricarboxylic acid cycle, fatty acid synthesis and oxidation, triglyceride synthesis and lipolysis and ketone body formation. Each pathway is treated in the same way, beginning with the elucidation of the regulatory enzymes, progressing through the theories of control of these regulatory enzymes and concluding with an appraisal of the physiological significance of the mechanism of regulation with regard to the proper functioning of the cell, the tissues and, where applicable, the animal as a whole. In this way we hope to provide such a unified approach to the subject of metabolic regulation that this book will be of use, not only to biochemistry students interested in the field of enzyme activity regulation, but also to students of physiology, medicine and biology. The book has been written with the aim of providing information about basic metabolism and its control and consequently it contains background information that may be of value to students, lecturers or research workers interested in physiological, pharmacological or clinical problems that are related to basic metabolic processes. Clinical aspects of regulation are stressed in relation to the role of the glucose/fatty acid cycle in diabetes mellitus, the role of fructose in hypertriglycerideamia, or the mechanism of mobilization of non-esterified fatty acids in response to stress and starvation. Intriguing physiological problems which are discussed include the control of fuel utilization by muscles during exercise and the control of heat production in brown adipose tissue. At a biochemical level, considerable space is given to a description of the delicate interplay between the various fuels for energy production (glucose, fatty acids, triglyceride and ketone bodies) which circulate simultaneously in the blood. The concept of the glucose/fatty acid cycle is developed to coordinate the roles and metabolic effects of these various fuels. Such a concept links the functions of several different tissues and therefore is discussed from different viewpoints in various chapters, with the aim of presenting a unified theory.

In general, this book is designed for second and third year undergraduates who have already received an introduction to the chemistry of metabolic pathways, but it should also be of some value to research students and lecturers who have to cover subjects related to metabolic regulation. The considerable amount of factual information, drawn from many different sources and presented in tabular form is supported by an extensive bibliography. Appendices have been placed at the end of certain chapters because they contain additional information relevant to the chapters in question which would have interrupted the flow of the subject matter if inserted in the body of the text.

Finally we have compiled a hormone index which deals in turn with each of the hormones whose functions are related to energy metabolism. This index was designed to aid students who need to study the various actions of an individual hormone for a particular study-project and it consists of a short description of each effect of the hormone, along with a reference to the section of the book in which the effect in question is described in greater detail.

This book could have been entitled 'Caloric Homeostasis'* since our discussion centres upon how the various fuels of respiration are made available to the major tissues under different conditions, how their concentrations in the blood are controlled, and how the rate of fuel utilization by a particular tissue is related to the needs of the tissue and to the availability of alternative fuels. However, our discussion is not confined to the physiological aspects but extends to biochemical regulation at all levels of organization from the individual enzyme to the animal as a whole. Therefore we decided that 'Regulation in Metabolism' was an apt title.

We wish to express our gratitude to our colleagues who have helped in various ways with the preparation of the material for this book. In particular, Dr B. Crabtree provided many helpful discussions, Dr D. H. Williamson provided much factual information and always at very short notice, and Dr A. R. Leech provided advice and technical expertise in the preparation of many of the Figures. Finally we would like to thank our typist, Mrs I. Mellor who produced an excellent typescript with the minimum of typographical error from our somewhat disorganized and, in parts, illegible manuscript.

---

* The term homeostasis has been defined by G. M. Hughes (1964) *Symp. Soc. Expt. Biol.*, **18**, vii, as follows:

Homeostasis in its widest context includes the coordinated physiological processes which maintain most of the steady states in organisms. Similar general principles may apply to the establishment, regulation and control of steady states for other levels of organization. It must be emphasized that homeostasis does not necessarily imply a lack of change, because the 'steady states' to which the regulatory mechanisms are directed may shift with time. But throughout the change they remain under more or less close control.

Such a concept can therefore be applied to organizations at cellular, organ system, individual and social levels. It may be considered in relation to time intervals ranging from milliseconds to millions of years. Its essential feature is the interplay of factors which tend to maintain a given state at a given time.

CONTENTS

CHAPTER 1

INTRODUCTION TO REGULATION IN METABOLIC PATHWAYS

A. INTRODUCTION

A metabolic pathway consists of a series of enzyme-catalysed reactions that convert a substrate into a product. The constituent reactions of many such pathways have been elucidated largely during the period 1930–1950 by the application of various techniques: the identification of intermediates which accumulate upon the addition of specific inhibitors of the pathway, the addition of possible intermediates of the pathway (since their conversion to the product confirms this role) and the addition of radioactively labelled substrate (or intermediates) and the study of the distribution of label in intermediates and product. The final stage has involved the separation of the enzymes of the pathway and the elucidation of the chemistry of each reaction in isolation. The results of these investigations have been collated into the metabolic maps which adorn the walls of many laboratories. The advent of such maps, in which metabolic pathways are presented rather like a wiring diagram for a piece of electronic apparatus, has served a useful purpose in providing a visual aid for understanding and memorizing complex pathways. However, these maps do not explain the process known as 'metabolism'. The more detailed study of the kinetic properties of individual enzymes in the period 1940–1960, together with the development of simple but specific enzymatic assays for metabolic intermediates, opened the way for an extension of research into the comparatively new field of metabolic control. There has been such an explosive increase in the amount of information in this field that an appraisal of the experimental facts and a discussion of current theories may help to clarify the situation. Such a discussion is attempted in this volume, especially in relation to the pathways involved in the storage, synthesis and utilization of various fuels for energy production in higher animals.

The biological necessity for a large number of enzymatic steps in a metabolic pathway probably stems from the limitation in the chemistry that can be performed by individual enzymes. The advantages of enzymatic catalysis include specificity and high turnover rate, but these are probably attained at the expense of chemical versatility. The chemistry involved in the individual steps is usually relatively simple. Consecutive steps in a pathway are related by the substrates and products of each reaction. However, it is possible for the reactions to be organized to a greater extent than this. Thus, enzymes catalysing individual reactions may be so structurally organized that the metabolic intermediates constituting the pathways are always bound to an enzyme surface and the products are handed on as substrates for the subsequent reactions. This situation is somewhat analogous to the production line in modern mass-production industry. One example of this type of enzymatic organization is the β-oxidation pathway for conversion of fatty acyl-CoA derivatives to acetyl-CoA. The fatty acyl-CoA molecule loses two hydrogens which are transferred to flavin adenine dinucleotide (FAD) by the enzyme fatty acyl-CoA dehydrogenase; a molecule of water is added across the carbon-carbon double bond by the enzyme enoyl hydrase, and the product, a β-hydroxyacyl-CoA, is dehydrogenated by the appropriate NAD^+-linked dehydrogenase. The resulting β-ketoacyl-CoA is cleaved thiolytically to produce one molecule of acetyl-CoA and one molecule of a fatty acyl-CoA whose hydrocarbon chain is two carbon atoms shorter than the original fatty acid (see Figure 1.1). The intermediates of this pathway, fatty enoyl-CoA,

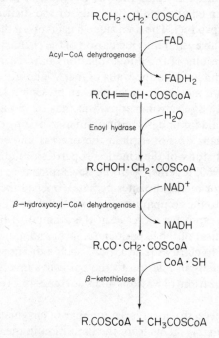

Figure 1.1. The β-oxidation pathway

β-hydroxyacyl-CoA and β-ketoacyl-CoA have not been isolated from tissues and this has led to the suggestion that they are all enzyme-bound. This would seem a satisfactory biological arrangement as these intermediates are not required for any process other than the β-oxidation system.

Although the β-oxidation pathway is not the sole example of an organized enzyme system, such systems are comparatively rare in metabolism. Metabolic pathways such as glycolysis, gluconeogenesis, the tricarboxylic acid (TCA) cycle, the pentose phosphate pathway and various aspects of amino acid metabolism do not appear to be organized to the extent of the above example. The intermediates of these pathways, although present at low concentrations in the tissue, are detectable by specific assay techniques. Indeed the interrelated nature of metabolism requires that a number of compounds function as intermediates and/or precursors for more than one metabolic pathway (for example, glucose-6-phosphate is a precursor for glycolysis, pentose phosphate pathway and glycogen synthesis). Such intermediates always have to be available for more than one pathway and the relative rates of these pathways may vary under different conditions. Therefore the intermediates cannot be exclusively enzyme-bound. Indeed, the apparent mobility of metabolic intermediates within the cell is employed for the purpose of metabolic regulation; certain compounds function both as metabolic intermediates and as metabolic regulators of key enzymes. A change in concentration of such an intermediate provides information about the state of metabolism at a particular position. The mobility of the intermediate allows it to relay information rapidly to regulatory enzymes which may be found in a different position in the cell.

The term 'organized' has been used to describe such pathways as fatty acid oxidation because of the structural organization of the enzymes involved. This must not imply that other pathways (such as glycolysis, TCA cycle) are disorganized. Although the enzymes which constitute such pathways are not *physically* organized, they are highly organized in a chemical sense. The concentrations of enzymes of the pathway are such that the catalytic activities of certain enzymes can limit the overall flux through the pathway, while other reactions can occur rapidly and are limited by the substrate (intermediate) or cofactor concentrations. This chemical organization is synonymous with metabolic regulation. As the details of these regulatory mechanisms are unfolded throughout this book they will emphasize that specific chemical catalysis is but one function of enzymes in a metabolic pathway and that, although not necessarily in physical contact, each enzyme is informed of the state of the remainder of the pathway by specific chemical signals (such as concentrations of substrate, product or specific regulators).

B. SOME THEORETICAL ASPECTS OF METABOLIC PATHWAYS

This section will discuss certain theoretical principles relating to the operation of metabolic pathways, since it is necessary to have some knowledge of these principles before attempting to understand the experimental approaches to metabolic control. In this book such principles are considered from an energetic rather than kinetic viewpoint.

1. Theoretical introduction to energy transfer

Energy transfer plays a fundamental role in all living organisms and therefore it has received a great deal of attention both experimentally and theoretically. Many books have been written on the theoretical aspects of energy transfer and it is not the desire of the authors to repeat detailed discussions and explanations of subjects that are dealt with elsewhere. Nonetheless, as energy considerations cannot be excluded from any discussion of metabolic regulation, particularly for an understanding of the experimental approaches, some important principles of energy transfer are described as briefly and as simply as possible. This section is not intended to be a comprehensive account of biological energetics. References 1–7 are recommended for students who wish to read more deeply into this fascinating subject.

One simple means of understanding some of the problems that arise in biological energetics is to divide energy transfer into three classes: chemical bond energy, heat energy and energy expended in work.

(a) Chemical bond energy

In the following reaction

$$A\text{–}B + C \underset{k_2}{\overset{k_1}{\rightleftarrows}} B\text{–}C + A$$

the chemical bond energy of the system (A–B + C), is redistributed in order to form a certain quantity of the system (B–C + A). If the concentrations (or more correctly the thermodynamic activities) of the reactants and products are such that no energy is lost (or gained) as heat during the reaction and no work is done, either by the reaction or on the reaction, then the system is at equilibrium. Under such conditions the rates of the forward and reverse reactions are identical and the concentrations of reactants and products remain constant, despite the fact that they are being rapidly interconverted. Although this is known as the stationary state, it must be emphasized that chemical bonds are being broken and formed and energy is being constantly redistributed. Since the system is at equilibrium, the transference of chemical bond energy occurs without any loss and is therefore 100 % efficient. When a chemical reaction is not at equilibrium, the approach to equilibrium occurs spontaneously and it is accompanied by a decrease in Gibbs free energy (ΔG). This means that the reaction system loses energy which may be released as heat, or may be used to perform useful work, or may be transferred as chemical bond energy into the components of another reaction to which it is coupled. The conservation of energy in the form of specific chemical bonds is the basis of energy transfer in living organisms. If the reaction A–B + C $\rightleftarrows$ B–C + A is displaced from equilibrium, some of the energy that is released as the process approaches equilibrium could be used to form

ATP by phosphorylation of ADP with inorganic phosphate (P_i). In other words, two reactions are coupled together and from the energetic point of view they can be considered as one reaction.

$$A\text{–}B + C \rightleftarrows B\text{–}C + A$$
$$P_i + ADP \quad ATP$$

If the overall reaction is at equilibrium, the transfer of energy for the phosphorylation of ADP is 100% efficient, but there is no *net* formation of ATP.

The Gibbs free energy (ΔG) of any chemical reaction is a measure of its capacity to do work. As the reaction proceeds spontaneously and the free energy decreases, so its capacity for performing useful work declines until at equilibrium it reaches zero, when there is no longer any change in free energy. Obviously the free energy of the system must in some way be related to the concentrations of reactants and products, since the free energy no longer changes once the equilibrium concentrations are attained. It can be shown (see references 2 and 3 or any standard text) that the relation between concentrations of reactants and products is described by the equation:

$$\Delta G = -RT \ln \left(\frac{\text{Product of equilibrium concentrations of products}}{\text{Product of equilibrium concentrations of substrates}} \right)$$
$$+ RT \ln \left(\frac{\text{Product of initial concentrations of products}}{\text{Product of initial concentrations of substrates}} \right)$$

Therefore

$$\Delta G = -RT \ln K + RT \ln \left(\frac{[\text{Product}]_{\text{initial}}}{[\text{Substrate}]_{\text{initial}}} \right)$$

where K is the equilibrium constant. (When the initial concentrations of products and reactants are 1·0 M, the term on the right, i.e.

$$RT \ln \left(\frac{[\text{Product}]_{\text{initial}}}{[\text{Substrate}]_{\text{initial}}} \right)$$

becomes zero, so that

$$\Delta G° = -RT \ln K.$$

$\Delta G°$ is a constant and is known as the *standard free energy change* of the reaction.) The higher the initial concentrations of A–B and C, and the lower the concentrations of B–C and A, the greater is the amount of energy released. The equation given above indicates the amount of energy that is released at an instant of time when the concentrations are as stated. As the reaction continues with the conversion of A–B and C into B–C and A, the equilibrium position will be approached so that RT ln ([products]/[substrates]) will approach the value of $RT \ln K$ (but with the opposite sign) and the amount of energy released will approach zero. In order to calculate the amount of energy released when certain concentrations of A–B and C are allowed to proceed to equilibrium, integration of the above equation between the limits of the initial and final concentrations of reactants and products will be necessary.

Calculations of the free energy changes in various biochemical reactions described in some textbooks are based on $\Delta G°$ values. Therefore, the amounts of energy that are calculated are only valid if all the components of the reaction are 1·0 M. Such concentrations are unlikely to occur in the living cell. To calculate more realistic energy changes the *actual* concentrations of the products and reactants within the cell must be taken into account, i.e. the equation

$$\Delta G = -RT \ln K + RT \ln \left(\frac{[\text{products}]}{[\text{reactants}]} \right)$$

must be used in any calculation and not $\Delta G° = -RT \ln K$. If ΔG is negative the reaction will proceed in the forward direction and if ΔG is positive the reaction will proceed in the reverse direction. Thus, by manipulating the concentrations of the products and reactants, the direction of the reaction can be changed.

However, in many metabolic reactions it is not even valid to calculate ΔG from these equations. The reason is that although the concentrations of reactants and products are usually maintained fairly constant, there is a continuous flux through the pathway (that is, a steady-state condition). The above equations for ΔG have been derived from equilibrium thermodynamics but in the steady-state condition, equilibrium thermodynamics no longer applies. The thermodynamics of the steady state is a complex subject which will not be discussed in this text; interested students should consult references 8 and 9 for information on steady-state or irreversible thermodynamics. Nonetheless, important qualitative information can still be obtained from the application of equilibrium thermodynamics to metabolic systems.

(b) Heat energy

Chemical bond energy can be converted into heat. When the reaction

$$A–B + C \rightarrow B–C + A + \text{heat}$$

proceeds from left to right, heat, which arises from some of the chemical bond energy of the system (A–B + C), is released. If loss of heat from the system is prevented, the reaction is described as a *closed adiabatic system*— i.e. there is no gain or loss of any component to the environment. Eventually in such a system the reaction will reach equilibrium in which the rate of the forward reaction, which liberates heat, equals the rate of the reverse reaction which absorbs heat. However, if a large proportion of this heat is lost to the environment, the reaction is described as an *open system* and will proceed until large quantities of B–C and A accumulate and very small quantities of A–B and C remain. Thus, chemical reactions which release a large amount of heat will have a large negative standard free energy change ($\Delta G°$). Of course, some of this energy which in one situation may be released as heat, can also be utilized to drive another chemical reaction. This process is known as coupling and, if all the available energy is coupled to the other reaction, no energy is lost as heat and the combined reaction is at equilibrium. (These discussions assume that there is no change in entropy.) If some of the available energy is released as heat which is dissipated to the environment, the reaction will be displaced from equilibrium. The greater the loss of heat, the greater will be the displacement from equilibrium. In biochemical systems, reactions which are displaced far from equilibrium are described as irreversible or non-equilibrium reactions.

From subsequent discussions on metabolic regulation it should become apparent that the importance of non-equilibrium reactions is that they are selected by the cell for the purpose of feedback regulation. Thus, the continuous transfer of chemical bond energy into heat is an absolute necessity in order to keep such reactions displaced far from equilibrium (see below).

(c) Energy for useful work

The reaction

$$A–B + C \rightleftarrows B–C + A$$

may be so organized that, as it takes place, A is translocated across a membrane against a concentration gradient. In this case some of the energy of the chemical bonds in the system (A–B + C) is used for osmotic work—that is, to reverse the spontaneous movement of A down a concentration gradient. In this situation chemical bond energy is transformed into the increased chemical potential of compound A. Similarly, if the energy released in this reaction was used for muscular contraction, it might result in the movement of an animal from a lower to a higher position (for example, from the ground to a branch in a tree). The animal would have done work against gravity and chemical bond energy would have been converted into potential energy stemming from the elevated position of the animal. In this case the amount of work performed by the animal can be calculated from the equation, work done = mgh, when m is the mass of the animal, g is the gravitational acceleration and h is the increase in height. Energy is of course expended in movement along a horizontal surface but in this case the energy is used to overcome frictional rather than gravitational forces.

2. The conditions of equilibrium, non-equilibrium and the steady state as applied to metabolic pathways

The terms, equilibrium, non-equilibrium and steady state will be used in various chapters throughout this book and it is essential that the meanings of these terms are clarified at this early stage.

(a) The equilibrium condition

In a process at equilibrium the rates of the forward and reverse reactions are identical: there is no net flux in either direction. Since there is no free energy change at equilibrium, this is the most stable condition for any reaction or process. Consequently, all reactions will proceed towards this stable state. The change in Gibbs free energy as a reaction proceeds spontaneously towards the equilibrium state is the driving force behind all biological and, for that matter, non-biological processes. Therefore the equilibrium state, of itself, is of no energetic value to an organism, since the release of energy, its conservation and its utilization are the manifestations of life itself. Metabolic processes constitute a dynamic system in which there is a net flux of both matter and energy, so that the overall process must always be removed from equilibrium. Of course, the direction of flux within a metabolic pathway is dictated by the position of equilibrium. These discussions must not be taken to imply that all reactions in the cell are removed far from equilibrium. Indeed some reactions appear to be very close to equilibrium, but the *overall* process must be non-equilibrium.

(b) The non-equilibrium condition

A process that is removed from equilibrium will undergo a negative free energy change as it proceeds towards the equilibrium state. This free energy may be lost as heat to the environment so that the reaction will proceed until a large proportion of the reactants are converted into the products. Thus the unidirectionality of a reaction or pathway depends on some of the available free energy being lost as heat. However, *all* the available energy need not be lost; some of it can be conserved for use by the cell. This is illustrated with reference to glycolysis which can be represented in a shorthand version as follows:

$$\text{glucose} \longleftrightarrow \text{lactate}$$
$$\text{ADP} + \text{P}_i \qquad \text{ATP}$$

If this pathway were at equilibrium (or very close to equilibrium), all the energy released from the conversion of glucose to lactate would be transferred to the ATP molecules and the process of energy transfer would be totally efficient. Unfortunately, at equilibrium there would be no net flux through the pathway and no net synthesis of ATP.

It is necessary for glycolysis to proceed in the direction of lactate formation and, in order to ensure such unidirectionality, the pathway must be displaced from equilibrium. This means that some of the chemical energy that is released when glucose is converted into lactate must be lost as heat. If all the energy were lost as heat, the non-equilibrium character of the pathway would be ensured, but it would be of little value to the organism. Therefore, a living organism must compromise by losing *some* of the available energy and conserving the remainder in a biologically useful form (usually ATP). Thus, in glycolysis only a proportion of the total energy is used in the synthesis of ATP (for every glucose molecule converted to lactate, two molecules of ATP are produced from ADP and P_i). Similarly, in a process which performs work, some of the available energy must be lost as heat in order to ensure that the production of work always occurs when this process is stimulated. For example, in the process of ion transport across a membrane (which requires ATP) some of the available energy from ATP hydrolysis must be lost as heat so that the ion-transport process is unidirectional. If the transport process were to approach equilibrium, any slight change in the concentration of the ions might cause ion transportation to change direction and result in ATP generation. The loss of heat in a metabolic pathway (or any other process) may be considered as the price the organism has to pay in order to ensure unidirectionality of the pathway (or process).

Although it is possible to consider the loss of heat as the 'driving force' of the process, it must not be assumed that the *rate* of the pathway will be governed by this degree of displacement from equilibrium. The flux is usually governed by other factors that are quantitatively unrelated to this displacement (for example, the activities of specific regulatory enzymes in the pathway or the concentration of a cofactor for the pathway—see Section D).

(c) The steady-state condition

How can processes such as glycolysis or the aerobic oxidation of glucose be maintained continually in the non-equilibrium state? This is only achieved by the constant exchange of matter and energy between living organisms and their environment. A system which exchanges matter and energy with its environment is described as an open system. Conversely a closed system does not exchange matter or energy with the environment and will therefore eventually reach equilibrium. The substrates of metabolic pathways are continually derived from the environment and end-products are continually returned to the environment (ultimately as CO_2, H_2O, etc.). The processes that constitute metabolism only attain the equilibrium state when the organism is dead. The condition in which the substrate is continually supplied and the products continually removed, so that the concentrations of the intermediates of the pathway remain constant despite a constant flux through the pathway, is known as the steady state. It can be described as a stable yet dynamic non-equilibrium condition.

(d) The steady-state condition and metabolic regulation

In the series of reactions that constitute a metabolic pathway the total loss of energy as heat could be divided fairly evenly between each of the individual reactions so that they are all somewhat displaced from equilibrium. This would appear to be the spontaneous situation in any non-equilibrium pathway. It is somewhat analogous to a river flowing downhill in which potential energy of the water is lost continuously and fairly evenly along the length of the river. The analogy between the steady-state condition of a river and that of a metabolic pathway is illustrated in Figure 1.2.

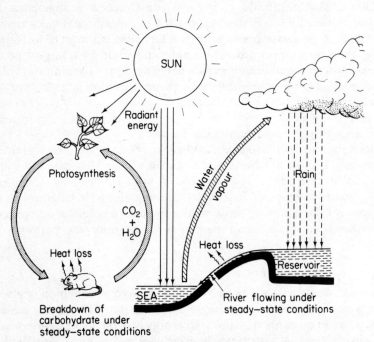

Figure 1.2. Maintenance of a steady-state condition. The elevated position of the water in the reservoir provides the source of the water for the river which links the reservoir and the sea. The difference in levels between the reservoir and the sea provides the potential energy for the flow of water. This difference is maintained by the evaporation of water from the sea, formation of clouds, and rainfall over the reservoir. The energy for maintenance of the steady state is obtained from the sun. The steady-state condition of carbohydrate oxidation in a living organism is maintained in an analogous manner. The chemical energy of the carbohydrate is released during the oxidative process, but the photosynthetic organisms resynthesize carbohydrate from CO_2 and H_2O with radiant energy obtained from the sun

If the rate of flow of water along a river is to be controlled, dams must be constructed at various stages along the length of the river. A dam produces a reservoir of water and the outflow from such reservoirs can be controlled by the level of the sluice gate at the dam. For example, if the gate is lowered, the potential of the water at the dam is increased and the water flows more rapidly downhill. In the series of reactions which constitute a metabolic pathway, a few may be displaced far from equilibrium, whereas the majority of reactions may be close to equilibrium (Figure 1.3). (It must be emphasized

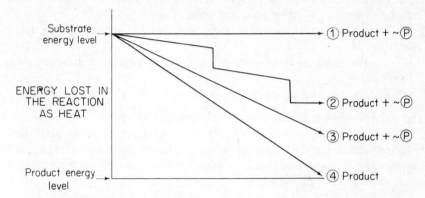

Figure 1.3. Simple energy diagram of metabolic pathways. (1) Pathway is at equilibrium so that no energy is lost: all the chemical energy released in the pathway is conserved in the energy-rich phosphate ($\sim \circled{P}$) bonds. (2) Pathway is non-equilibrium and energy loss occurs at two discrete steps. Some energy is conserved in $\sim \circled{P}$ bonds. (3) Pathway is non-equilibrium and energy loss occurs all along the length of the pathway. Some energy is conserved in $\sim \circled{P}$ bonds. (4) All chemical energy available in the pathway is lost as heat along the length of the pathway

that a reaction cannot be at equilibrium if a flux occurs through that reaction; it can, however, be very close to equilibrium.) This is not a spontaneous situation. The non-equilibrium reactions have a similar function to a dam in that they restrict the flux at that position of the pathway.[10] Consequently they provide potential control points.

C. EXPERIMENTAL APPROACHES TO METABOLIC CONTROL

The complexity of metabolism makes it difficult to understand how information on the regulation of enzyme activity can ever be obtained. Nevertheless, major advances in knowledge of metabolic regulation in higher animals have been made over the past ten years and these have stemmed from improvements both in techniques and in experimental approach. The latter is based on a theoretical understanding of the energetics and dynamics of metabolic pathways and it represents a logical procedure for investigating regulation, once details of the biochemistry and physiology of the pathway are available. The approach outlined below is not intended to cover comprehensively all aspects of regulation of enzyme activity, but it should provide a broad basis for reviewing the regulation of metabolic pathways.

The basic principles which have been discussed in detail in a review article[11] are as follows:

(a) The enzymes which play a specific role in the regulation of a metabolic pathway are identified by certain criteria.

(b) The properties of such regulatory enzymes are investigated in detail *in vitro*.

(c) On the basis of these properties a theory of metabolic control is formulated.

(d) The theory, or predictions which arise from the theory, are tested.

The theory is modified, extended or rejected accordingly.

Although the relationship between points (b), (c) and (d) varies according to the particular enzyme under consideration, the identification of regulatory enzymes (a) is an exercise that is similar for all metabolic pathways and it poses some general problems (see reference 12).

1. Identification of non-equilibrium reactions

One of the first problems in metabolic control is to understand how, when presented with a pathway consisting of a large number of intermediate reactions (glycolysis, for example, contains at least 11 reactions between glucose and pyruvate), the regulatory enzymes can be identified. The theoretical principles discussed above were designed to provide background information for this experimental approach. The first step is to classify the intermediary reactions as near-equilibrium (equilibrium) or far-removed from equilibrium (non-equilibrium). The two main experimental approaches that have been used to identify non-equilibrium reactions are the comparison of equilibrium constants with mass-action ratios and the measurement of maximal enzyme activities.

(a) *Comparison of equilibrium constants and mass-action ratios*

The equilibrium constant of a reaction

$$A + B \rightleftarrows C + D$$

is defined by

$$K' = \frac{[C][D]}{[A][B]}$$

In most experiments the equilibrium constant is calculated from the concentrations of substrates and products when these are *not* at infinite dilution, so that the calculated constant is termed the *apparent* equilibrium constant (K'). The thermodynamic equilibrium constant (K_{eq}) is obtained if the concentrations approach those at infinite dilution or if the thermodynamic activities of the substrates and products are calculated from the concentrations and inserted into the equation in place of the concentrations. Some experimental methods for the determination of K' are given in Appendix 1.1.

An enzyme is a catalyst and therefore cannot alter the position of equilibrium of a reaction. If an enzyme catalyses an equilibrium (or near-equilibrium) reaction in the cell, the concentration ratio Products/Substrates should approximate to K' of that reaction. The contents of substrates and products of a reaction can be measured within a tissue and the ratio Products/Substrates, which is termed the mass-action ratio (Γ), can be calculated. If the value of Γ is similar to that for K' then it can be concluded that this reaction is near-equilibrium in the cell. However, if Γ is found to be markedly smaller than K' then this suggests that the reaction is displaced far from equilibrium—that is, the enzyme catalyses a non-equilibrium reaction in the cell.

The measurement of the mass-action ratio poses a number of problems, some of which are only apparent when the details of the experimental technique are fully understood. The measurement of a mass-action ratio and a discussion of some of the problems that arise in the interpretation of mass-action ratio data are described in Appendix 1.2.

(b) *The measurement of maximal enzyme activities*

A non-equilibrium reaction in a metabolic pathway arises because the enzyme which catalyses this reaction is not sufficiently active to bring the substrates and products to equilibrium. The preceding and subsequent enzymes possess much higher catalytic capacities for formation of the substrate and removal of the product than the 'non-equilibrium' enzyme has for their interconversion. This situation provides a second method of identifying non-equilibrium reactions in a metabolic pathway. The maximum activities of all the enzymes in the pathway are measured *in vitro* and on the basis of these results the enzymes are classified into low- and high-activity groups. The enzymes in the low-activity group are considered to catalyse non-equilibrium reactions in the cell. Meaningful results can be obtained from such a study only if the enzymes are assayed under optimal conditions and consequently some preliminary information on the properties of each enzyme is essential before this method is attempted. It is preferable to measure enzyme activities in crude homogenates since purification can lead to a loss of activity; but in certain cases some degree of purification may be necessary in order to obtain a satisfactory assay.

In general it has been found that the difference in activities of these two groups of enzymes is 10- to 1,000-fold. When such a difference exists the identification of non-equilibrium reactions is straightforward since it is unlikely that enzymes will have been wrongly classified owing to poor recovery or inadequate assay conditions. In the interpretation of enzyme activity data it should be made clear that if an enzyme is found to be of high activity it need not necessarily catalyse an equilibrium reaction *in vivo*: it may be inhibited to a very great extent in the cell. Consequently such data should be supported, if possible, by mass-action ratio measurements. Also an enzyme may catalyse an equilibrium reaction under one set of conditions but under other conditions it may be inhibited 95–99% and therefore catalyse a non-equilibrium reaction. Ideally the two methods of identification of non-equilibrium reactions should provide a similar classification. Indeed the mass-action ratio method should reflect the relative enzyme activities *in situ*, since the non-equilibrium character of a reaction is due to a low catalytic activity in relation to enzymes catalysing other reactions.

These two techniques have been used extensively in the study of most of the metabolic pathways which have been examined to date. However, two other possible approaches to the problem of identifying non-equilibrium reactions should be mentioned.

(c) Supplementation experiments

Potential regulatory reactions can occasionally be indicated by measuring the rate of synthesis of the product from a variety of intermediates of the pathway. Thus for a pathway

$$S \rightleftarrows A \rightarrow B \rightleftarrows C \rightleftarrows D \rightleftarrows P$$

P will be synthesized more rapidly from B than from A or S, if $A \rightarrow B$ is a non-equilibrium reaction. On a practical level, the difficulty with supplementation experiments is the relative impermeability of whole cells (or cell organelles) to the intermediates of the pathway. Therefore P may be formed faster from C than from B, simply because the cell is more permeable to C, and a non-equilibrium reaction at the interconversion of B and C may be falsely indicated. It is also important to realize that if a substrate is used which is not an intermediate *per se*, but which can give rise to an intermediate, then its entry into the pathway could occur via a non-equilibrium reaction. For example, in the pathway

$$\begin{array}{c} E \\ \downarrow \\ S \rightleftarrows A \rightarrow B \rightleftarrows C \rightleftarrows D \rightleftarrows P \end{array}$$

if C gives rise to P faster than E gives rise to P, this does not indicate that $B \rightarrow C$ is non-equilibrium, since the rate of conversion of $E \rightarrow B$ could be limiting.

(*d*) *General considerations*

Finally, it may be possible to assess which reactions would be suitable regulatory reactions on the basis of their position in a pathway. In general, the most efficient control of the utilization of a substrate would be effected by a reaction at the beginning of the pathway, possibly even at the level of transport into the cell. Other likely control points occur immediately after a branch point in a pathway. Obviously such general considerations merely provide a guideline in the initial stages of the investigation and, if they support the experimental findings, they may inspire confidence in the results at the end of the investigation.

2. Identification of regulatory enzymes

The above discussions have dealt with the identification of enzymes which catalyse non-equilibrium reactions. What is the relationship between a 'non-equilibrium' enzyme and a regulatory enzyme? One difficulty in understanding the problem of metabolic control lies in the definition of a regulatory enzyme. To some extent the activities of all the enzymes in a metabolic pathway are regulated : when the flux through the pathway changes, the activities of *all* the enzymes must change. The crucial question is, which is the enzyme which responds to the original metabolic signal and thereby initiates subsequent changes in the activities of the remaining enzymes? Since the nature of the metabolic signal remains unknown until the regulatory enzyme has been identified, postulated mechanisms of control cannot be used to indicate regulatory enzymes. This problem is resolved by the precise definition of the term 'regulatory enzyme'.

It is possible to define a regulatory enzyme simply as 'an enzyme which catalyses a non-equilibrium reaction'. (Although under certain conditions reactions which are close to equilibrium may be regulatory—see Section D.2.) A 'non-equilibrium' enzyme possesses a low catalytic activity and for this reason it will limit the flux through the pathway. The activity of this enzyme could be regulated solely by changes in substrate concentration. In this case the investigation would then be directed towards factors responsible for the modification of substrate concentration. A feedback-inhibition type of control mechanism operates if the enzyme is controlled by factors other than the substrate concentration. Therefore a regulatory enzyme may be defined as 'an enzyme which catalyses a non-equilibrium reaction and whose activity is controlled by factors other than the substrate concentration'. This second definition is more restrictive than the first but both are applicable —there can be no absolute definition of the term 'regulatory enzyme'. The two definitions given above are operational in that they suggest experimental approaches to the problem of identifying regulatory enzymes. The experimental approaches that can be used in the identification of non-equilibrium reactions have already been described. The approach that can be employed for the identification of regulatory enzymes (according to the second more restrictive definition) is described below.

(a) Changes in substrate concentration of a non-equilibrium reaction

The identification of a non-equilibrium reaction requires that the pathway is in a steady-state condition but the knowledge of the flux through the pathway is not required. However, for identification of a regulatory enzyme the flux through the pathway must be perturbed in order that changes in the steady-state concentrations of the substrates of the 'non-equilibrium' enzymes can be measured. If the substrate concentration of a 'non-equilibrium' enzyme changes in the opposite direction to the flux (for example, flux increased and the substrate concentration decreased), this indicates that the enzyme is regulatory. The rationale behind this approach is very simple : a change in substrate concentration in the opposite direction to the change in catalytic activity is inconsistent with control by substrate concentration. It must be stressed that the reason for the change in substrate concentration is unimportant and in no way interferes with the interpretation of the data.

There are two important points to note in the interpretation of the data from such experiments. First, it is not possible to conclude that the enzyme is *not* regulatory (according to the second definition); if the flux and substrate concentration change in the same direction, this *cannot* be interpreted as regulation only by substrate concentration. It is possible for an enzyme to be regulated both by a change in substrate concentration and by a specific regulator. Second, when the term 'substrate' is used in this definition, it refers only to the *pathway substrate* and not to a cofactor or alternative substrate (such as ATP or NAD^+). The *pathway substrate* may be defined as that substrate which is modified by the enzyme and which represents the flow of matter through the pathway.

(b) The significance of the crossover theorem in metabolic control

The use of changes in flux and steady-state levels of intermediates to identify positions of regulation or inhibition was first discussed in detail by Chance et al.[13] in the study of electron transport and oxidative phosphorylation. These workers proposed the 'crossover theorem' which states that when a pathway is inhibited at a specific reaction, the substrate concentration will increase and the product concentration will decrease and vice versa. This is indeed the case in the respiratory chain where the components change, not in terms of concentration, but in the state of oxidation. Consequently, if the oxidized form is increased, it follows that the reduced form must be decreased. The concept of the crossover theorem was then applied to the identification of regulatory enzymes but in this case the change in the product concentration is irrelevant. All that is required in this analysis of regulatory enzymes is to establish the non-equilibrium character of the reaction and to show that the substrate of this reaction changes in the opposite direction to the flux (see reference 12).

3. Study of the properties of regulatory enzymes

A positive indication that a 'non-equilibrium' enzyme is indeed regulatory (that is, its activity is modified by factors other than the pathway substrate) inspires confidence that it will be possible to identify the metabolic regulator(s) in a systematic *in vitro* study of the properties of the enzyme. Initially, the effects of substrate, product, cofactors, etc., are tested, but after this it is necessary to search for effector molecules which may bear no chemical relationship to either substrate or product. Often this is a process of trial and error, although the nature of the effector may be predicted by intelligent assessment of the pathway and its association with other pathways.

The experimental conditions for the assays of regulatory enzymes depend upon the particular enzyme under investigation. The enzyme is normally extracted from the tissue in a medium in which it retains maximum catalytic activity. However, it is difficult to assess how much purification of the initial crude extract is necessary, or desirable, before the properties of the enzyme can be studied. A suitable compromise has to be reached between the use of crude extracts, in which the properties of the enzyme that are relevant to metabolic control are more likely to be preserved, and purification of the enzyme to facilitate accurate assays for a detailed kinetic analysis. Excessive purification may distort, or even remove, important control properties. Therefore the enzyme should be investigated initially in as crude a system as allows satisfactory assay of activities.

4. Formulation of a theory of metabolic control

Once the regulatory enzymes have been identified and their properties investigated, it is possible to postulate a theory of control. There are two points concerning the formulation of theories which are elementary but which are often overlooked. First, the theory should give rise to predictions that are experimentally testable since there is little value in suggesting a theory of metabolic regulation which cannot be tested, either because it is too complex or because the practical problems are insuperable. Second, the theory has to accommodate itself to most of the accepted physiological facts relating to the particular metabolic pathway.

The major drawback of this general approach to metabolic control is that the theory is based upon the extrapolation of properties of isolated enzymes to the unknown conditions of the intact cell: it is assumed that factors that influence the activity *in vitro* will have a similar effect inside the cell.

In many cases the enzymes are studied *in vitro* at concentrations of approximately 1 μg/ml whereas in the living cell their concentrations may be as high as 1 mg/ml. The methods currently available for enzyme assays are designed to operate over a period of several minutes and with these methods it is not possible to measure activities of enzymes at such high concentrations. In order to tackle such problems experimentally it may be necessary to apply stop-flow techniques. Incubations could be precisely controlled for tenths of seconds with these techniques so that the properties of higher concentrations of enzyme could be investigated. So far such techniques have not been used in the study of the properties of regulatory enzymes.

5. Testing the theory of metabolic control

The theory may be tested by experimental manipulations that result in variations in the concentrations of factors which are thought to regulate the enzyme activity. These are correlated with effects on the rate of the metabolic pathway. The most decisive experiments are usually those performed on intact tissue preparations. If the theory is to be substantiated, and particularly if criticism of the extrapolation from *in vitro* systems is to be answered, changes in factors which are considered to regulate the enzyme should be observed in the intact tissue. Unfortunately, compartmentation within the cell means that a negative result does not necessarily disprove the theory. It is not possible to test the hypothesis directly because of the difficulties of measuring changes in the concentrations of proposed regulators at the site of the enzyme (see reference 14).

The relationship between the properties of the enzyme, the proposal of a theory and examination of its predictions varies with each particular problem. If the initial theory does not appear satisfactory after such examination, it may be necessary to investigate in more detail the properties of the enzyme. Individual examples of the methods of applying stages (b), (c) and (d) of the approach to the study of metabolic control will be discussed in detail in the appropriate chapters.

D. A CLASSIFICATION OF METABOLIC CONTROL SYSTEMS

In living organisms the rates of metabolic processes may be varied in response to changing environmental conditions in at least two ways. There exists a rapid mechanism (operating within seconds or minutes) for the regulation of enzyme activity and this depends upon changes in the catalytic activity of individual enzyme molecules. There also exists a somewhat slower mechanism (operating within hours or days) that is dependent upon an increase in the number of enzyme molecules through modification of the rate of synthesis or degradation (see reference 15 for a review). The material in this book will be concerned primarily with changes in catalytic activity which are *not* dependent upon synthesis or degradation of the enzyme. There are several general mechanisms for modifying the activity of an enzyme and these mechanisms may be divided into various classes. The classification presented here is by no means complete and it may be necessary to further subdivide the individual classes. However, the classification should prove useful for clarification of the term *regulatory* and for reference purposes when mechanisms of regulation are described in subsequent chapters.

1. Four classes of metabolic control

Four factors which could be responsible for controlling fluxes through metabolic pathways are as follows:

(*a*) Substrate availability.
(*b*) Cofactor availability.
(*c*) Product removal.
(*d*) Feedback regulation.

Such an arbitrary classification has no physiological significance; its value lies in the simplification of the complex problem of metabolic control. The general properties and advantages of each control mechanism will be mentioned only briefly at this point. Specific examples, for which there is favourable evidence, will be described in more detail in the subsequent chapters.

(*a*) Substrate availability

Any metabolic pathway could, in theory at least, be regulated very simply by the availability of substrate. A reduction in substrate concentration will decrease the activity of an enzyme (provided it is not saturated with substrate) and this could result in a decreased flux through the pathway. Similarly an increase in substrate concentration could stimulate the pathway. In general, however, the constancy of the internal environment of both the animal and the cell, as regards the substrates of metabolic pathways (such as blood glucose and intracellular glycogen), implies that such regulatory mechanisms are not common in higher animals. There is, however, at least one important example of control by substrate availability which will be discussed in detail in Chapters 3 and 5: the concentration of plasma fatty acids appears to play a fundamentally important role in the regulation of their oxidation by various tissues, and in turn their oxidation can modify the rate of carbohydrate utilization by the animal. In such situations, if the substrate concentration can be shown to be regulatory, the investigational emphasis shifts from the metabolic pathway *per se* to the factors responsible for the changes in substrate concentration. The factors responsible for the regulation of the plasma level of fatty acids are discussed in Chapter 5.

It should be emphasized that substrate availability must remain a potential regulatory mechanism for almost any pathway even if it is regulated by a feedback inhibition mechanism. Stimulation of a metabolic pathway may reduce the concentration of its substrate and minimize the extent of the stimulation that can occur. However, the complex organization of metabolic regulation at both physiological and biochemical levels usually ensures that an increase in substrate supply is provided either simultaneously or immediately prior to the increase in flux through a pathway, so that, despite a very high rate of substrate utilization, its concentration is not a limiting factor.

(b) Cofactor availability

A regulatory mechanism based upon availability of a cofactor is somewhat similar to control by substrate availability. However, substantial inhibition of enzyme activity (and therefore the rate of the metabolic pathway) could be achieved only if the concentration of the cofactor was reduced to very low levels. This may only be possible if the cofactor is specific for the particular pathway in question and is not required for other pathways. Such specificity is uncommon, although carnitine, which is a cofactor involved in fatty acid oxidation, may be a possible example. Fatty acids are activated by an enzyme, fatty acyl-CoA synthetase, to produce fatty acyl-CoA and this reaction occurs

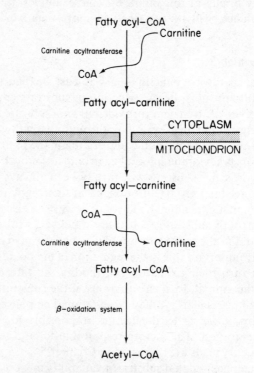

Figure 1.4. The role of carnitine in fatty acid oxidation. The fatty acyl-CoA in the cytoplasm may be derived from exogenous fatty acids or from endogenous triglyceride

outside the mitochondrion. The β-oxidation of fatty acids occurs inside the mitochondrion and therefore the fatty acyl-CoA has to traverse the mitochondrial membranes. There is a substantial body of evidence which suggests that one of the mitochondrial membranes (probably the inner membrane) is impermeable to fatty acyl-CoA and, in order to overcome this barrier, fatty acyl-CoA must be converted into fatty acyl-carnitine by the enzyme carnitine acyltransferase. Fatty acyl-carnitine is able to traverse the membrane. The enzyme carnitine acyltransferase is also present inside the mitochondrion so that the fatty acyl-carnitine is converted back to fatty acyl-CoA and thus provides substrate for β-oxidation (Figure 1.4). Therefore, theoretically, it is possible that variations in the concentration of carnitine could regulate the rate of fatty acid oxidation without affecting other metabolic processes.

Another possible example of control by cofactor availability is the regulation of electron transport and oxidative phosphorylation in the mitochondria. Inside the mitochondria the adenine nucleotides are required primarily for ATP synthesis by the electron-transport chain. This is an example of specificity in cofactor requirement provided by intracellular compartmentation. The availability of cofactors may regulate the process of electron transport and this is discussed in some detail below.

Cofactors can become limiting in vitamin-deficient diseases, but this is of course not a physiological control mechanism. Although vitamin-deficient diseases can be explained on the basis of lack of specific cofactors, the symptoms of the diseases cannot as yet be precisely explained on the basis of the known biochemical functions of these cofactors.

(c) Product removal

If a pathway substrate is converted to the pathway product by a series of reactions, which are all at equilibrium (or close to equilibrium), the removal of the product could control the rate of its formation from the substrate. However, most pathways of major physiological importance appear to be controlled at non-equilibrium reactions, so that product removal will be unimportant in control of the pathway. Minor pathways or perhaps specific portions of some metabolic pathways may be controlled by such a mechanism. For example, the conversion of pyruvate to lactate in muscle which is catalysed by lactate dehydrogenase, and the movement of lactate from the muscle to the blood (diffusion) are thought to be equilibrium processes: an increased flow of blood through the muscle will increase the rate of product removal which could therefore increase the rate of the conversion of pyruvate to lactate. (It is not expected that under normal physiological conditions the rate of conversion of pyruvate to lactate and its diffusion into the blood will limit the rate of glycolysis in muscle.) Another possible example is the utilization of acetoacetic acid by extrahepatic tissues (see Chapter 7, Section D.2).

(d) Feedback regulation

Feedback regulation of enzyme activity is the most flexible and biologically widespread mechanism of metabolic control (for a general review see reference 16). Several types of control systems which may be included under this general heading are discussed from a theoretical standpoint in the next chapter and some biochemical examples are discussed in detail in Chapters 3 to 7. Feedback control in metabolic systems operates solely through the regulation of the activity of enzymes that catalyse non-equilibrium reactions. In the hypothetical pathway

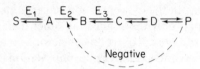

it is assumed that the conversion of A to B is non-equilibrium so that the activity of enzyme E_2 limits the overall flux from S to P. Therefore if the catalytic activity of the enzyme E_2 is inhibited by P, this provides a feedback inhibition mechanism for regulation of the flux through the pathway.

The extension of this concept of feedback regulation to include feedforward activation and, in its widest sense, to include any specific regulation of enzyme activity by factors other than the pathway substrate, leads to the conclusion that control of 'non-equilibrium' enzymes provides a very flexible means of control for the cell or organism. During the course of evolution the enzymes that catalyse non-equilibrium reactions can develop the specific regulatory properties that result in the most biologically efficient regulation. The chemistry of the reaction or the pathway provides no limitation on the mechanism of control: any compound may modify the activity of the regulatory enzyme and hence control the rate of flux through the pathway.

The four classes of metabolic regulation described above may in fact all play some role in the regulation of a single metabolic pathway. This emphasizes the semantic problem arising from the term 'pathway'. For example, glycolysis, the TCA cycle and the electron-transport chain may all be considered either as one pathway or as three separate pathways. When considered as a single overall pathway, control must obviously occur at non-equilibrium reactions by a feedback mechanism. However, sections of this overall pathway, which can be considered as separate pathways, may be regulated by the availability of substrate and/or cofactor, or by the removal of product. For example, when a muscle fibre contracts, the rate of ATP utilization is increased and therefore the rate of metabolism must increase to provide more ATP. The rate of glycolysis is increased by a mechanism

dependent upon specific feedback regulation from the change in the concentration of ATP (see Chapter 3). As a consequence of the increase in
glycolysis, the rate of formation of acetyl-CoA which is the substrate for the
TCA cycle is increased. The flux through the TCA cycle is also increased by
specific feedback mechanisms dependent upon the changes in concentrations
of ATP and ADP. The increased rate of the cycle provides more NADH as
substrate for electron transport which is also increased by a specific regulatory mechanism. In fact the latter is one of the best examples of equilibrium
control in metabolism: for this reason it is discussed in some detail below.

2. Control of electron transport at equilibrium reactions

If an enzyme catalyses a reaction which is very close to equilibrium, a
change in catalytic activity (caused by factors other than substrates and
products) cannot regulate the flux through that reaction (unless the enzyme
is so strongly inhibited that the reaction becomes non-equilibrium). However,
the flux in any one direction can be limited by the concentration of substrate
or cofactor, so that changes in these factors could modify the flux through
this reaction and hence through the pathway as a whole.

Consider a series of reactions which are close to equilibrium and which
constitute a metabolic pathway in which A is converted to P,

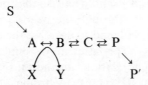

The assumptions implicit in this model are as follows:

(*a*) All the reactions between A and P are close to equilibrium and the
rate of each reaction depends on the concentration of substrate (for
example, B limits B → C, C limits C → P).
(*b*) The product P is removed to P′ by a non-equilibrium reaction at a rate
which is proportional to the concentration of P.
(*c*) The compound A is produced by a non-equilibrium reaction (S → A)
which is controlled in such a way that the concentration of A remains
constant.

In this hypothetical pathway the compounds X and Y are cofactors for the
reaction A ⇌ B such that the total cofactor concentration (X + Y) remains
constant. If the concentration of X is increased and that of Y correspondingly
decreased, this should result in a decrease in the concentration of A and an
increase in the concentration of B. (This is because the enzyme catalyses a
near-equilibrium situation between the participants of the reaction such that
$K' = [B][Y]/[X][A]$.) However, the concentration of A is kept constant by

the reaction $S \rightarrow A$, and therefore the rate of the forward reaction $A + X \rightarrow B + Y$ will be increased (owing to the increased concentration of X) so that the concentration of B will remain increased. This will increase the conversion of B to C, etc., and the rate of the whole pathway A to P will be increased. Obviously the overall pathway is non-equilibrium owing to reactions $S \rightarrow A$ and $P \rightarrow P'$ and these play an important role in the regulation of the overall flux. Nonetheless the reaction that has responded to the change in regulator concentrations (X and Y) is near-equilibrium.

One example of this type of equilibrium-control may be provided by the mitochondrial electron transport/oxidative phosphorylation system. There is accumulating evidence that the reactions that occur between the level of the pyridine nucleotides and cytochrome-c are easily reversed and therefore, under some conditions at least, they must be close to equilibrium.[17] Thus, at the first phosphorylation site, ATP hydrolysis can be used to cause the reduction of NAD^+ by reduced flavoprotein,

$$NADH + FP_{ox} \leftrightarrow NAD^+ + FP_{red}$$
$$P_i + ADP \qquad ATP$$

Any process that increases the rate of ATP utilization will increase the concentrations of ADP and P_i and decrease that of ATP. These changes in adenine nucleotides and P_i, through the near-equilibrium reaction at the first phosphorylation site, will tend to decrease the concentration of NADH and increase that of FP_{red}. The latter may stimulate the flow of electrons towards the second phosphorylation site and thus lead to an increase in the flow of electrons from NADH to the cytochromes. The supply of NADH for the electron-transport chain is derived from the TCA cycle which is therefore analogous to the $S \rightarrow A$ reaction in the hypothetical scheme described above. The increase in the rate of ATP utilization may specifically stimulate the TCA cycle which is a non-equilibrium process. As a result the rate of reduction of NAD^+ to NADH will increase at the same time as the rate of NADH oxidation has increased. Consequently, the ratio $NAD^+/NADH$ will remain constant despite the increase in flux through the pathway.

Since reversibility of the second phosphorylation site has been demonstrated, it is probable that this reaction is close to equilibrium. Therefore changes in the concentration of ATP, ADP and P_i may control the flux through this reaction also. Up to the present time reversibility of electron transport at the terminal phosphorylation site has not been demonstrated although it has been postulated to be a near-equilibrium reaction.[18] If all three phosphorylation steps are close to equilibrium, this would provide a concerted mechanism of control along the electron-transport chain to ensure an effective increase in electron transport as the levels of ATP, ADP and P_i are changed. Nevertheless the overall process of electron transfer (and therefore oxidative phosphorylation) must be non-equilibrium in order to ensure an adequate flow of electrons and net ATP formation. Such non-equilibrium character may be provided by the supply of NADH (for example, from the TCA cycle) and also by the final non-equilibrium reaction in the chain: this may be either the terminal phosphorylation reaction or a final stage of electron transport (for example, the cytochrome oxidase reaction). In the latter case all three phosphorylation sites may be close to equilibrium. Whatever the identity of the final non-equilibrium reaction, it fulfils the requirements of reaction $P \rightarrow P'$ in the hypothetical pathway $A \rightarrow P$.

There are other examples of equilibrium control which have been studied less intensively than the non-equilibrium control systems. In general, equilibrium control must play a subservient role to non-equilibrium control in that, once the specific feedback signal has informed the non-equilibrium reaction to increase, the remainder of the pathway will respond in accord through equilibrium control mechanisms.

An advantage of equilibrium control is that reactions which are close to equilibrium can provide efficiency of energy transfer approaching 100%. In the case of respiratory chain phosphorylation this means that a large pro-portion of the energy released during the transfer of electrons along the respiratory chain may be conserved as chemical bond energy in ATP. Obviously the overall process of electron transport cannot approach 100% efficiency since it has to be non-equilibrium. However, the importance of the fact that all the phosphorylation sites may be close to equilibrium is probably related to the efficiency of energy transfer. Since there are three phosphoryla-tion sites in series in the electron-transport chain, non-equilibrium control at each site would cause considerable loss of energy. If these three phos-phorylation reactions are close to equilibrium, energy loss may only occur in the non-equilibrium reactions at the beginning and end of the electron-transport chain (possibly NADH generation and the cytochrome oxidase reaction). Thus, if the electron-transport chain *as a whole* is maintained far from equilibrium, via the initial and terminal reactions of the process, equilibrium control of the three phosphorylation sites may involve the loss of less energy than non-equilibrium control of these phosphorylation reactions. One could speculate that the requirement for equilibrium control of the major energy-producing reactions in the cell is one factor underlying the evolutionary development of respiratory chain phosphorylation as opposed to substrate-level phosphorylation. A large number of substrate-level phosphorylation reactions could provide the same amount of ATP as that obtained from respiratory chain phosphorylation but this would of course increase the complexity of intermediary metabolism. If the rate of catabolism is to be regulated precisely to fulfil the energy needs of the cell, these numerous substrate-level phosphorylation reactions would all require regulation by feedback inhibition. Such a large number of non-equilibrium reactions would necessitate an excessive loss of energy in the form of heat. The efficiency of energy conservation provided by an oxidative process in which all phosphorylation reactions are close to equilibrium may have been one of the driving forces of natural selection that ensured the successful development of the electron-transport chain within the mitochondria.

In summary, the advantages of equilibrium control are simplicity and efficiency in energy transfer. The disadvantage is the lack of flexibility: the substrates and products of the reaction are the only factors by which it can be regulated. Conversely, control at non-equilibrium reactions suffers the disadvantage of inefficiency in energy transfer, but has the great advantage of flexibility.

An interesting point arises from this difference. Equilibrium control may bear no direct quantitative relationship to the actual rate of the pathway and for this reason it may be termed an 'open-loop' system of control by analogy to control in engineering systems.[19] For example, the rate of flow of water through a tube could simply be controlled by a valve connected to a dial (Figure 1.5). The dial settings would be calibrated initially so that for a given

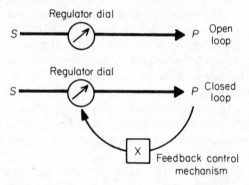

Figure 1.5. Diagrammatic representation of open and closed loops in feedback regulation. In the open-loop system the flux $(S \to P)$ is regulated only by the position of the regulator dial. If the dial setting is incorrect the flux will be incorrect for a given situation. In the closed-loop system the setting of the regulator dial is determined by the actual rate of formation of P via the feedback control mechanism, X. Thus, X measures the flux through the pathway and conveys this information to the regulator dial

dial setting a given flux of water should result. However, there is no ability to relate the dial settings to factors that might modify the flux of water (such as pressure of water or damage to the valve mechanism). On the other hand in a 'closed-loop' system, feedback information from the flow of water at the end of the tube would control the operation of the valve (Figure 1.5). The closed-loop system is of course analogous to non-equilibrium control and in this case there is a precise, quantitative control over the rate of flow of water according to the demands of the system.

APPENDIX TO CHAPTER 1

APPENDIX 1.1. METHODS FOR DETERMINING EQUILIBRIUM CONSTANTS

There are several ways of carrying out a practical determination of the apparent equilibrium constant (K') for an enzyme-catalysed reaction. The simplest and most widely employed method is to mix the substrate(s) of the reaction with the appropriate purified enzyme and allow the reaction to reach equilibrium. If there are no side reactions which produce or remove either substrate(s) or product(s) (that is, the added enzyme is sufficiently pure), the closed system will, in time, reach equilibrium. At this point the ratio of the concentrations of products and reactants (K') will always be the same (at this particular temperature) no matter what ratios of substrates or products were present initially (that is, the enzyme does not alter the position of equilibrium). After a suitable interval of time the reaction is inhibited by addition of a protein precipitant (such as perchloric acid) and the concentration of substrates and products measured so that K' can be calculated.

For example, the equilibrium constant of phosphoglucoisomerase (PGI) which catalyses the interconversion of glucose-6-phosphate and fructose-6-phosphate, is measured as follows. A preparation of the enzyme (PGI) is added to a solution of glucose-6-phosphate (G6P) and after two separate time intervals, hydrochloric acid is added to inactivate the enzyme. The concentrations of glucose-6-phosphate and fructose-6-phosphate (F6P) are measured. Equilibrium is attained if the concentrations are the same at the two time intervals. The experiment is repeated using various initial concentrations of G6P and also in the reverse direction with various initial concentrations of F6P. Using this method, an average value of 0·36 for K' has been obtained.[20]

Recent advances in the techniques for the rapid and accurate measurement of concentrations of metabolites have made this type of experimental determination of K' possible for a wide variety of biochemical reactions. However, for reactions which involve a large standard free energy change $\Delta G°$ (that is, where the reaction proceeds almost to completion in one direction), K' is extremely large. At equilibrium the concentrations of substrates will be exceedingly small and therefore difficult to measure. In such cases it may be possible to calculate K' from either kinetic or thermochemical data.

The kinetic data necessary to calculate K' for an enzyme-catalysed reaction (single substrate enzyme) is the maximum catalytic activity in both directions (V_{max}) and the K_m values of the enzyme for substrate and product. From this data K' can be calculated using the Haldane relationship.[21] For the reaction, $A \rightleftarrows B$

$$K' = \frac{[A]}{[B]} = \frac{V_{max}^{A \rightarrow B} K_m^B}{V_{max}^{B \rightarrow A} K_m^A}$$

It is also possible to calculate K' from the change in free energy involved in a reaction using the equation

$$\Delta G = \Delta G^\circ + RT \ln \left(\frac{[Products]}{[Reactants]} \right)$$

At equilibrium,

$$\frac{[Products]}{[Reactants]} = K' \quad \text{and} \quad \Delta G = 0$$

(i.e. at equilibrium there is no change in free energy). Therefore

$$\Delta G^\circ = -RT \ln K'$$

For example, in the case of the phosphofructokinase (PFK) reaction, ΔG° was calculated from the combination of the standard free energy of hydrolysis of ATP and the (indirectly calculated) standard free energies of formation in aqueous solution of fructose-6-phosphate and fructose diphosphate (see reference 22). The ΔG° for the PFK reaction is -4.2 kcal/mol.
Since $\Delta G^\circ = -RT \ln K'$,

$$-4,200 = -1.98 \times 310 \times 2.303 \log_{10} K'$$

$$\log K' = \frac{4,200}{1,413} = 2.974$$

$$K' = 940 \quad \text{at pH 7.0 and 37 °C.}$$

Thus the apparent equilibrium constant for PFK at 37 °C and pH 7.0 is approximately 10^3.

The determination of heat changes in experiments involving biological compounds is often difficult since vast quantities of these compounds are required in order to give a temperature change which can be accurately measured. The introduction of microcalorimetry (which allows the measurement of temperature changes of the order of 10^{-6} °C) will no doubt remedy this situation in the future.

Using microcalorimetry it is possible to calculate the equilibrium constant *directly* from the heat evolved (Q_1) when the equilibrium is approached by addition of enzyme to the substrate and for the heat absorbed $(-Q_2)$ when the equilibrium is approached by the addition of enzyme to the product. In each case the ratio $Q_1/\Delta H$ or $-Q_2/\Delta H$ represents the proportion of the reactant converted to product as equilibrium is reached. Therefore,

$$K' = \frac{Q_1/\Delta H}{-Q_2/\Delta H} = \frac{Q_1}{Q_2}$$

Thus the equilibrium constant can be found from just two heat measurements in dilute solution (for example, see reference 23).

APPENDIX 1.2. MEASUREMENT OF MASS-ACTION RATIOS

The practical measurement of a mass-action ratio demands an intact physiological tissue preparation. This could be whole cells (such as yeast cells or ascites tumour cells), a perfused preparation (such as muscle or liver), an incubated tissue slice preparation (such as kidney cortex or cerebral cortex), or the actual tissue *in situ* (such as the liver of an anaesthetized animal). The first step is to freeze the whole preparation as rapidly as possible so that the enzyme-catalysed reactions are all simultaneously stopped and the concentrations of all the metabolic intermediates remain the same as they were in the physiologically functional tissue. This is achieved by freeze-clamping the tissue; that is, rapidly compressing it between large aluminium plates precooled to the temperature of liquid nitrogen $(-190\,°C)$. This is necessary because the rate of freezing after dropping a piece of tissue into liquid nitrogen is surprisingly slow. A thermocouple placed 1 mm inside the ventricle of a guinea-pig heart showed that the tissue cooled from 37 to 0 °C in 16 seconds.[24] As the tissue cools a bubble of nitrogen gas is produced and surrounds the tissue so that it is partially insulated from the liquid nitrogen. No such insulation occurs with the aluminium clamps when the tissue can be shown to cool from 37 to $-80\,°C$ in less than 0·1 second. After freeze-clamping, the frozen tissue must be deproteinized rapidly at a low temperature. This is accomplished by powdering the frozen tissue at temperatures well below freezing point (for example, $-70\,°C$) and thoroughly mixing the powder with a frozen protein precipitant such as perchloric acid. As the powder thaws, the enzymes are almost immediately inactivated and form a protein precipitate which can be removed by centrifugation. The supernatant is neutralized and analysed for the metabolites by specific enzymatic measurements. The advantage of enzymatic analysis is that it permits precise and specific measurements of individual metabolites in a complex biological mixture, without the necessity of tedious and laborious separations.

Such an analysis allows the calculation of the tissue content in terms of μmol of metabolite contained in each gram of tissue. An extrapolation of this value to the actual concentration of the metabolite within the intracellular water is possible, provided that the total water content of the tissue is known (measured by weighing the tissue when fresh and when completely dry) and provided that the extracellular volume is measured (using some compound which is known not to penetrate into the cell—see Chapter 3, Appendix 3.5). This gives rise to an apparent intracellular concentration which assumes that the metabolite is evenly distributed throughout the whole of the intracellular water.

Thus, for the PFK reaction

$$F6P + ATP \rightarrow FDP + ADP$$

the mass-action ratio would be

$$\frac{[FDP][ADP]}{[F6P][ATP]}$$

as measured in the freeze-clamped tissue. The tissue contents of these metabolites in the isolated rat heart perfused with a 5 mM glucose solution are given in Table 1.1, from which a mass-action ratio of 0·029 is computed.

Table 1.1. Measurement of the mass-action ratio of the PFK reaction in the isolated perfused heart[25]

Metabolite	Tissue content (μmol/g dry tissue)	Apparent concentration (mM) (μmol/ml intracellular H_2O)
fructose-6-phosphate	0·154	0·087
fructose diphosphate	0·042	0·022
ATP	21·70	11·52
ADP	2·49	1·32

$$\Gamma = \text{mass-action ratio} = \frac{[FDP][ADP]}{[F6P][ATP]} = \frac{0·022 \times 1·32}{0·087 \times 11·52} = 0·029$$

Since the apparent equilibrium constant for this reaction has been shown to be of the order of 10^3 (see above), it appears that this reaction is non-equilibrium in the cell.

This reaction has been chosen because it demonstrates clearly the principles involved and because it is quite easy to draw a definite conclusion from the results. However, there are at least two main criticisms of this approach which in some cases can pose major problems in the interpretation of experimental data. First, it is possible that the measured content of the metabolite, which is used to calculate Γ, bears no relation to the actual concentration of the metabolite within the immediate environment of the enzyme in question. This may be due to physical compartmentation (mito-chondrial or cytoplasmic, for example) or chemical compartmentation (as in adsorption of the metabolite onto protein). If a considerable portion of the ATP of the cell was not available for PFK (for example, if 99·9 % of the measured ATP was in the mitochondria whereas PFK was in the cytoplasm), Γ would closely approach K' and PFK might catalyse an equilibrium re-action. It is very unlikely that a cell could specifically localize 99·9 % of the ATP without having any effect on the distribution of ADP. This would require a highly selective transport process and it would consume large amounts of energy. Secondly, the interpretation of the quantitative difference between Γ and K' can be difficult. In any metabolic pathway in which there is a finite flux, the reactions cannot be at equilibrium. However, some reactions may be close to equilibrium (for example, 10 % removed) and some reactions may be far removed (for example, the PFK reaction). How large does the difference between Γ and K' have to be in order to define a reaction as non-equilibrium? There appears to be only an arbitrary division such that reactions which exhibit a difference of 20-fold or greater between Γ and K' are probably non-equilibrium (see reference 12). If the difference is smaller than this it is difficult to conclude that the reaction is non-equilibrium without other lines of evidence (such as maximum enzyme activities) to support this conclusion.

REFERENCES FOR CHAPTER 1

1. Lehninger, A. L. (1965). *Bioenergetics*. New York: W. A. Benjamin.
2. Spanner, D. C. (1964). *Introduction to Thermodynamics*. London & New York: Academic Press.
3. Linford, J. H. (1966). *An Introduction to Energetics*. London: Butterworths.
4. Wyatt, P. A. H. (1967). *Energy and Entropy in Chemistry*. London: Macmillan.
5. Klotz, I. M. (1967). *Energy Changes in Biochemical Reactions*. New York & London: Academic Press.
6. Krebs, H. A. & Kornberg, H. L. (1957). *Ergebnisse der Physiologie*, **49**, 212.
7. Morowitz, H. J. (1970). *Entropy for Biologists*. London & New York: Academic Press.
8. Denbigh, K. G. (1965). *The Thermodynamics of the Steady State*. London: Methuen.
9. Katchalsky, A. & Curran, P. F. (1965). *Nonequilibrium Thermodynamics in Bio-physics*. Cambridge, Mass.: Harvard University Press.
10. Bücher, Th. & Rüssman, W. (1964). *Angew. Chem. Internat. Edit.* **3**, 421.
11. Newsholme, E. A. & Gevers, W. (1967). *Vitamins & Hormones*, **25**, 1.
12. Rolleston, F. S. (1972). In *Current Topics in Cellular Regulation*, vol. 5, p. 47. Ed. B. L. Horecker & E. W. Stadtman. London & New York: Academic Press.
13. Chance, B., Holmes, W., Higgins, J. J. & Connelly, C. M. (1958). *Nature, Lond.* **182**, 1190.
14. Sols, A. & Marco, R. (1970). In *Current Topics in Cellular Regulation*, vol. 2, p. 227. Ed. B. L. Horecker & E. W. Stadtman. London & New York: Academic Press.
15. Schimke, R. T. (1969). In *Current Topics in Cellular Regulation*, vol. 1, p. 77. Ed. B. L. Horecker & E. W. Stadtman. London & New York: Academic Press.

16. Stadtman, E. W. (1966). *Adv. Enzymol.* **28,** 41.
17. Klingenberg, M. (1964). *Angew. Chem. Internat. Edit.* **3,** 54.
18. Slater, E. C. (1969). In *Energy Level and Metabolic Control in Mitochondria*, p. 255. Ed. S. Papa, J. M. Tager, E. Quagliariello & E. C. Slater. Bari: Adriatica Editrice.
19. Wilkins, B. R. (1966). In *Regulation and Control in Living Systems*, p. 12. Ed. H. Kalmus. London: John Wiley.
20. Kahana, S. E., Lowry, O. H., Schulz, D. W., Passonneau, J. V. & Crawford, E. J. (1961). *J. biol. Chem.* **235,** 2178.
21. Haldane, J. B. S. (1930). *Enzymes.* London: Longmans Green.
22. Burton, K. & Krebs, H. A. (1953). *Biochem. J.* **54,** 94.
23. Kitzinger, C. & Benzinger, T. H. (1960). *Methods in Biochem. Analysis*, **8,** 309.
24. Wollenberger, A., Ristau, O. & Schoffa, G. (1960). *Pflügers Archiv. ges Physiol.* **270,** 399.
25. Williamson, J. R. (1965). *J. biol. Chem.* **240,** 2308.

CHAPTER 2

MOLECULAR MECHANISMS IN THE REGULATION OF ENZYME ACTIVITY

A. INTRODUCTION TO ALLOSTERIC ENZYMES

1. The discovery of feedback inhibition in bacteria

The story of the development of the concept of allosteric proteins in metabolic regulation probably begins with the work of Roberts and his colleagues which was published in 1955.[1] They were studying the growth of *Escherichia coli* on a medium containing ^{14}C-glucose as the sole source of carbon in order to label all the cell constituents with ^{14}C. The addition of an amino acid to such a growth medium resulted in complete inhibition of incorporation of label into that particular amino acid. Such effects were observed with all amino acids synthesized by specific biosynthetic pathways (such as histidine, proline and tryptophan), but not with amino acids which could be produced by simple transamination reactions (such as aspartate and glutamate). Thus, a specific biosynthetic pathway was necessary in order to observe this inhibitory effect and the theory was proposed that this represented end-product inhibition of the pathway. Following these early discoveries, many other pathways in bacteria were found to be specifically inhibited by their end-products.

In 1956 Umbarger reported that the enzyme, threonine deaminase, which catalyses an early reaction in the biosynthetic pathway leading to isoleucine (Figure 2.1), was inhibited by this compound *in vitro*.[2] In the same year Gerhart and Pardee reported that aspartate transcarbamylase (ATCase), which catalyses the first reaction of the pathway for the biosynthesis of pyrimidines, was inhibited *in vitro* by the end-product of its pathway, CMP, although later it was established that CTP (Figure 2.2) was an even more effective inhibitor.[3] These discoveries provided a biochemical explanation for the end-product inhibition observed in intact bacterial cells. The physiological significance of these inhibitions was emphasized by the fact that the end-product did not inhibit any other enzyme of the pathway, nor were the other intermediates of the pathway effective in causing inhibition of the enzyme *in vitro*. From 1956 onwards many other enzymes of biosynthetic pathways were investigated with a view to discovering end-product inhibitors. The wealth of information made available by these studies between 1956 and 1963 provided the factual basis for the allosteric theory developed by Monod, Changeux and Jacob in 1963.[4]

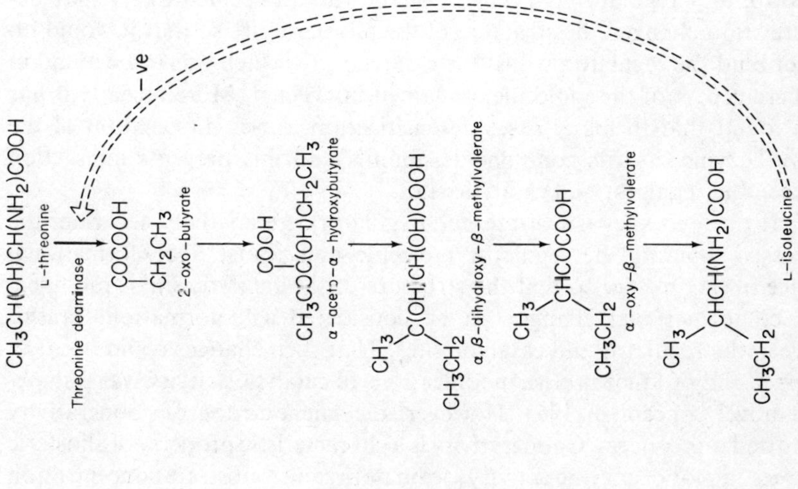

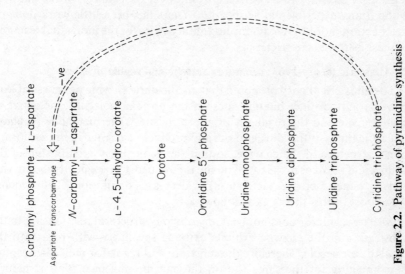

Figure 2.2. Pathway of pyrimidine synthesis

Figure 2.1. Pathway of isoleucine synthesis

The relative simplicity of these biosynthetic pathways in bacteria permitted regulatory enzymes to be detected from direct observation of the pathway without any experimental verification. There has been little work done on mass-action ratios or maximum enzyme activities for the individual reactions of these pathways in bacteria.

2. Allosteric theory 1963: separate catalytic and regulator sites

The allosteric theory proposed that an allosteric enzyme possesses at least two spatially distinct binding sites on the protein molecule: the active or catalytic site and the regulator or allosteric site.[4] The metabolic regulator molecule binds at the allosteric site and produces a change in the conformational structure of the enzyme, so that the geometrical relationship of the amino acid residues in the catalytic site is modified. Consequently the enzyme activity either increases (activation) or decreases (inhibition). The evidence in support of this theory is as follows.

(a) The regulator does not bear any obvious structural relationship to the substrate and the enzyme exhibits extreme specificity with regard to the regulator molecule. Therefore the substrate and regulator molecules cannot be competing for the same site on the enzyme molecule. This structural dissimilarity gave rise to the term 'allosteric'.

(b) Treatment of the allosteric enzyme with agents or conditions that exert a mild denaturing effect can result in loss of sensitivity to the effects of the regulator molecule without changing the catalytic activity. This process of desensitization can be effected by mercurials (such as mercuric chloride), urea or by gentle heating. When this theory was first put forward desensitization provided the strongest evidence for the existence of separate sites for substrate and regulator molecules. At the time it seemed likely that desensitization changed the structure of the allosteric site so that it would no longer bind the regulator, whilst the catalytic site, which was to be found in a different part of the molecule, remained unaffected. More recently it has been found that in many cases desensitization causes dissociation of the native enzyme into its component subunits and this prevents interaction between the regulator and catalytic sites.

(c) If the two sites (substrate and regulator) are spatially separate, the process of binding the regulator molecule must cause a conformational change in the protein so that the structure of the catalytic site is modified. This conformational change can be considered as information transfer between the regulator and catalytic sites. That such changes could occur in enzymes and produce precise modifications of catalytic activity was a somewhat novel concept in 1963. However, the phenomenon of cooperativity supported this concept. Cooperativity is a characteristic property of allosteric enzymes: a plot of enzyme activity (ordinate) against substrate concentration (abscissa) is S-shaped or sigmoid rather than hyperbolic (see Figure 2.3).

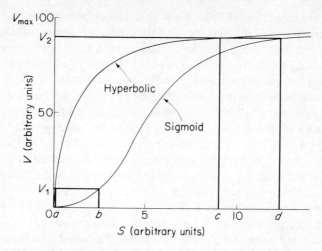

Figure 2.3. Hyperbolic and sigmoid plots of enzyme activity against substrate concentration. A change in activity from V_1 to V_2 (i.e. 10% to 90% of the maximal activity) requires a change in substrate from a to c for the hyperbolic plot and from b to d for the sigmoid plot

One possible explanation for the occurrence of these sigmoid kinetics is that each molecule of enzyme possesses more than one catalytic site to which the substrate can be bound. The binding of substrate at one site could somehow affect the binding of subsequent molecules of substrate at the remaining sites; that is, there must be some form of information transfer between binding sites. Evidence that cooperativity is not a direct effect but is transmitted through the conformational structure of the protein was to be found in studies on haemoglobin. This protein exhibits cooperativity in the binding of oxygen: a plot of the amount of oxygen bound to haemoglobin against the partial pressure of oxygen (equivalent to substrate concentration for an enzyme) is sigmoid rather than hyperbolic. There are known to be four binding sites for oxygen on each molecule of haemoglobin, so that cooperativity can be explained if the binding of an oxygen molecule to one of the haem groups causes an increase in the affinity of the remaining haem groups for oxygen (see later for various molecular explanations). However, the three-dimensional structure of haemoglobin, which had been published by Perutz and coworkers in 1960, showed that the four haem groups were completely spatially separate in the molecule and that direct interaction between the haem groups was impossible. This provided a precedent for the involvement of protein conformation in relaying information between various sites on the protein molecule.

The importance of the 1963 paper was that it assembled convincing evidence for the separation of the two sites (catalytic and regulatory) on the enzyme molecule. Furthermore, such a separation offered an advantage for the process of natural selection: the two sites could develop quite independently of one another so as to provide the most efficient system for both catalytic activity and metabolic regulation. No restrictions need be placed on the regulatory mechanism by the nature of the catalytic process, and selection of regulators for the metabolic pathway could be based on advantages for the metabolism of the cell as a whole rather than on the individual reaction or pathway *per se*. In addition, any mutation which resulted in a change in the amino acid sequence of a region of the polypeptide chain, which was not involved in binding either substrate or regulator, might modify the degree of interaction between the two sites. Such a mutation could be important for improving the regulatory properties of the enzyme and consequently would be acted upon by natural selection. Therefore allosteric enzymes provide an extremely flexible system from an evolutionary point of view.

B. DERIVATION OF EQUATIONS DESCRIBING THE PROCESS OF EQUILIBRIUM BINDING

Following the publication of these ideas on allosteric enzymes in 1963, various model systems were proposed which attempted to explain the sigmoidal variation of enzyme activity with substrate concentration. These models may be classified into two groups. The first group consists of models that depend upon multiple binding sites on a single protein with some form of interaction between the sites. The binding of the substrate molecules and the various conformational changes of the enzyme that result are the basis of the cooperative effect. These changes are considered to occur so rapidly with respect to the actual catalysed reaction that the various conformational states are in equilibrium with each other. The second group consists of kinetic models in which the cooperativity arises from the actual kinetics of the enzyme-catalysed reaction. In this type of model conformational changes are considered to occur relatively slowly with respect to the overall catalysed reaction, so that various conformational states are not in equilibrium but reach steady-state concentrations. The cooperativity arises out of the actual kinetics of the reaction pathway and could occur in a monomeric as well as a polymeric protein. The experimental finding that some enzymes which exhibit cooperativity are oligomeric (that is, they consist of a number of identical subunits or protomers) has led to emphasis upon the multiple-binding-site models. The basic differences between these two types of models will be explained in detail later in this chapter. Before the various models are discussed, a brief description of the derivation of the basic equations for multiple-binding-site models is useful.

1. Equilibrium binding to monomeric proteins

Before considering the mathematics of the binding of a ligand (small molecule) to allosteric enzymes (that is, multiple binding sites), it is instructive to consider the binding of a ligand, S, to a monomeric protein, Pr.

At equilibrium the process can be represented as follows,

$$\text{Pr} + \text{S} \underset{k_{-1}}{\overset{k_1}{\rightleftarrows}} \text{PrS}$$

Let $\overline{Y}_s$ be the fractional saturation of the protein with S (that is, the fraction of the total number of binding sites for S which are occupied by S) and $(1 - \overline{Y}_s)$ be the fraction of unoccupied sites,

$$\text{Rate of association} = \overset{\bullet}{k}_1 . [S](1 - \overline{Y}_s)$$

$$\text{Rate of dissociation} = k_{-1} . \overline{Y}_s$$

At equilibrium these two processes occur at equal rates so that,

$$k_{-1} . \overline{Y}_s = k_1[S](1 - \overline{Y}_s)$$
$$= k_1[S] - k_1[S]\overline{Y}_s$$

Dividing through by $\overline{Y}_s$

$$k_{-1} = \frac{k_1[S]}{\overline{Y}_s} - k_1[S]$$

Therefore

$$\overline{Y}_s = \frac{k_1[S]}{k_{-1} + k_1[S]}$$

$$= \frac{[S]}{(k_{-1}/k_1) + [S]}$$

Since $k_{-1}/k_1 = K_d$ (the dissociation constant)

$$\overline{Y}_s = \frac{[S]}{K_d + [S]}$$

$$= \frac{[S]/K_d}{1 + [S]/K_d} \tag{2.1}$$

In terms of the binding constant K_b which is given by k_1/k_{-1} or $1/K_d$

$$\overline{Y}_s = \frac{K_b[S]}{1 + K_b[S]} \tag{2.2}$$

Equations 2.1 and 2.2 are of the type that describe a rectangular hyperbola. Therefore a plot of fractional saturation of the protein ($\overline{Y}_s$) against substrate concentration [S] is hyperbolic (Figure 2.3).

However, in the case of an enzyme which not only binds substrate but also catalyses a specific reaction, the plot of initial velocity against substrate concentration will be hyperbolic only if the overall velocity depends upon the concentration of the enzyme-substrate complex, PrS: in this case the latter is dependent upon the equilibrium binding process.

$$\text{Pr} + \text{S} \underset{k_{-1}}{\overset{k_1}{\rightleftarrows}} \text{PrS} \overset{k_2}{\rightarrow} \text{Pr} + \text{Product}$$

If k_2 is complex (that is, a number of intermediate reactions occur) or if the enzyme catalyses a reaction involving more than one substrate, this simple relationship may not hold and hyperbolic curves may not be obtained (see Section E).

2. Equilibrium binding to polymeric proteins

In the case of a protein that has several binding sites for the same ligand on each molecule, the interaction between the ligand and the protein can be described by equation 2.1 *provided that all the sites are identical and there is no interaction between them*, that is, the binding of the first substrate molecule has no effect upon the affinity for the second substrate molecule, etc. In the case of a tetrameric protein with four substrate-binding sites, the following four equilibria are considered to exist:

Reaction	Apparent binding constant
$\text{Pr}_4 + \text{S} \rightleftarrows \text{Pr}_4\text{S}$	K_{b1}
$\text{Pr}_4\text{S} + \text{S} \rightleftarrows \text{Pr}_4\text{S}_2$	K_{b2}
$\text{Pr}_4\text{S}_2 + \text{S} \rightleftarrows \text{Pr}_4\text{S}_3$	K_{b3}
$\text{Pr}_4\text{S}_3 + \text{S} \rightleftarrows \text{Pr}_4\text{S}_4$	K_{b4}

If there is no interaction between the binding sites, the microscopic (or intrinsic) binding constant, K_b, is the same for each monomer and is statistically related to the apparent binding constants, K_{b1}, K_{b2}, etc., by the number of empty binding sites available on the protein molecule.*

For a monomeric protein described by the reaction $\text{Pr} + \text{S} \underset{k_{-1}}{\overset{k_1}{\rightleftarrows}} \text{PrS}$ the binding constant (K_b) is as follows:

$$K_b = \frac{k_1}{k_{-1}} \tag{2.3}$$

---

* The difference between the microscopic and the apparent binding constants for binding sites on monomers within polymeric proteins is sometimes difficult to understand. If the constant could be measured on each monomer in the absence of the binding sites on the other monomers the microscopic binding constant would be obtained. However, in practice the binding constants for each site vary according to the number of available binding sites in each polymer, that is the microscopic and apparent binding constants are statistically related. For example in the reaction governed by K_{b1} there are four sites available for binding S but only one site from which bound S can dissociate. Therefore K_{b1} is 4-fold greater than K_b. Similarly $K_{b2} = \frac{3}{2}K_b$, $K_{b3} = \frac{2}{3}K_b$ and $K_{b4} = \frac{1}{4}K_b$.

However, for the tetrameric protein, Pr_4, the reactions and the binding constants are as follows:

Reaction	Binding constant	
$Pr_4 + S \underset{k_{-1}}{\overset{k_1}{\rightleftharpoons}} Pr_4S$	$K_{b1} = \dfrac{4k_1}{k_{-1}} = 4K_b$	(2.4)
$Pr_4S + S \underset{k_{-2}}{\overset{k_2}{\rightleftharpoons}} Pr_4S_2$	$K_{b2} = \dfrac{3k_2}{2k_{-2}} = \dfrac{3}{2}K_b$	(2.5)
$Pr_4S_2 + S \underset{k_{-3}}{\overset{k_3}{\rightleftharpoons}} Pr_4S_3$	$K_{b3} = \dfrac{2k_3}{3k_{-3}} = \dfrac{2}{3}K_b$	(2.6)
$Pr_4S_3 + S \underset{k_{-4}}{\overset{k_4}{\rightleftharpoons}} Pr_4S_4$	$K_{b4} = \dfrac{k_4}{4k_{-4}} = \dfrac{1}{4}K_b$	(2.7)

In a reaction between a polymeric protein and a ligand, all species of intermediates may be present (that is, Pr_4, Pr_4S, Pr_4S_2, Pr_4S_3 and Pr_4S_4). Therefore the fractional saturation of the protein Pr_4 with S, which is defined as the total amount of S bound divided by the total number of sites available, is given by the following expression

$$\bar{Y}_s = \frac{[Pr_4S] + 2[Pr_4S_2] + 3[Pr_4S_3] + 4[Pr_4S_4]}{4([Pr_4] + [Pr_4S] + [Pr_4S_2] + [Pr_4S_3] + [Pr_4S_4])}$$

(In the numerator, for each molecule in the Pr_4S_2 state, two sites are filled with substrate and therefore Pr_4S_2 must be multiplied by 2, similarly for Pr_4S_3 and Pr_4S_4. In the denominator, the total number of sites available is obtained from summing the total species of molecules that are present and multiplying by 4, since the protein is tetrameric.) However, the concentrations of all the intermediate species, Pr_4S, Pr_4S_2, etc., may be expressed in terms of free Pr_4, free S, and the four apparent binding constants K_{b1}, K_{b2}, etc.

Reaction	Apparent binding constant	Concentration of intermediate species
$Pr_4 + S \leftrightarrows Pr_4S$	K_{b1}	$[Pr_4S] = K_{b1}[Pr_4][S]$
$Pr_4S + S \rightleftharpoons Pr_4S_2$	K_{b2}	$[Pr_4S_2] = K_{b2}[Pr_4S][S]$
		but substituting for $[Pr_4S]$ from above
		$[Pr_4S_2] = K_{b1}K_{b2}[Pr_4][S]^2$
$Pr_4S_2 + S \rightleftharpoons Pr_4S_3$	K_{b3}	$[Pr_4S_3] = K_{b3}[Pr_4S_2][S]$
		$= K_{b1}K_{b2}K_{b3}[Pr_4][S]^3$
$Pr_4S_3 + S \leftrightarrows Pr_4S_4$	K_{b4}	$[Pr_4S_4] = K_{b4}[Pr_4S_3][S]$
		$= K_{b1}K_{b2}K_{b3}K_{b4}[Pr_4][S]^4$

It is now possible to substitute for these intermediate concentrations in the expression for fractional saturation which is given above.

$$\bar{Y}_s = \frac{\begin{aligned}K_{b1}[Pr_4][S] + 2K_{b1}K_{b2}[Pr_4][S]^2 + 3K_{b1}K_{b2}K_{b3}[Pr_4][S]^3 \\ + 4K_{b1}K_{b2}K_{b3}K_{b4}[Pr_4][S]^4\end{aligned}}{\begin{aligned}4\{[Pr_4] + K_{b1}[Pr_4][S] + K_{b1}K_{b2}[Pr_4][S]^2 + K_{b1}K_{b2}K_{b3}[Pr_4][S]^3 \\ + K_{b1}K_{b2}K_{b3}K_{b4}[Pr_,][S]^4\}\end{aligned}}$$

The $[Pr_4]$ values now cancel out so that

$$\bar{Y}_s = \frac{K_{b1}[S] + 2K_{b1}K_{b2}[S]^2 + 3K_{b1}K_{b2}K_{b3}[S]^3 + 4K_{b1}K_{b2}K_{b3}K_{b4}[S]^4}{4\{1 + K_{b1}[S] + K_{b1}K_{b2}[S]^2 + K_{b1}K_{b2}K_{b3}[S]^3 + K_{b1}K_{b2}K_{b3}K_{b4}[S]^4\}}$$

(2.8)

If all four binding sites are identical and there is no interaction between them, K_{b1}, K_{b2}, K_{b3} and K_{b4} may all be expressed in terms of the microscopic binding constant K_b (equations 2.4 to 2.7). (For example, $K_{b1} = 4K_b$ and $K_{b2} = \frac{3}{2}K_b$ so that $2K_{b1}K_{b2}[S]^2$ is the same as $2 \times 4K_b \times \frac{3}{2}K_b[S]^2$ which equals $12K_b^2[S]^2$.) The equation for fractional saturation now simplifies to

$$\bar{Y}_s = \frac{4K_b[S] + 12K_b^2[S]^2 + 12K_b^3[S]^3 + 4K_b^4[S]^4}{4\{1 + 4K_b[S] + 6K_b^2[S]^2 + 4K_b^3[S]^3 + K_b^4[S]^4\}}$$

$$= \frac{K_b[S](1 + 3K_b[S] + 3K_b^2[S]^2 + K_b^3[S]^3)}{1 + 4K_b[S] + 6K_b^2[S]^2 + 4K_b^3[S]^3 + K_b^4[S]^4}$$

$$= \frac{K_b[S](1 + K_b[S])^3}{(1 + K_b[S])^4} \quad \text{(N.B. } (1 + K_b[S])^3 = 1 + 3K_b[S] + 3K_b^2[S]^2}$$
$$+ K_b^3[S]^3)$$

$$= \frac{K_b[S]}{1 + K_b[S]}$$

(2.9)

Therefore, with the provision that binding sites are identical and there are no interactions, equation 2.9 is obtained which is exactly the same as that derived for a monomeric protein (equation 2.2) and it describes a hyperbolic curve.

C. EARLY MATHEMATICAL MODELS TO EXPLAIN SIGMOID BINDING OF OXYGEN TO HAEMOGLOBIN

One of the first oligomeric proteins whose binding characteristics were examined in detail was haemoglobin. As early as 1904 it was shown that the fractional saturation of haemoglobin with oxygen when plotted against the partial pressure of oxygen gas (equivalent to the concentration) was not hyperbolic but was strongly sigmoidal.[5] That such a departure from normality might result from a multiplicity of binding sites (i.e. that one haemoglobin molecule was capable of binding more than one oxygen molecule) was discussed by Barcroft and Hill in 1909.[6] At this time it was known that each haem group bound only one oxygen molecule but it was not known how many haem groups each haemoglobin molecule possessed.

1. The model of Hill, 1909

This model proposed very simply that if there were n binding sites for oxygen per haemoglobin molecule, the reaction between haemoglobin and oxygen could be described by the following equation.

$$Hb + nO_2 \rightleftarrows Hb(O_2)_n$$

for which the equilibrium constant (or binding constant), K_b, was given by

$$K_b = \frac{[Hb(O_2)_n]}{[Hb]pO_2^n} \tag{2.10}$$

where pO_2 is the partial pressure of oxygen, or

$$[Hb(O_2)_n] = K_b pO_2^n [Hb] \tag{2.11}$$

In equation 2.10 (which is based on the reaction $Hb + nO_2 \rightleftarrows Hb(O_2)_n$) the assumption was made that only two species of haemoglobin exist, Hb and $Hb(O_2)_n$: the possibility of stable intermediates (such as $Hb(O_2)_{n-1}$ or $Hb(O_2)_{n-2}$) was not considered. The fractional saturation, $\overline{Y}_s$, was derived in terms of the binding constant K_b and the partial pressure of O_2,

$$\overline{Y}_s = \frac{[Hb(O_2)_n]}{[Hb] + [Hb(O_2)_n]} \quad \text{by definition}$$

Substituting for $[Hb(O_2)_n]$ from equation 2.11,

$$\overline{Y}_s = \frac{K_b pO_2^n [Hb]}{[Hb] + K_b pO_2^n [Hb]}$$

$$= \frac{K_b pO_2^n}{1 + K_b pO_2^n} \tag{2.12}$$

If $n = 1$ (that is, there is only one O_2-binding site per protein molecule), this equation reduces to

$$\overline{Y}_s = \frac{K_b pO_2}{1 + K_b pO_2} \tag{2.13}*$$

* The oxygen-binding protein which occurs in muscle tissue is called myoglobin and this is a monomeric protein which contains one haem group per molecule. The binding of oxygen to this protein is described by a hyperbolic curve which is explained by equation 2.13.

Equation 2.13 is identical to equation 2.2 and describes a hyperbolic curve. From equation 2.11 it can be seen that

$$\frac{[Hb(O_2)_n]}{[Hb]} = K_b pO_2^n$$

Taking logarithms of both sides of this equation,

$$\log\left(\frac{[Hb(O_2)_n]}{[Hb]}\right) = \log K_b + n \log pO_2$$

or in a more general form for the fractional saturation $\overline{Y}_s$ of a protein with substrate S

$$\log\left(\frac{\overline{Y}_s}{1 - \overline{Y}_s}\right) = \log K + n \log [S] \tag{2.14}$$

Equation 2.14 is known as the Hill equation and a plot of $\log\left(\dfrac{\overline{Y}_s}{1 - \overline{Y}_s}\right)$ against $\log [S]$ is referred to as a Hill plot.

In the case of an enzyme-catalysed reaction in which the velocity of the reaction is determined by the concentration of enzyme-substrate complex, a fractional saturation of unity is equivalent to the maximum velocity (V_{max}) and thus a Hill plot consists of a plot of $\log\left(\dfrac{v}{V_{max} - v}\right)$ against $\log [S]$, where v is the initial velocity at a given substrate concentration.

In developing equation 2.12 Hill made the assumption that only two species of haemoglobin exist (Hb and $Hb(O_2)_n$). This assumption predicts that a plot of $\log\left(\dfrac{[Hb(O_2)_n]}{[Hb]}\right)$ against $\log pO_2$ should be linear with a slope of n, where n is equal to the total number of binding sites for O_2 on haemoglobin (from equation 2.14). However, the experimentally determined value of n for haemoglobin is 2·8 whereas it is now known that the haemoglobin molecule possesses 4 sites for binding oxygen (4 haem groups). Therefore the mathematical model proposed by Hill to explain the sigmoidicity of the reaction between oxygen and haemoglobin is invalid. Consequently, Hill plots for enzymes (that is, plots of $\log\left(\dfrac{v}{V_{max} - v}\right)$ against $\log [S]$), even if they are linear, do not necessarily have a slope which is equal to the number of substrate binding sites. Instead the slope gives some indication of the degree of interaction between the subunits; see Section D.3.

2. The model of Adair, 1925

The obvious improvement on the Hill model was to include all the possible intermediates of the reaction between haemoglobin and oxygen. In 1925

Adair[8] put forward the intermediate-compound hypothesis which took into account the possible existence of $Hb(O_2)$, $Hb(O_2)_2$, $Hb(O_2)_3$, etc. Adair considered that the binding of O_2 to Hb occurred in a stepwise fashion as follows.

Reaction	*Apparent binding constant*
$Hb + O_2 \rightleftarrows HbO_2$	K_{b1}
$HbO_2 + O_2 \rightleftarrows Hb(O_2)_2$	K_{b2}
$Hb(O_2)_2 + O_2 \rightleftarrows Hb(O_2)_3$	K_{b3}
$Hb(O_2)_3 + O_2 \rightleftarrows Hb(O_2)_4$	K_{b4}

This is analogous to the binding of S to Pr_4 and the equation for fractional saturation of Hb with O_2 can be expressed in terms of the free concentrations of Hb and pO_2, as developed above (Section B.2).

$$\bar{Y}_s = \frac{K_{b1}pO_2 + 2K_{b1}K_{b2}pO_2^2 + 3K_{b1}K_{b2}K_{b3}pO_2^3 + 4K_{b1}K_{b2}K_{b3}K_{b4}pO_2^4}{4(1 + K_{b1}pO_2 + K_{b1}K_{b2}pO_2^2 + K_{b1}K_{b2}K_{b3}pO_2^3 + K_{b1}K_{b2}K_{b3}K_{b4}pO_2^4)}$$

(2.15)

This equation was developed by Adair in 1925. According to this equation, if $K_{b1} < (8/3)K_{b2}$, $K_{b2} < (9/4)K_{b3}$, $K_{b3} < (8/3)K_{b4}$, sigmoidal curves of $\bar{Y}_s$ against pO_2 are obtained. (As described in Section B.2, if the microscopic binding constant is the same for each monomer, the apparent binding constants, K_{b1}, K_{b2}, etc., are simply related to the microscopic binding constant, K_b, by the number of empty sites available ($K_{b1} = 4K_b$, $K_{b2} = (3/2)K_b$, $K_{b3} = (2/3)K_b$, $K_{b4} = (1/4)K_b$), and the equation simplifies to that of a hyperbolic curve.

D. EQUILIBRIUM BINDING MODELS TO EXPLAIN SIGMOID BEHAVIOUR

The models of Hill and Adair were basically equations describing the binding of a ligand to a polymeric protein and the Adair equation showed that a difference in the binding constants for the various intermediate reactions between haemoglobin and oxygen could explain sigmoidicity. The problem of explaining sigmoidicity of binding was now transferred to a molecular understanding of why the microscopic binding constants should be different. The publication of the three-dimensional structure of haemoglobin in 1960[9] showed that the haem groups were completely separate in the haemoglobin molecule and therefore precluded any explanation based upon direct interactions. Furthermore, the three-dimensional model showed that the environments of the haem groups in the individual subunits were very similar, so that differences in the binding constants for oxygen would be produced only upon the binding of an oxygen molecule.

The molecular interpretation of sigmoid behaviour received a stimulus in 1963 when Monod et al.[4] noted that many regulatory enzymes exhibited sigmoidicity in their initial rate plots (initial velocity against substrate concentration). The field of interest had now moved from haemoglobin to the regulatory enzymes, although any model system must include haemoglobin. The importance of discussing haemoglobin is that it provides a historical account of sigmoidicity and a factual basis with which to view the molecular models of sigmoidicity.

In 1965, Monod, Wyman and Changeux[10] published their classic paper in which they proposed a molecular model to explain cooperative behaviour in allosteric proteins. An alternative model was proposed by Koshland and coworkers[11] somewhat later, in 1966, but since the Koshland model is a development of the Adair intermediate-compound hypothesis, discussion of this model follows logically, if not chronologically, at this point. The Monod–Wyman–Changeux model is discussed later (Section D.2).

1. The Koshland model

The intermediate-compound hypothesis of Adair has been extended by Koshland and coworkers to explain the cooperative effect exhibited by allosteric enzymes.[11] The theory was developed from the original 'induced fit' theory proposed by Koshland in 1958 in order to explain enzyme specificity. It was suggested that the binding of substrate to an enzyme induces a localized structural change in the active site and this creates the correct three-dimensional arrangement of the amino acid residues in the active centre for catalysis.[12] Thus, the structure of the substrate was important not only for binding but also for creating the 'catalytic conformation' of the enzyme. Such a theory could be extended to polymeric enzymes with the additional proposal that a conformational change induced by substrate binding in one subunit could modify the conformation of another subunit, which had not bound the substrate. This implies that binding of a substrate molecule by one subunit produces a conformational change that is transferred to another subunit so that the latter is able to bind substrate more easily. The binding of the second substrate molecule stabilizes this conformation in the second subunit and this will influence the conformation of a third subunit. The binding of substrate should therefore become progressively easier. In the case of a tetrameric protein this sequential process can be described diagrammatically as follows:

If the circle is termed the A conformation and the square the B conformation, the situation may be described by $A_4 \rightleftarrows A_3BS \rightleftarrows A_2B_2S_2 \rightleftarrows A_1B_3S_3 \rightleftarrows B_4S_4$. The four equilibria are governed by constants K_{b1}, K_{b2}, K_{b3} and K_{b4}. A saturation function $(\overline{Y}_s)$ can be derived which is exactly analogous to that of Adair and which has the form:

$$\overline{Y}_s = \frac{K_{b1}[S] + 2K_{b1}K_{b2}[S]^2 + 3K_{b1}K_{b2}K_{b3}[S]^3 + 4K_{b1}K_{b2}K_{b3}K_{b4}[S]^4}{4(1 + K_{b1}[S] + K_{b1}K_{b2}[S]^2 + K_{b1}K_{b2}K_{b3}[S]^3 + K_{b1}K_{b2}K_{b3}K_{b4}[S]^4)}$$

The equations show that if there is no interaction between the binding sites, the apparent binding constants are statistically related to each other $(K_{b1} = (8/3)K_{b2}$, etc.) and a curve of $\overline{Y}_s$ against $[S]$ is hyperbolic. If $K_{b1} < (8/3)K_{b2}$, etc., sigmoid curves result. The model of Koshland attempts to explain why these constants should have different values.

Each equilibrium constant can be considered to have three components:
(a) An equilibrium constant K_t, for the conformation change $A \rightleftarrows B$,

$$K_t = \frac{[B]}{[A]}$$

(b) A binding constant K_s for the process $B + S \rightleftarrows BS$

$$K_s = \frac{[BS]}{[B][S]}$$

(c) An interaction constant which depends upon the degree of stability that one subunit confers upon the resultant complex.

	Reaction	Interaction constant
	$A + B \leftrightarrows AB$	$K_{AB} = \dfrac{[AB]}{[A][B]}$
Also	$A + A \leftrightarrows AA$	$K_{AA} = \dfrac{[AA]}{[A][A]}$
	$B + B \leftrightarrows BB$	$K_{BB} = \dfrac{[BB]}{[B][B]}$

For example, the ratio K_{BB}/K_{AA} compares the stabilities of the two complexes, AA and BB. In the Koshland model K_{AA} is assigned as unity so that if $K_{AB} > 1$, the interaction between A and B is more favourable than between A and A. In this case interaction will stabilize the complex AB and will therefore increase the binding of the substrate. If $K_{AB} < 1$, the interaction between A and B will decrease the stability of AB and decrease the binding of S.

The involvement of these three constants can best be explained by reference to a reaction involving a dimeric protein

$$\text{AA} + S \rightleftharpoons \text{ABS}$$

The equilibrium constant for this reaction is the product of K_t and K_s, multiplied by the change in the subunit interaction K_{AB}/K_{AA}

$$K = \frac{2K_t K_s K_{AB}}{K_{AA}}$$

The statistical factor 2 must be included as there are two forms of intermediate complex (A.BS and BS.A) and only one form of AA.

Similarly, for the binding of a second molecule of substrate

$$\text{ABS} + S \rightleftharpoons \text{BBS}_2$$

$$K = \frac{K_t K_s K_{BB}}{2K_{AB}}$$

As $K_{AA} = 1$ (convention of Koshland), the binding of the second molecule of S will occur more readily than the first if $2K_{AB}/K_{AA} < \frac{1}{2}K_{BB}/K_{AB}$ (positive cooperative effect): if $K_{AB}/K_{AA} > K_{BB}/K_{AB}$ then binding of the second molecule of S will occur less readily than the first (negative cooperative effect—see Section D.3(b)).

However, the interaction constant (such as K_{AB}) is even more complicated in a polymeric molecule. In the case of a tetramer the interactions can be described as tetrahedral, square or linear. These terms only classify the subunit interactions and do not correspond necessarily to the spatial structure of the protein. In the tetrahedral model each subunit interacts with the other three (see Figure 2.4a). In the square model, each subunit interacts with two of its neighbours (diagonal interactions are assumed to be negligible). In the linear model the two external subunits interact with one neighbour each, while the two internal subunits interact with two neighbours each (Figure 2.4a). For each model it is possible to derive expressions for the fractional saturation of protein with substrate in terms of the various Koshland constants in exactly the same way as Adair derived the expression for $\overline{Y}_s$ for haemoglobin in 1925 (see Section B.2).

(a) Saturation function for the tetrahedral model

This is derived in an analogous way to that of Adair, only the process is somewhat more complicated.

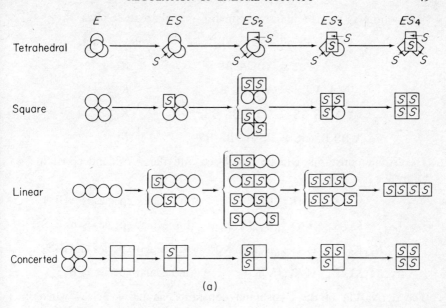

(a)

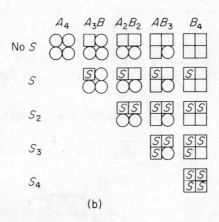

(b)

Figure 2.4. (a) The four types of interaction models described by Koshland. Conformation A is denoted by circles and conformation B by squares.[11] (b) Schematic illustration of possible molecular species for a general model involving four subunits, exclusive binding, and two possible conformations per subunit. Species with identical number of subunits in B conformation, vertical columns. Species with identical numbers of ligand molecules bound, horizontal rows[13]

Reactions of the Koshland tetrahedral model are as follows.

Reactions	*'Adair constants'*
A A A A $\rightleftarrows$ A A A BS	K_{b1}
A A A BS $\rightleftarrows$ A A BS BS	K_{b2}
A A BS BS $\rightleftarrows$ A BS BS BS	K_{b3}
A BS BS BS $\rightleftarrows$ BS BS BS BS	K_{b4}

The 'Adair constants' can be translated into the 'Koshland constants' as follows

$$K_{b1} \text{ is } 4K_{AB}^3 K_S K_t \qquad \text{(molecular species is } A_3BS)$$

$$K_{b1} K_{b2} \text{ is } 6K_{AB}^4 K_{BB}(K_S K_t)^2 \qquad \text{(molecular species is } A_2B_2S_2)$$

$$K_{b1}K_{b2} K_{b3} \text{ is } 4K_{AB}^3 K_{BB}^3 (K_S K_t)^3 \qquad \text{(molecular species is } AB_3S_3)$$

$$K_{b1}K_{b2}K_{b3} K_{b4} \text{ is } K_{BB}^6 (K_S K_t)^4 \qquad \text{(molecular species is } B_4S_4)$$

The derivation of the 'Koshland constants' should be clear when it is realized that there are 4 equivalent ways to bind one molecule of S, 6 equivalent ways to bind two molecules of S, 4 equivalent ways to bind three molecules of S and only one way to bind four molecules of S. Also the number of interacting subunits is 3 A–B and 3 A–A for the A_3BS species and therefore the constants K_{AA} and K_{AB} are raised to the third power (as K_{AA} is unity this is omitted from the expression); for the $A_2B_2S_2$ species the number of interacting subunits will be one B–B, 4 A–B and one A–A; for the AB_3S_3 species the number of interacting subunits will be 3 B–B, and 3 A–B; and finally for the B_4S_4 species the number of interacting subunits will be 6 B–B. Thus, by substituting the 'Koshland constants' in the original Adair equation the following expression is obtained.

$$\overline{Y}_s = \frac{K_{AB}^3(K_s K_t[S]) + 3K_{AB}^4 K_{BB}(K_s K_t[S])^2 + 3K_{AB}^3 K_{BB}^3(K_s K_t[S])^3 + K_{BB}^6(K_s K_t[S])^4}{1 + 4K_{AB}^3(K_s K_t[S]) + 6K_{AB}^4 K_{BB}(K_s K_t[S])^2 + 4K_{AB}^3 K_{BB}^3(K_s K_t[S])^3 + K_{BB}^6(K_s K_t[S])^4}$$

$$(2.16)$$

Similarly $\overline{Y}_s$ can be derived for the square and linear models and these are simpler than the tetrahedral model.

(b) A general sequential model

The sequential model of Koshland was introduced by reference to the 'induced fit' idea of enzyme specificity. In this case the binding of substrate actually initiates a conformational change which can affect the binding of substrate molecule by other subunits. This is not a necessary prerequisite of the sequential model. A variation on this model assumes that two or more conformations of each subunit can exist even in the absence of substrate. This situation is described diagrammatically in Figure 2.4b.

The extreme case, in which the hybrid intermediates A_1B_3, A_2B_2, etc., are unstable, has been termed the 'concerted model' by Koshland[13] since it is considered that in this case there is simultaneous (concerted) transition of all four subunits from the A conformation to the B conformation. (It will be seen that this version of the sequential model is similar to the model of Monod, Wyman and Changeux.)

In this concerted model in which all subunit interactions change concomitantly with conformational changes, the equilibrium constant for the conformational change, K_t, and the various interaction constants, K_{AA}, K_{AB}, etc., are all incorporated into a single constant, K_{tc}. The fractional saturation is given by

$$\bar{Y}_s = \frac{[B_4S_1] + 2[B_4S_2] + 3[B_4S_3] + 4[B_4S_4]}{4\{[A_4] + [B_4] + [B_4S_1] + [B_4S_2] + [B_4S_3] + [B_4S_4]\}}$$

The concentrations of the intermediate compounds, $[B_4S_1]$, $[B_4S_2]$, etc., can all be expressed in terms of the substrate concentration [S], the concentration of free enzyme $[A_4]$, the microscopic binding constant K_s and the equilibrium constant K_{tc}. The statistical factors for the number of types of each species and the number of interacting subunits must also be taken into account (as for the tetrahedral model described in Section D.1(a)).

$$[B_4] = K_{tc}^4[A_4]$$

$$[B_4S_1] = 4K_s[S][B_4] = 4K_s[S]K_{tc}^4[A_4]$$

$$[B_4S_2] = 6K_s^2[S]^2[B_4] = 6K_s^2[S]^2K_{tc}^4[A_4]$$

$$[B_4S_3] = 4K_s^3[S]^3[B_4] = 4K_s^3[S]^3K_{tc}^4[A_4]$$

$$[B_4S_4] = K_s^4[S]^4[B_4] = K_s^4[S]^4K_{tc}^4[A_4]$$

Substituting these expressions into the equation for fractional saturation,

$$\bar{Y}_s = \frac{4K_s[S]K_{tc}^4[A_4] + 12K_s^2[S]^2K_{tc}^4[A_4] + 12K_s^3[S]^3K_{tc}^4[A_4] + 4K_s^4[S]^4K_{tc}^4[A_4]}{4\{A_4 + K_{tc}^4[A_4] + 4K_s[S]K_{tc}^4[A_4] + 6K_s^2[S]^2K_{tc}^4[A_4] + 4K_s^3[S]^3K_{tc}^4[A_4] + K_s^4[S]^4K_{tc}^4[A_4]\}}$$

$$= \frac{4K_s[S]K_{tc}^4[A_4](1 + 3K_s[S] + 3K_s^2[S]^2 + K_s^3[S]^3)}{4K_{tc}^4[A_4]\{K_{tc}^{-4} + (1 + 4K_s[S] + 6K_s^2[S]^2 + 4K_s^3[S]^3 + K_s^4[S]^4)\}}$$

$$= \frac{K_s[S](1 + 3K_s[S] + 3K_s^2[S]^2 + K_s^3[S]^3)}{K_{tc}^{-4} + (1 + 4K_s[S] + 6K_s^2[S]^2 + 4K_s^3[S]^3 + K_s^4[S]^4)}$$

Since

$$(1 + 3K_s[S] + 3K_s^2[S]^2 + K_s^3[S]^3) = (1 + K_s[S])^3$$

and

$$(1 + 4K_s[S] + 6K_s^2[S]^2 + 4K_s^3[S]^3 + K_s^4[S]^4) = (1 + K_s[S])^4$$

$$\bar{Y}_s = \frac{K_s[S](1 + K_s[S])^3}{K_{tc}^{-4} + (1 + K_s[S])^4} \tag{2.17}$$

Equation 2.17 is identical to equation 2.19 which describes the Monod, Wyman and Changeux model.

If all the interaction constants, K_{AA}, K_{AB}, K_{tc}, etc., are set to unity (that is, if there is no subunit interaction), the equations for fractional saturation all simplify to equations which describe a hyperbolic curve.

The usefulness of these models is that values can be assumed for the various constants (K_{AA}, K_{AB}, K_s, etc.) and substituted into the equations for $\bar{Y}_s$ (or $\bar{N}_s$, which is defined by Koshland as the average number of molecules of substrate bound per protein molecule: for a tetramer, $\bar{N}_s = 4\bar{Y}_s$). Theoretical curves can be constructed from these equations and compared to experimental curves. The goodness of fit of the experimental curves with the theoretical curves will provide an indication of the best model (square, concerted, etc.) for the enzyme in question.

It is difficult to prove experimentally that any particular enzyme conforms to a specific type of sequential model. The kinetic data on the behaviour of an enzyme may *support* one of these types of models but it cannot yet be proved conclusively that the enzyme conforms to such a model rather than to some other model which may not even have been proposed.

2. The model of Monod, Wyman and Changeux

A somewhat simpler system than that described by Koshland was proposed in 1965 by Monod, Wyman and Changeux.[10] This model (MWC model) can be considered as an extreme case of the general Koshland model shown in Figure 2.4b, in which only the completely symmetrical states are considered to be stable. The theory set out to explain not only the sigmoid behaviour of these enzymes but also the effects of allosteric inhibitors and activators. This is explained by referring to ATCase as an example of an allosteric enzyme: a plot of initial velocity against substrate concentration is sigmoid and the effect of the inhibitor (CTP) is to increase the sigmoidicity of this plot, whereas the effect of the activator (ATP) is to decrease the sigmoidicity (Figure 2.5). Thus, the effects of the inhibitor and activator appear to be achieved through the cooperative phenomenon, so that if the molecular basis of cooperativity could be understood, the mechanisms of inhibition and activation could be readily explained.

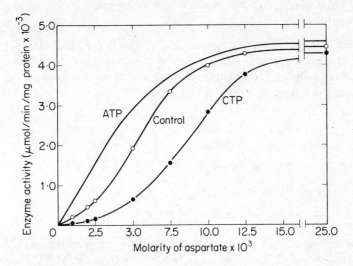

Figure 2.5. The effects of CTP (inhibitor) and ATP (activator) on the plot of the activity of aspartate transcarbamylase against the concentration of aspartate[3]

(a) Description of the model

The symmetrical model can be described by the following statements.

(a) Allosteric proteins are oligomers (that is, they are comprised of a number of separate protein subunits) whose protomers (individual subunits which in combination with one another constitute the oligomer) are associated in such a way that they all occupy equivalent positions in the native protein. Therefore the protein possesses at least one axis of symmetry.

(b) Each protomer possesses one stereospecific site for each ligand. The binding sites within the molecule for any particular ligand are all equivalent to one another.

(c) The conformation of each protomer is constrained by its association with the other protomers. In other words, the ability of the protomer to bind the substrate is reduced by the association of the protomers in the oligomeric protein.

(d) At least two conformations of the oligomeric protein exist in the absence of substrate and these conformational states are in equilibrium with each other. These states differ in their inter-protomer bonding and therefore in the constraint imposed on the conformation of the protomers and their ability to bind the substrate.

(e) It follows from (d) that the transition from one form to the other results in a change in the affinity for a ligand.

(*f*) Molecular symmetry of the oligomeric protein is conserved during this transition.

The two conformational states are called the R (relaxed) and T (tensed) states and each consists of a number of identical protomers. Consider the case of an oligomer consisting of four identical protomers: the model proposes the following situation to apply:

$$R_4 \rightleftarrows T_4$$

$$R_4 + S \rightleftarrows R_4S_1 \qquad T_4 + S \rightleftarrows T_4S_1$$

$$R_4S_1 + S \rightleftarrows R_4S_2 \qquad T_4S_1 + S \rightleftarrows T_4S_2$$

$$R_4S_2 + S \rightleftarrows R_4S_3 \qquad T_4S_2 + S \rightleftarrows T_4S_3$$

$$R_4S_3 + S \rightleftarrows R_4S_4 \qquad T_4S_3 + S \rightleftarrows T_4S_4$$

The two essential differences between this symmetrical model and the simple sequential model (Figure 2.4) are as follows. First, in the MWC model, only the symmetrical forms of the proteins are stable, so that the protein is always either in the R_4 or T_4 state. The intermediates R_3T, R_2T_2 and RT_3 are asymmetrical and therefore unstable. Thus, in the absence of substrate, an equilibrium exists between the state R_4 and T_4 and this is governed by an equilibrium constant L termed the allosteric constant. Second, the microscopic dissociation constant K_R for the dissociation of the substrate-enzyme complex is the same for all the binding sites irrespective of whether S is bound at other sites on the protein. The apparent dissociation constants K_{d1}, K_{d2}, etc., for the four reactions $R + S \rightleftarrows RS_1$, $RS_1 + S \rightleftarrows RS_2$, etc., are all statistically related to K_R (see Appendix 2.1). Similarly the apparent dissociation constants for the reactions $T + S \rightleftarrows TS_1$; $TS_1 + S \rightleftarrows TS_2$, etc., are all statistically related to the microscopic dissociation constant K_T. In the simple sequential model of Koshland, sigmoid curves result because, for example, K_{b4} is larger than $(1/16)K_{b1}$ but in the MWC model K_{d4} is equal to $16K_{d1}$ (K_{d1} and K_{d4} are dissociation constants).

(*b*) *Mathematical explanation for sigmoidicity*

The fractional saturation of the protein with the substrate can be expressed in terms of the substrate concentration, the dissociation constants K_T and K_R, and the allosteric constant L. The equation describing the fractional saturation for a tetrameric molecule is as follows:

$$\overline{Y}_s = \frac{\dfrac{[S]}{K_R}\left(1 + \dfrac{[S]}{K_R}\right)^3 + L\dfrac{[S]}{K_T}\left(1 + \dfrac{[S]}{K_T}\right)^3}{\left(1 + \dfrac{[S]}{K_R}\right)^4 + L\left(1 + \dfrac{[S]}{K_T}\right)^4} \tag{2.18}$$

The algebraic details for the derivation of this equation are given in Appendix 2.1.

If it is assumed that the substrate binds only to the R state of the protein (exclusive binding to one state), K_T is infinitely large and the functions containing K_T on the right-hand side of the equation approach zero. The equation for fractional saturation simplifies to

$$\bar{Y}_s = \frac{\dfrac{[S]}{K_R}\left(1 + \dfrac{[S]}{K_R}\right)^3}{L + \left(1 + \dfrac{[S]}{K_R}\right)^4} \tag{2.19}$$

This equation is identical to equation 2.17 which was derived from the Koshland concerted model. The constant K_{tc}^{-4} in equation 2.17 is equivalent to the allosteric constant L. Since K_s in the Koshland model is a binding constant whereas K_R in the MWC model is a dissociation constant,

$$K_s[S] = \frac{[S]}{K_R}$$

The MWC model is obviously not restricted to tetrameric proteins but where there are n substrate binding sites the variation of fractional saturation with substrate concentration is given by

$$\bar{Y}_s = \frac{\dfrac{[S]}{K_R}\left(1 + \dfrac{[S]}{K_R}\right)^{n-1}}{L + \left(1 + \dfrac{[S]}{K_R}\right)^n} \tag{2.20}$$

Theoretical curves have been constructed by Monod *et al.*; the effect of variation in allosteric constant L upon the relationship between fractional saturation and substrate concentration is shown in Figure 2.6 for the situation in which there is exclusive binding of the substrate to the R state (that is,

Figure 2.6. Theoretical curves of the fractional saturation ($\bar{Y}_s$) against α, where $\alpha = [S]/K_R$. The allosteric constant L is varied as shown, n is 4 and K_R/K_T is zero. The equation

$$\bar{Y}_s = \frac{\dfrac{[S]}{K_R}\left(1 + \dfrac{[S]}{K_R}\right)^3}{L + \left(1 + \dfrac{[S]}{K_R}\right)^4}$$

(i.e. equation 2.19) is used to calculate the fractional saturation[10]

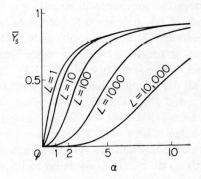

$K_R/K_T = 0$). Thus the model predicts the existence of the substrate cooperative effect which is the more pronounced the greater is the value of the
allosteric constant L (that is, the greater the proportion of the enzyme in the
T state in the absence of substrate). As L approaches zero (that is, the proportion of enzyme in the R state approaches 100%) the curve approaches
the hyperbolic. This can readily be seen by putting $L = 0$ in equation 2.20
when

$$\bar{Y}_s = \frac{\dfrac{[S]}{K_R}\left(1 + \dfrac{[S]}{K_R}\right)^{n-1}}{\left(1 + \dfrac{[S]}{K_R}\right)^n}$$

$$= \frac{\dfrac{[S]}{K_R}}{1 + \dfrac{[S]}{K_R}} \tag{2.21}$$

Equation 2.21 is exactly the same as equation 2.1 (Section B.1) and describes
a rectangular hyperbola (see Appendix 2.1).

Similarly if the substrate binds with equal affinity to both states ($K_R = K_T$),
the model once more reverts to a hyperbolic system (see Appendix 2.1) as
is also the case when the protein is a monomer with only one substrate
binding site (that is, $n = 1$).

(c) Qualitative description of the model

In purely descriptive terms the differences between a hyperbolic and a
sigmoid curve are two-fold: the initial binding of substrate to the enzyme is
small in comparison to the hyperbolic curve, and the rate of binding increases
at higher substrate concentrations so that the curve has a point of inflexion.
The first point is easily explained by the symmetrical model. In the absence
of substrate the equilibrium R/T is in favour of T, so that at low substrate
concentrations there will be only a very small amount of R to bind the substrate (if L is 10^3 only 0·1% of the enzyme is in the R form in the absence of
substrate). The concentration of R limits the formation of RS_1, etc. However,
once the substrate reaches a concentration at which it can have a significant
effect on the formation of RS_1, RS_2, etc., there will be an effect of substrate
on all the reactions with the result that R will be converted into RS_1, RS_2,
RS_3, and RS_4. The effect of this will be to remove R from the equilibrium
$R \rightleftharpoons T$ so that some T will be converted into R, which will be able to react
with more substrate. Thus to some extent the $R \rightleftharpoons T$ equilibrium can be
considered as a buffer system for maintaining the concentration of R fairly
constant despite its conversion to RS_1, RS_2, etc.

The effects of activators and inhibitors can be explained very simply by this model (for mathematical theory see Appendix 2.3). Thus, the inhibitor is considered to bind preferentially (or even exclusively in the extreme case) to the T state and therefore to stabilize this state. This will have the effect of increasing the allosteric constant L and therefore the sigmoidicity of the curve will be increased. Similarly, if the activator binds preferentially (or exclusively) to the R state this will have the effect of reducing the allosteric constant and the curve will become less sigmoid.

The symmetrical model explains in a simple, elegant and aesthetically pleasing way how the kinetics of allosteric enzymes could arise. Aesthetics should not prejudice the scientific investigator and it is therefore not surprising that many experiments have been performed in order to discover whether or not symmetry does tend to be conserved in allosteric enzymes generally, whether this model applies to some enzymes and not others, or whether the more general sequential model of Koshland is a more valid method of describing allosteric systems. A detailed discussion of such experiments would not only provide the material for another book but would also be of little value to the general reader. However, an outline of the types of experimental approach which can be used to distinguish between the symmetrical and sequential models will be given.

There are three types of experiment whose results may confirm or refute the symmetry theory. These are (a) the demonstration of 'Hill-type' kinetics, (b) the demonstration of negative cooperativity, and (c) the study of relaxation kinetics. In addition, a fourth type of investigation may be used to confirm or refute the simple induced fit sequential theory of Koshland and this involves the relationship between conformational changes and substrate binding.

3. Experimental differentiation between the two models

(a) 'Hill-type' kinetics

The symmetrical model of allosteric proteins can be considered to be a special case of the sequential model, in the same way that the Hill model is a special case of the more general Adair model. A necessary assumption of the Hill model is that only two species of protein exist, completely free of substrate or fully saturated. The equation which describes the fractional saturation under these conditions is the same as equation 2.12 (the Hill equation),

$$\overline{Y}_s = \frac{K[S]^n}{1 + K[S]^n}$$

Under certain conditions, the equation which describes the MWC model reduces to one similar to the Hill equation. If the substrate binds only to the

R state,

$$\overline{Y}_s = \frac{\dfrac{[S]}{K_R}\left(1 + \dfrac{[S]}{K_R}\right)^{n-1}}{L + \left(1 + \dfrac{[S]}{K_R}\right)^n}$$

If the allosteric constant L is very large (that is, if most of the enzyme is in the form which does not bind S), $[S]/K_R \gg 1$ for most of the range of $\overline{Y}_s$ when plotted against [S] and the equation reduces to

$$\overline{Y}_s = \frac{\left(\dfrac{[S]}{K_R}\right)^n}{L + \left(\dfrac{[S]}{K_R}\right)^n}$$

Dividing top and bottom lines on the right-hand side by L,

$$\overline{Y}_s = \frac{\dfrac{[S]^n}{K_R^n L}}{1 + \dfrac{[S]^n}{K_R^n L}}$$

But $1/K_R^n L = $ constant (K')
Therefore

$$\overline{Y}_s = \frac{K'[S]^n}{1 + K'[S]^n}$$

which is the Hill equation.

In some allosteric proteins very large values for L can be produced by addition of the allosteric inhibitor, which binds exclusively to the T state and whose effect is to increase L. Under such conditions, very little of the R form would be present and almost all the available R would be saturated with substrate, even at low substrate concentrations; that is, only T and RS_n would exist: this is precisely the Hill assumption. Therefore, under such conditions, a plot of log $\overline{Y}_s/(1 - \overline{Y}_s)$ against the log of the concentration of S (or for an enzyme, $\log v/(V_{max} - v)$ against $\log[S]$) should be linear with a slope equal to the number of binding sites. However, the number of binding sites (which is sometimes denoted by q) must be measured in an independent experiment. In other words, if it can be shown that a 'Hill plot' has a slope which is equal to the independently determined number of binding sites for S, then the symmetrical model is proved. This experimental test can only be used positively: lack of correlation between n and the number of binding sites does not exclude the symmetrical model (for example, the binding of S may not be exclusive; the allosteric constant may not be sufficiently great even in the presence of high concentrations of inhibitor).

'Hill type' kinetics have been demonstrated for donkey spleen deoxy-cytidine monophosphate deaminase[14] which catalyses the reaction

$$dCMP + H_2O \rightarrow dAMP + NH_3$$

The enzyme shows sigmoid kinetics towards dCMP and the sigmoidicity is increased by the inhibitor dTTP. In the presence of dTTP, the slope of the Hill plot (i.e. n) is 4. The number of substrate binding sites has been estimated from the binding of the substrate analogues, dGMP and dAMP, to the enzyme (binding of the substrate cannot be investigated directly because of the catalytic activity of the enzyme). This study infers that there are 4 binding sites for the substrate (i.e. $q = 4$). This provides very strong evidence that the symmetrical model is correct for this enzyme.

A note upon the physical significance of Hill's n, in conditions where the Hill assumption does not apply, may be helpful here. It has been shown[15] that n which is defined by

$$n = \frac{d \log \left(\dfrac{\overline{Y}_s}{1 - \overline{Y}_s} \right)}{d \log [S]}$$

is a measure of the interaction between the binding sites (that is, the co-operativity). A complete plot over the whole range of $\overline{Y}_s$, for a protein exhibiting positive cooperativity, is shown in Figure 2.7.

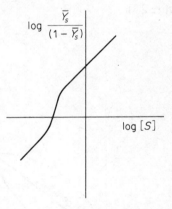

Figure 2.7. Diagrammatic representation of a Hill plot for the saturation of a protein exhibiting positive cooperativity. As the two extremes (i.e., $\overline{Y}_s = 0$ and $\overline{Y}_s = 1$) are approached, the slope of the curve approaches unity. Experimental points usually centre around $\overline{Y}_s = 0.5$ when the slope (i.e. n) is greater than one[16]

At the two extremes $\overline{Y}_s = 0$ and $\overline{Y}_s = 1$, $n = 1$, i.e. there is no cooperativity since as $\overline{Y}_s \rightarrow 0$, almost all the protein molecules have no substrate bound, and as $\overline{Y}_s \rightarrow 1$, almost all the protein molecules are fully saturated with substrate. In the intermediate range, n reaches a maximum and, since the experimental points are often collected in the region $\overline{Y}_s = 0.5$, the Hill plot often looks roughly linear with $n > 1$. For further discussion on the significance of n, see reference 16.

(b) Negative cooperativity

In the sequential model, sigmoidicity of the saturation curve is explained by the increasing values for the apparent binding constants K_{b1}, K_{b2}, K_{b3} and K_{b4}. This is induced by the binding of the first molecule of substrate, which causes interactions in the other protein subunits that increase the value of the binding constants. However, it is equally plausible that binding of the substrate to the first subunit could cause interactions between the subunits that result in the binding constants being decreased (the binding of the first substrate molecule makes it more difficult for the second and subsequent substrate molecules to bind). For example, if $K_{b1} < (8/3)K_{b2}$, etc., a positive cooperative effect is obtained, if $K_{b1} = (8/3)K_{b2}$, etc., a hyperbolic response is obtained, and if $K_{b1} > (8/3)K_{b2}$, etc., a negative cooperative effect is obtained.

In the latter case, the plot of $\overline{Y}_s$ or v against [S] would rise more steeply at low concentrations of S than the hyperbolic curve and would rise more slowly at high concentrations of S. This form of plotting the experimental results means that it is difficult to interpret such a curve by visual observation, as indeed it is for sigmoid curves which exhibit only minimum deviations from the hyperbolic. The interpretation is made easier by a double reciprocal plot (i.e. $1/\overline{Y}_s$ or $1/v$ against $1/[S]$): the hyperbolic curve becomes linear, positive cooperativity is shown by a curve which is concave upwards and negative cooperativity is shown by a curve which is concave downwards (see Figure 2.8).

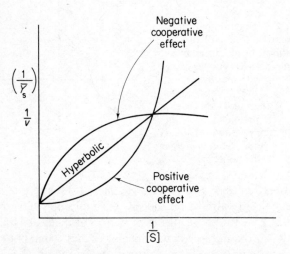

Figure 2.8. Diagrammatic double reciprocal plot demonstrating positive and negative cooperative effects

The symmetrical model (which is a configurational rather than an inter-action model) predicts only positive cooperativity: negative cooperativity is not permitted. An increase in the substrate concentration should always result in shifting of the R $\rightleftarrows$ T equilibrium in favour of the state to which the substrate preferentially binds (i.e. T → R). It has been shown mathematically that negative interaction cannot be obtained from the symmetrical model.[17] Hence the cooperative effect should always be positive. Therefore if negative cooperativity can be demonstrated, it provides strong evidence in favour of the simple sequential model.

Rabbit muscle glyceraldehyde 3-phosphate dehydrogenase[18] and beef-liver glutamate dehydrogenase[19] both exhibit negative interactions in respect of the binding of the pyridine nucleotide cofactor to the enzyme. The binding constants for NAD^+ for rabbit muscle glyceraldehyde 3-phosphate dehydro-genase have been measured by equilibrium dialysis studies. The values reported are as follows: $K_1 = 2.5 \times 10^{-5}$ M; $K_2 = 3.0 \times 10^{-7}$ M; $K_3 =$ approx. 10^{-9} M; $K_4 =$ approx. 10^{-11} M. The results of these studies support the simple sequential model, at least for these two enzymes.

(c) Relaxation kinetics

These studies involve perturbation of a reaction which is at equilibrium. The kinetics of the reaction are followed as a new equilibrium is approached, a process known as relaxation. The equilibrium between an enzyme and its substrate can be studied only if catalysis is prevented—for example, by omission of one substrate in the case of a two-substrate reaction. The relaxation experiment is performed as follows: an enzyme and substrate are allowed to reach equilibrium and the system is perturbed extremely rapidly (for example, by passing a high voltage through the solution when the temperature can be raised by 10 °C in as little as 1 μsec: this is known as the 'temperature-jump' technique). The transition to a new equilibrium is followed by rapid-reaction techniques. Each individual step in the overall reaction takes a characteristic time which is a function of the rate constant of this individual step.

Kirschner and coworkers[20] have applied this technique to yeast glycer-aldehyde 3-phosphate dehydrogenase which possesses 4 binding sites for NAD^+. An equilibrium between NAD^+ and the enzyme was established, the system was perturbed by a 'temperature jump', and the change in the NAD^+-binding was measured by the change in absorption at 360 nm. The time course of relaxation to a new equilibrium could be separated into three different time scales (10^{-3}, 10^{-2} and 1 second) and from each of these times individual rate constants for the three processes could be calculated ($k_1 = 7,000$ s^{-1}, $k_2 = 690$ s^{-1}, $k_3 = 0.2$ s^{-1}). The slowest rate constant was affected neither by the protein nor by the NAD^+ concentration, whereas the other two rate constants were decreased with increasing concentrations of

NAD^+. These data could be explained as follows: the two fast rate constants indicate binding of NAD^+ to two states of the protein (i.e. R and T) whereas the slowest rate constant can be attributed to the process of interconversion between these two states (i.e. $R \rightleftarrows T$ transformation). This latter process would be expected to be independent of the protein and the NAD^+ concentration. These results strongly favour the symmetrical model since the sequential model would predict at least four separate relaxation times which would all be dependent upon the NAD^+ concentration. Furthermore, from these results it was possible to calculate all three constants for the MWC model (i.e. K_R, K_T and L) and to construct a curve of $\bar{Y}_s$ against $[NAD^+]$. This theoretical curve fitted extremely well with the experimentally determined curve.

(d) Relationship between conformation and fractional saturation

In the induced-fit (simple sequential) model, the binding of the substrate induces a change in the conformation of the protein. Therefore the fraction of the protein in the substrate-binding form (that is, the degree of conformation change) is dependent upon the fractional saturation of the protein by substrate. However, in the general sequential model (extended Koshland model, see Figure 2.4) which includes the symmetry model as an extreme case, the change in conformation is not directly dependent upon substrate binding so that the degree of conformational change need not be proportional to the fractional saturation. This is apparent from the equations derived for the symmetrical model. For a tetrameric molecule, fractional saturation is given by equation 2.18.

$$\bar{Y}_s = \frac{\dfrac{[S]}{K_R}\left(1 + \dfrac{[S]}{K_R}\right)^3 + L\dfrac{[S]}{K_T}\left(1 + \dfrac{[S]}{K_T}\right)^3}{\left(1 + \dfrac{[S]}{K_R}\right)^4 + L\left(1 + \dfrac{[S]}{K_T}\right)^4}$$

and the proportion of protein in the R state (that is, degree of conformational change) is given by the following equation (see Appendix 2.2)

$$\bar{R} = \frac{\left(1 + \dfrac{[S]}{K_R}\right)^4}{\left(1 + \dfrac{[S]}{K_R}\right)^4 + L\left(1 + \dfrac{[S]}{K_T}\right)^4}$$

Thus $\bar{R}$ and $\bar{Y}_s$ will vary independently especially when the factor $L\dfrac{[S]}{K_T}\left(1 + \dfrac{[S]}{K_T}\right)^3$ is large.

Studies have been performed on the change in the conformational state of haemoglobin when oxygen is bound.[21] The data for $\overline{Y}_s$ are obtained from the oxygen binding to haemoglobin and the data for $\overline{R}$ are acquired using a spin resonance probe. The changes in $\overline{Y}_s$ and $\overline{R}$ are not similar and therefore haemoglobin would not appear to fit the simple Koshland model. Similarly, work with ATCase, in which $\overline{Y}_s$ was measured by the binding of a substrate analogue, succinate, and $\overline{R}$ was measured either by reactivity of sulphydryl groups or by sedimentation studies, shows that the conformational change can be much larger than the change in fractional saturation.[22,23]

4. Summary

The properties of the two types of configurational model which have been proposed to explain cooperativity may be summarized as follows. The symmetry model of Monod, Wyman and Changeux is based upon the postulate that at least two symmetrical conformational states of the protein (R and T) exist in equilibrium in the absence of any ligand and this equilibrium favours the T state. The binding of substrate to any of the protomers in a particular state in no way influences the binding of substrate to the remaining protomers in that state (that is, the microscopic binding constants for the reaction between R-type protomers and substrate are all identical). Positive cooperativity is explained by the conversion of the T state to the R state (to which S binds preferentially or even exclusively) so that the equilibrium between the two states is altered in the direction of the preferred substrate-binding state (i.e. R).

The simple sequential model of Koshland requires the existence of only one state of the protein in the absence of ligand. Symmetry is not conserved during ligand binding since the protomer to which the ligand is bound is present in a different conformational state from the remaining protomers. The ligand-saturated protomer interacts with the remaining protomers such that the microscopic binding constants are either increased (positive cooperativity) or decreased (negative cooperativity).

The occurrence of negative cooperativity precludes the operation of the symmetry model whereas the occurrence of Hill kinetics precludes the operation of the simple sequential model. The variation in the conformational change of the protein $\overline{R}$ on binding the substrate must be identical to the variation in the fractional saturation of the protein $\overline{Y}_s$ in order to comply with the simple sequential model, whereas they may vary independently for the symmetry model. The study of relaxation times may also distinguish between the two models by providing evidence for the existence of reactions which are independent of ligand and protein concentrations (symmetrical model) or by the demonstration that all reactions are dependent upon the ligand concentration (simple sequential model).

E. KINETIC MODELS TO EXPLAIN SIGMOID BEHAVIOUR

The two models described above have assumed that the sigmoid nature of the plot of initial velocity versus substrate concentration is due to non-hyperbolic binding of the substrate to the enzyme protein. In the case of the reaction between oxygen and haemoglobin there is no doubt that the actual binding of the four oxygen molecules to one haemoglobin molecule is sigmoidal. However, in an enzymatic reaction, the initial velocity measurements follow the conversion of substrate to product and it is frequently assumed that the velocity is directly related to the amount of substrate bound to the enzyme—that is, it is assumed that the free enzyme and substrate are in equilibrium with the enzyme-substrate complex and it is merely the concentration of the latter which determines the rate of the overall reaction. The problem is emphasized as follows

$$Hb + O_2 \underset{k_{-1}}{\overset{k_{+1}}{\rightleftarrows}} HbO_2$$

$$E + S \underset{k_{-1}}{\overset{k_{+1}}{\rightleftarrows}} ES \overset{k_{+2}}{\longrightarrow} E + P$$

Thus, for comparison with haemoglobin, only the enzyme-substrate reaction should be measured, whereas in almost all cases of the analysis of cooperative effects in enzymes, it is the overall conversion of substrate to product that is measured. If the reaction $E + S \rightleftarrows ES$ is very close to equilibrium and if the rate of product formation is dependent simply and directly upon the concentration of the ES complex, cooperativity (as measured by the rate of product formation) can be interpreted as cooperative binding of substrate. However, if the breakdown of ES to form $E + P$, which is governed by k_{+2}, is complex (as when it is comprised of more than one reaction), this kinetic complexity may give rise to sigmoid rate curves in the absence of cooperative substrate binding.

1. The Rabin model

Perhaps the simplest kinetic model has been suggested by Rabin.[24] This model is represented in Figure 2.9. The initial reaction is the formation of the enzyme-substrate complex E′S, which isomerizes to give the complex E″S, in which the enzyme has undergone a conformational change. The E″S complex then reacts further to give E″ and the product P of the reaction. There are thus two conformational isomers of the enzyme, E′ and E″, of which the former is thermodynamically more stable. The rate-limiting step (that is, the slowest step in the whole reaction sequence) is assumed to be the conversion of E′S to E″S governed by the rate constant k_{+2}. The conversion of E″ to E′ is also assumed to occur relatively slowly. Thus the genera-

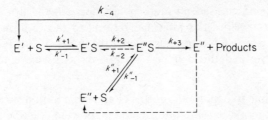

Figure 2.9. A diagrammatic representation of
the Rabin model to explain cooperativity[24]

tion of free E″ and the direct combination of this E″ with S, bypasses the slowest step (E′S → E″S) in the reaction pathway. The free energy for the conversion of E′ to E″ is derived from the overall reaction of substrate conversion to product. If the velocity constant $k_{+2} \gg k_{-2}$ (that is, if the conversion of E′S to E″S is essentially irreversible), it is a thermodynamic consequence that the affinity of E″ for S is very much greater than E′ for S ($k''_{-1}/k''_{+1} \ll k'_{-1}/k'_{+1}$), otherwise it would be possible to proceed from E′ (via E′S, E″S and E″) back to E′ without any chemical change taking place but with a net change in $\Delta G°$. This would violate the first law of thermodynamics.

At low substrate concentrations, the concentration of E′S will be low and consequently the rate of conversion of E′S to E″S (which is dependent upon the concentration of E′S) will be very slow in comparison to the rate of conversion of E″ to E′ (i.e. k_{-4}). Thus the number of molecules in the E″ conformation at any given time will be very small. Consequently the catalytic rate will be low. At higher concentrations of substrate, the concentration of E′S will be higher, the rate of conversion of E′S to E″S will be greater and the number of molecules in the E″ conformation will be larger. The probability that E″ will react with a molecule of S before being converted back to E′ is correspondingly greater so that the rate of catalysis increases to a greater extent than the increase in substrate concentration. A sigmoid activity curve results.

Perhaps the best description of the operation of the Rabin model has been provided by Whitehead[16] and the following is a quotation from his paper in which the symbols have been changed to be consistent with the present discussion.

A molecule as long as it stays in the state E″ could be said to conserve the 'memory' of the fact that it has combined with a molecule of S and effected a catalytic event. Since E″ and E′ have different properties towards S, we could say that the protomer recognizes S differently according to whether or not it has within a certain probable time past met S and catalysed S → P, in other words, there is an interaction or cooperation between the first

S molecule and the second (and indeed between the first and any subsequent ones) before the molecule returns to the E'-form and 'forgets'
S—the S in this scheme are thus interacting in pairs. This is an interaction
that is transmitted through *time* instead of, as in the equilibrium case,
through *space*.

It is also possible to explain the effects of allosteric inhibitors and activators
on this kinetic model: an inhibitor would favour the reaction in which E" is
converted to E' (that is, increase the value of the rate constant k_{-4}) which is
the thermodynamically favoured state. On the other hand an activator
would increase the rate of the reaction E'S $\rightarrow$ E"S, so that even at very low
substrate concentrations a large number of molecules would exist in the
E" conformation and the response curve would become more hyperbolic.

It is interesting that this model requires the existence of two conformational
states (at least) of the enzyme which have different affinities for the substrate
(compare with the symmetrical MWC model). In the equilibrium binding
models the conformational states of the enzyme are in equilibrium whereas
in the kinetic model they are in steady state. Furthermore the kinetic model
has no requirement for more than one substrate binding site per protein
molecule and therefore the protein could be monomeric. Neither is there any
requirement for symmetry in the structure of the protein. However, if the
enzyme was a regulatory enzyme controlled by feedback inhibition, it would
need specific sites for the binding of the regulator molecules and specific
conformational changes to produce modifications in the geometry of the
protein molecule at the 'centres' which govern the conversions of E" to E'
and E'S to E"S.

2. Two-substrate enzymes

Enzymes which catalyse reactions involving more than one substrate may
possess intrinsic characteristics which provide a basis for a kinetic theory
of the cooperative effect. The essential point about two-substrate reactions
is that the kinetics can be much more complex than single-substrate reactions
and such complexity can give rise to a sigmoid response (or more correctly
deviations from linear double-reciprocal plots). This complexity was first
emphasized by Dalziel[25] and its relationship to the sigmoid response of
enzymes was developed by Ferdinand.[26] The model system is described in
Figure 2.10. It is necessary that the enzyme follows a random order mechanism (that is, it can bind either substrate irrespective of the binding of the other
substrate). Therefore alternative pathways to the ternary complex (ES_1S_2)
are available. It is assumed that the pathway

$$E \rightleftarrows ES_1 \rightleftarrows ES_1S_2 \rightarrow E + \text{Products}$$

is kinetically preferred (i.e. that $k_{+1}k_{+3} > k_{+2}k_{+4}$) and that the affinity of

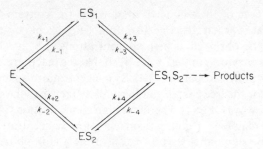

Figure 2.10. A diagrammatic representation of the Ferdinand model to explain cooperativity in two-substrate enzymes[26]

E for S_2 is less than that of ES_1 for S_2. It can be shown that the initial rate equation for such a system is as follows

$$r = \frac{A[S_1] + B[S_1]^2}{C + D[S_1] + E[S_1]^2} \qquad (2.22)$$

where A, B, C, D and E are constants involving the second substrate, S_2 (they are complex functions of the rate constants). This equation applies when the concentration of substrate S_1 is varied and that of S_2 is held constant. This equation is of the Adair type (equation 2.15) and Ferdinand shows that when $CB > DA$ sigmoid kinetics will be observed.

A more qualitative interpretation of this kinetic model is as follows. If S_2 is kept at a fixed concentration (invariant substrate) and S_1 is increased from very low concentrations, at first most of S_1 will react with ES_2 which will be present at a much higher concentration than E. Consequently the reaction will proceed by the slower pathway, $E \rightleftarrows ES_2 \rightleftarrows ES_1S_2$. However, as the concentration of S_1 is increased further, the amount of S_1 which reacts with free E will be greater and ES_1 will begin to be formed. Loss of E to form ES_1 will cause ES_2 to dissociate into E and S_2 so that more E is available to react with S_1. As the variable substrate concentration is increased, more of the enzyme will be in the form ES_1 and the rate of formation of the products will increase. A sigmoid response curve will result. As in the case of the Rabin model, two different conformational states of the enzyme exist and the proportion of each depends upon the concentration of the substrate. Changes in the extent of preference for one pathway produced by binding molecules other than the substrate (i.e. regulators) could either exaggerate (inhibition) or minimize (activation) the sigmoidicity of the curve. From the point of view of regulation, such a mechanism would appear to be simpler than the equilibrium-binding models. The sigmoidicity is an intrinsic part of the catalytic process and does not demand any modifications in protein structure (with the exception of specific regulator sites).

Another aspect of this model is that when the converse experiment is performed (that is, when the concentration of S_1 is kept constant), substrate inhibition can be observed at high concentrations of S_2. At low concentrations of S_2, the enzyme is in the form ES_1 so that the reaction is forced through the kinetically preferred pathway. As S_2 concentration is increased, it competes with S_1 for the free enzyme and gradually increases the contribution of the slower pathway (via ES_2). Therefore high concentrations of S_2 will inhibit the catalysed reaction in comparison with low concentrations. This is of interest because sigmoidicity with one substrate and inhibition by the other substrate are the characteristic properties of phosphofructokinase (see Chapter 3).

At the present time there is only sufficient information to distinguish between these types of kinetic models and the equilibrium-binding models for a very small number of the enzymes. It should be borne in mind that the question, 'Which model is correct?' is probably not valid because different enzymes will very likely conform to different models and therefore all models may be partially applicable. One simple way of differentiating between the kinetic models and the equilibrium-binding models is by studying the binding of the substrate to the enzyme. In the case of the symmetrical and sequential models, the actual binding of the substrate to the enzyme must be sigmoid but for the kinetic models it could be hyperbolic. Thus, hyperbolic binding and sigmoidal rate curves would strongly indicate a kinetic model. Of course binding studies with substrate in the absence of the complete reaction are exceedingly difficult to perform. Sometimes analogues of the substrate, which are thought to bind at the same site as the substrate, can provide useful information, although conclusions must then be tentative. In cases of two-substrate enzymes with a random order mechanism, binding can be studied by omitting one of the substrates whilst estimating the extent of binding of the second substrate.

F. THE PHYSIOLOGICAL SIGNIFICANCE OF SIGMOID BEHAVIOUR

So far in this chapter the sigmoid curve has been discussed in terms of molecular mechanisms that have attempted to explain such behaviour. This discussion emphasizes that sigmoid behaviour is not a spontaneous result of interaction between a protein and a ligand, but requires considerable complexity of protein structure. It would be unlikely that an organism would increase the complexity of some of its proteins for no purpose. What then are the advantages of sigmoid behaviour to a cell or organism in comparison to the more usual hyperbolic behaviour? The advantages of sigmoid behaviour are related to the physiological functions of specific proteins in the organism. One example which clearly illustrates this point is the sigmoid binding of oxygen to haemoglobin which improves the function of this protein as an oxygen carrier in the blood. Another example of the advantages of sigmoid behaviour is the increase in sensitivity of enzymes to changes in the concentrations of substrates and metabolic regulators.

1. Haemoglobin

Haemoglobin releases oxygen in the capillaries from where it diffuses into the tissue cells. In muscle cells the pigment, myoglobin, transfers oxygen to the cytochrome oxidase of the mitochondria and thus it acts as a sort of 'middle-man', between the primary producer (haemoglobin) and the consumer (cytochrome oxidase). Myoglobin is a monomeric protein which possesses only one haem group and which binds oxygen in a hyperbolic manner. At an early stage of evolutionary development it probably performed the role of an oxygen-transporting pigment in the blood. However, in the course of evolution the monomeric protein was converted into a tetrameric protein, haemoglobin, which binds oxygen in a cooperative manner. Since this cooperativity is advantageous to the animal it has been favoured by natural selection.

The obvious question that must be asked is, what is the advantage of sigmoid binding over hyperbolic binding in relation to the transport of oxygen in the blood, but not in relation to intracellular oxygen transport? Both pigments are fully saturated with oxygen at the partial pressures which occur in the lungs. However, haemoglobin releases most of its bound oxygen at much higher partial pressures than myoglobin owing to the threshold response of the sigmoid curve. These higher partial pressures are in fact found in the capillaries within muscle and other tissues and therefore haemoglobin is capable of discharging most of its oxygen in the capillaries. At these comparatively high partial pressures of oxygen, myoglobin would release only a small proportion of its bound oxygen. The relatively high partial pressure of oxygen in the capillaries is necessary in order to provide a sufficient gradient for its rapid diffusion between capillaries and tissue cells (that is, across the interstitial space). The rate of diffusion of any compound is dependent upon the concentration gradient. If myoglobin was the oxygen carrier in the blood, the partial pressure in the capillaries would have to be very low for efficient discharge of oxygen. Consequently the rate of diffusion to the muscle would be very low and oxidative metabolism would be severely limited. Thus the biological advantage of haemoglobin as the transport pigment for oxygen is that its dissociation properties permit a greater rate of supply of oxygen to the tissue so that aerobic metabolism can proceed at a high rate.

2. Enzymes

Certain specific metabolic intermediates, which occur at important positions in metabolism (such as a pathway end-product; a precursor for two or more pathways) can relay information, usually by changes in concentration, to key regulatory enzymes concerning the state of metabolism at that particular position in the pathway. These metabolic regulators perform two roles: they act both as intermediates for metabolic pathways and as specific regulators for key enzymes which may constitute part of another pathway. This duality of function is at least part of the reason for sigmoid behaviour of regulatory enzymes. At first sight it may seem that these two roles of a metabolic intermediate are somewhat incompatible since large changes in concentration might be necessary in order to relay sufficient information to the regulatory enzyme, whereas such changes might be difficult to produce in a complex steady-state situation of a metabolic pathway (see Chapter 1). Moreover, large concentration changes might interfere in the basic enzymology of metabolism (for example, they may produce unwanted substrate or product inhibition or they may initiate non-specific side-reactions). Some indication of the change in concentration of regulator that is necessary to change the activity of an enzyme can be obtained from the model systems that have been described in this chapter. Thus, in the symmetrical or sequential models the fractional saturation of enzyme with ligand can be described mathematically and the effect of variations in ligand concentration upon the fractional saturation can be analysed theoretically.

If the interaction between an enzyme and a regulator molecule is described by a hyperbolic curve, a change in enzyme activity (that is, fractional saturation) from 10 to 90% requires a change in regulator concentration of about 80-fold (Table 2.1). The range 10 to 90% is chosen because it might represent a reasonable change in enzyme activity when a tissue responds metabolically to a change in physiological state. It should be stressed that an increase in

Table 2.1. The change in concentration of regulator that is necessary to increase the fractional saturation of an allosteric enzyme from 0·1 to 0·9 (see also Figure 2.3)

Allosteric constant	Concentration of regulator providing fractional saturation* of		Increase in concentration of regulator necessary to increase fractional saturation from 0·1 to 0·9
	0·1	0·9	
0 (hyperbolic)	0·11	9·0	81·0
1	0·18	8·0	44·4
100	1·20	9·8	9·2
500	2·00	11·5	5·7
1,000	2·60	12·6	4·8
10,000	5·00	19·6	3·9
100,000	9·60	32·6	3·4

* Fractional saturation is calculated according to the model of Monod, Wyman and Changeux assuming exclusive binding (equation 2.19). It is assumed that n has a value of 4.

enzyme activity from zero to 100% would demand an infinite change in concentration of regulator. As has been implied, even an 80-fold change is metabolically unlikely: it would take a long time to establish such a change and it could interfere non-specifically in metabolism or produce metabolic side effects (for example, an 80-fold change in the concentration of ATP or citrate, i.e. 0·2–16 mM, could cause marked ionic changes in the cell due to their chelation properties). However, if the response between the enzyme and its regulator is sigmoid, it can be calculated (using the simple model of Monod *et al.*, i.e. equation 2.19) that a change in enzyme activity from 10 to 90% may require a change in regulator concentration of only four-fold (for an exaggerated sigmoid curve—see Table 2.1). Hence the significance of the sigmoid behaviour is that it minimizes the change in regulator concentration that is necessary to modify sufficiently the catalytic activity of the enzyme. The role of sigmoid behaviour may be termed 'amplification'.

Thus the physical chemistry of equilibrium binding effectively limits the sensitivity of enzymes to changes in concentrations of regulator molecules. Whether such a system can provide an adequate control mechanism depends on the extent of the physiological response required by the organisms and the total change in concentration of regulators that the cell can either produce or withstand. For example, an increase in enzyme activity from 10 to 90% is not very large and a total change in regulator concentration of four-fold is perhaps metabolically acceptable. However, the situation may be different if the required response is from 1 to 99%, since the total concentration change for the regulator molecules will need to be much greater than four-fold (perhaps even 100-fold). In this condition simple feedback inhibition, which depends upon equilibrium-binding, may not be satisfactory and such a physiological situation will demand modifications in the control mechanism.

At least two mechanisms may exist for improving the response between the change in concentration of regulator and the enzyme activity. The first amplification mechanism, *substrate cycling*, retains the simplicity of equilibrium binding of the regulator molecule to the regulatory enzyme, whereas the second mechanism, the occurrence of *enzymatically interconvertible forms of an enzyme*, involves a completely different and more complicated system.

(*a*) *Amplification mechanisms in enzyme activity regulation*

(*i*) *Substrate cycles.* Consider a pathway in which the non-equilibrium reaction B → C is opposed by another separate non-equilibrium reaction which results in a conversion C → B. These two separate reactions are catalysed by enzymes E_1 and E_2 as follows.

$$S \rightarrow A \rightleftarrows B \overset{E_1}{\underset{E_2}{\rightleftharpoons}} C \rightleftarrows D \rightarrow P$$

As the reaction $B \rightarrow C$ is non-equilibrium (that is, energy is lost as heat), the reaction $C \rightarrow B$ must involve other reactants so that energy is also lost in the reaction (for example, $ATP + C \rightarrow B + ADP$). It is assumed that a regulator X activates the enzyme E_1 and inhibits the enzyme E_2 by equilibrium-binding mechanisms and that in the control situation both these enzymes (E_1 and E_2) are catalytically active. Thus a *substrate cycle* is established between B and C and the activities of both enzymes are involved in the regulation of the rate of the overall pathway S to P. This improves the effective response of the enzyme system to a change in concentration of the regulator X. The actual response will depend primarily on the rate of cycling compared with the overall flux through the pathway. This is illustrated in Table 2.2, where the effect on the overall flux of a twofold increase in the activity of

Table 2.2. Effects of a twofold increase in the activity of the 'forward enzyme' ($B \rightarrow C$) and a twofold decrease in the activity of the 'reverse enzyme' ($C \rightarrow B$) on the flux through a metabolic pathway.* Both enzymes are simultaneously catalytically active and thus constitute a *substrate cycle*

Initial flux through pathway (S → P) in arbitrary units	Rate of substrate cycling in arbitrary units	New flux through pathway (S → P) in arbitrary units (after twofold enzyme activity changes)	Percentage increase in flux due to effects of regulator
0·1	0·1	0·35	350
0·1	0·2	0·50	550
0·1	0·5	0·95	950
0·1	1·0	1·70	1,700
0·1	2·0	3·20	3,200
0·1	5·0	7·70	7,700

* The pathway in which compound S is converted to compound P can be described as follows :

$$S \rightleftarrows A \rightleftarrows B \overset{E_1}{\underset{E_2}{\rightleftarrows}} C \rightleftarrows D \rightleftarrows P$$

The rate of conversion of B to C, which depends upon the activities of the 'forward enzyme' (E_1) and the 'reverse enzyme' (E_2), limits the overall flux through the pathway. Thus E_1 and E_2 are regulatory enzymes for the pathway and it is assumed that a specific regulator can increase the activity of E_1 and decrease that of E_2. A twofold increase in activity of E_1 and a twofold decrease in activity of E_2 are produced by a small change in the regulator concentration (perhaps a 50% increase in concentration). The initial flux through the pathway (before the increase in regulator concentration) is 0·1 arbitrary units. In other words, if the rate of cycling is 0·1, E_1 catalyses B → C at a rate of 0·2 and E_2 catalyses C → B at a rate of 0·1 arbitrary units: the difference provides the net flux through the pathway. Similarly, at a cycling rate of 5·0 and flux of 0·1, E_1 has activity of 5·1 and E_2 an activity of 5·0 arbitrary units. In the absence of a *substrate cycle* an increase of 50% in concentration of the regulator could produce a change in flux through the pathway of about twofold (the calculations are similar to those in Table 2.1), since it will modify the activity of the 'forward enzyme' (E_1) only. However, if substrate cycling occurs at a rate which is 10 times greater than the flux through the pathway, this 50% increase in regulator concentration can produce a 17-fold increase in net flux through the pathway, S → P.[29]

enzyme E_1 and a twofold decrease in the activity of enzyme E_2 is shown at various rates of substrate cycling. In essence the response of the enzyme system to the regulator is proportional to the ratio $\dfrac{\text{cycling rate}}{\text{overall flux}}$: the larger is the value of this ratio, the greater is the amplification produced by the substrate cycle.

The basic limitation of allosteric regulation has been overcome by substrate cycling, since there is no theoretical limit to the extent of amplification that can be produced. However, a price must be paid for the amplification: this price is the energy which is lost as a result of cycling. In any substrate cycle, energy must be continually utilized in order to maintain the cycle.

In Chapters 3 and 6 evidence will be presented for the existence of a substrate cycle between fructose-6-phosphate and fructose diphosphate catalysed by the simultaneous activities of phosphofructokinase (PFK) and fructose diphosphatase (FDPase). In this example one molecule of ATP is hydrolysed for each turn of the cycle. Obviously the cycling rate should not be too great because of this energy loss. Since the response is dependent upon the ratio $\dfrac{\text{cycling rate}}{\text{overall flux}}$, the net flux through the pathway must be low if the system is to provide greater amplification than a non-cycling system without excessive loss of energy. This suggests that substrate cycling as a means of improving the response between enzyme activity and regulator concentration will only be found in metabolic situations in which the overall flux through the pathway is relatively small. Examples of such a mechanism are the regulation of glycolysis at the level of fructose-6-phosphate phosphorylation in resting skeletal muscle (see Chapter 3) and the regulation of glucose metabolism in liver (see Chapter 6).

(ii) *Enzymatically interconvertible forms of enzymes.* This type of control mechanism has three important properties. First, the regulatory enzyme of the pathway exists in two forms, one of which is catalytically active; the other is inactive (or much less active). Second, the active form is enzymatically converted into the inactive form by a reaction which has a large equilibrium constant (that is, it is not readily reversed); the inactive form is enzymatically converted into the active form by another reaction which has a large equilibrium constant. Third, the regulator X modifies the activities of the interconverting enzymes (not the pathway enzyme) in opposite directions by the process of equilibrium binding. These properties are summarized in Figure 2.11.

The essential difference between this type of mechanism and the allosteric mechanism is that the conversions of the active form to the inactive form and vice versa are thermodynamically 'primed' so that when the interconverting enzyme is active, the equilibrium position of the reaction which it catalyses includes a high percentage of the active (or inactive) form of the pathway

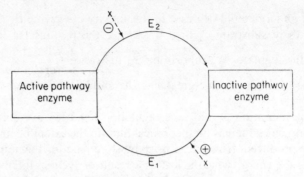

Figure 2.11. Regulation of enzyme activity via interconvertible forms. The active pathway enzyme catalyses
a regulatory reaction in a metabolic pathway. The reaction
(and consequently the pathway) is regulated by factor X.
However, X does not affect the pathway enzyme *per se*,
but modifies the activities of the two enzymes E_1 and
E_2 that interconvert the pathway enzyme between its
active and inactive forms. The reaction catalysed by E_1
is unidirectional, as is the reaction catalysed by E_2

regulatory enzyme (see Table 2.3). Also the role of the regulatory molecule X
has changed from that of a direct participant in the activation (and inactivation) of the pathway enzyme to that of a specific regulator of the interconverting enzymes. This system of control provides amplification as explained
below. In one physiological condition the activity of E_2 is much greater than
that of E_1 (Table 2.3) so that the reaction catalysed by E_2 will approach
equilibrium (about 99% of the enzyme is in the inactive form Pr). As the
concentration of X is increased, E_1 will be stimulated and E_2 inhibited. When
the activity of E_1 exceeds that of E_2, Pr will be converted to the other form
of the enzyme, Pr*, and this reaction will approach equilibrium (that is,
approximately 99% Pr*). For example, a four-fold increase in [X] will
inhibit E_2 and stimulate E_1 such that E_1 becomes dominant and Pr is
rapidly converted into Pr*. Since the equilibrium position of the reaction
catalysed by E_1 may be 99% in favour of Pr* a four-fold change in concentration of X, through this control system, can modify the activity of the pathway
regulatory enzyme from 1% to 99% of its maximum activity.

Moreover it can be seen from Table 2.3 that a change in [X] of less than
20% could cause a change in the domination between the activities of E_1
and E_2 which could result in a complete change in the distribution between
Pr and Pr*. Since the difference in activities between E_1 and E_2 would be
very small, the time taken for the reactions to approach equilibrium (that is,
99% Pr or 99% Pr*) could be reasonably large. Thus the larger the change
in [X] and the greater the difference between E_1 and E_2, the more rapidly

by enzymatic interconversions

Concentration of regulator X	Fractional saturation of enzymes E_1 and E_2 with X	Maximum activity of E_1 is 100 Maximum activity of E_2 is 100			Maximum activity of E_1 is 100 Maximum activity of E_2 is 10		
		Activity of E_1	Activity of E_2	Major form of pathway enzyme present	Activity of E_1	Activity of E_2	Major form of pathway enzyme present
0·0	0·00	0·0	100	Inactive (Pr)	0·0	10·0	Inactive (Pr)
1·0	0·01	1·0	99	Inactive	1·0	9·9	Inactive
2·0	0·05	5	95	Inactive	5	9·5	Inactive
3·0	0·15	15	85	Inactive	15	8·5	Active (Pr*)
4·0	0·31	31	69	Inactive	31	6·9	Active
5·0	0·47	47	53	Inactive	47	5·3	Active
6·0	0·60	60	40	Active (Pr*)	60	4·0	Active
8·0	0·77	77	23	Active	77	2·3	Active
12·0	0·89	89	11	Active	89	1·1	Active

The pathway enzyme exists in two forms, inactive (Pr) and active (Pr*). The inactive form is converted to the active form by a reaction which is catalysed by an enzyme E_1,

$$A + Pr \xrightarrow{E_1} Pr* + B$$

The active form is converted to the inactive form by a reaction which is catalysed by an enzyme E_2,

$$C + Pr* \xrightarrow{E_2} Pr + D$$

The energy released by the conversions A to B and C to D ensures that the reactions catalysed by E_1 and E_2 are unidirectional. This is achieved by the maintenance of satisfactory steady-state levels of A, B, C and D in the cell (that is, the concentrations of A and C are high, and those of B and D are low). The result of the unidirectionality is that, when the activity of E_1 far exceeds that of E_2, as much as 99% of the protein is in the active form (Pr*), whereas in the converse situation ($E_2 \gg E_1$) as much as 99% is in the inactive form (Pr). In the known examples of control by interconvertible forms of enzymes, the hydrolysis of ATP (to ADP or AMP) is used to provide the energy for the unidirectionality of the interconverting reactions.

A numerical example has been calculated in order to illustrate these properties of the system. The results of the calculation, which are presented in this table, have no real significance. They merely serve to illustrate the efficiency of response of the system to changes in the concentration of regulator.

For these theoretical calculations several assumptions are necessary. It is assumed that E_1 is inactive and that E_2 is maximally active in the absence of a specific regulator X and that at saturating concentrations of X, E_1 is maximally active and E_2 is inactive. The activities of E_1 and E_2 are calculated according to the model of Monod, Wyman and Changeux assuming exclusive binding (equation 2.19). The allosteric constant L is arbitrarily assigned a value of 10^3 and n a value of 4. Finally, it is assumed that the change in enzyme activity is proportional to the fractional saturation with X and that both enzymes have the same affinity for X.

will the equilibrium of the reaction catalysed by the dominant enzyme be approached. In the allosteric mechanism of regulation the basic limitation between response of enzyme and concentration change of regulator was one of thermodynamics: in the mechanism of regulation based on enzymatically interconvertible forms of enzymes the limitation is not one of thermodynamics but of kinetics. Is the change in [X] large enough to produce a sufficiently rapid conversion of one form of the enzyme to the other? This will of course depend upon the particular physiological situation and the enzyme involved.

There are now six definite examples of enzymes which are regulated by this type of mechanism: glutamine synthetase of *E. coli*, the pyruvate dehydrogenase complex, glycogen phosphorylase, phosphorylase *b* kinase, UDPG-glucosyltransferase and triglyceride lipase. The glutamine synthetase system is described in reference 27 and Figure 2.12. The pyruvate dehydrogenase system will be described in Chapter 3, and the phosphorylase system and glucosyltransferase will be described in Chapter 4, where the physiological reasons for this form of control will be discussed. The triglyceride lipase interconversion system will be discussed in Chapter 5.

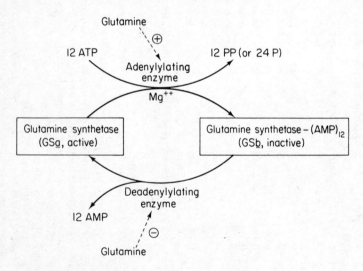

Figure 2.12. Regulation of glutamine synthetase by enzymatic interconversions. This figure has been taken from reference 27 and modified slightly

APPENDIX TO CHAPTER 2

APPENDIX 2.1. DERIVATION OF A SATURATION FUNCTION FOR THE MONOD–WYMAN–CHANGEUX MODEL

The allosteric protein is considered to exist in two conformational states, R and T, which are in equilibrium. The equilibrium is governed by the allosteric constant, L. In order to simplify the derivation of the saturation function, a tetrameric protein ($n = 4$) is considered. The microscopic dissociation constant, K_R, which describes the affinity of the R state for the ligand, is identical for all the binding sites. Similarly in the T state, K_T is identical for all the binding sites.

The situation is described as follows

$$R_0 \rightleftarrows T_0$$

$R_0 + S \rightleftarrows R_1$	$T_0 + S \rightleftarrows T_1$
$R_1 + S \rightleftarrows R_2$	$T_1 + S \rightleftarrows T_2$
$R_2 + S \rightleftarrows R_3$	$T_2 + S \rightleftarrows T_3$
$R_3 + S \rightleftarrows R_4$	$T_3 + S \rightleftarrows T_4$

The notation adopted by Monod et al.[10] is used here for ease of reference. This notation differs slightly from that used in Section D.2 which was chosen to be more consistent with the derivation of the Adair equation.

The apparent dissociation constants for the four reactions involving the R state are K_{d1}, K_{d2}, K_{d3} and K_{d4}, and for the T state they are K'_{d1}, K'_{d2}, K'_{d3} and K'_{d4}. These apparent dissociation constants are statistically related to the microscopic dissociation constants, K_R and K_T, respectively, as described below.

The saturation function, $\bar{Y}_s$ is defined below as the fraction of the total number of ligand-binding sites that are filled.

$$\bar{Y}_s = \frac{(R_1 + 2R_2 + 3R_3 + 4R_4) + (T_1 + 2T_2 + 3T_3 + 4T_4)}{4\{(R_0 + R_1 + R_2 + R_3 + R_4) + (T_0 + T_1 + T_2 + T_3 + T_4)\}} \quad (2.23)$$

(The brackets [ ] to denote concentration have been omitted from the appendices for the sake of simplicity.) However, R_1, R_2, etc., can be expressed in terms of R_0 and the apparent dissociation constants of the four reactions involving the R state (i.e. K_{d1}, K_{d2}, etc.).

Thus,

$$R_1 = \frac{R_0 S}{K_{d1}}$$

$$R_2 = \frac{R_1 S}{K_{d2}} = \frac{R_0 S^2}{K_{d1} \cdot K_{d2}}$$

$$R_3 = \frac{R_2 S}{K_{d3}} = \frac{R_0 S^3}{K_{d1} \cdot K_{d2} \cdot K_{d3}}$$

$$R_4 = \frac{R_3 S}{K_{d4}} = \frac{R_0 S^4}{K_{d1} \cdot K_{d2} \cdot K_{d3} \cdot K_{d4}}$$

These dissociation constants are statistically related to the microscopic dissociation constant K_R, as follows.

$$K_{d1} = \tfrac{1}{4} K_R$$

This should be clear when it is realized that there are four chances of the ligand binding to the protein R_0, for every one chance of ligand dissociating from R_1. Similarly,

$$K_{d2} = \tfrac{2}{3} K_R$$

$$K_{d3} = \tfrac{3}{2} K_R$$

$$K_{d4} = 4 K_R$$

Substituting for these dissociation constants in the above expressions

$$R_1 = \frac{4 R_0 S}{K_R}$$

$$R_2 = \frac{6 R_0 S^2}{K_R^2}$$

$$R_3 = \frac{4 R_0 S^3}{K_R^3}$$

$$R_4 = \frac{R_0 S^4}{K_R^4}$$

In an analogous way, expressions for T_1, T_2, etc., can be derived in terms of

T_0, S and the microscopic dissociation constant, K_T.

$$T_1 = \frac{4T_0S}{K_T}$$

$$T_2 = \frac{6T_0S^2}{K_T^2}$$

$$T_3 = \frac{4T_0S^3}{K_T^3}$$

$$T_4 = \frac{T_0S^4}{K_T^4}$$

These expressions for R_1, R_2, etc., and T_1, T_2, etc., can be substituted in equation 2.23.

$$\bar{Y}_s = \frac{\dfrac{4R_0S}{K_R} + \dfrac{12R_0S^2}{K_R^2} + \dfrac{12R_0S^3}{K_R^3} + \dfrac{4R_0S^4}{K_R^4} + \dfrac{4T_0S}{K_T} + \dfrac{12T_0S^2}{K_T^2} + \dfrac{12T_0S^3}{K_T^3} + \dfrac{4T_0S^4}{K_T^4}}{4\left\{\left(R_0 + \dfrac{4R_0S}{K_R} + \dfrac{6R_0S^2}{K_R^2} + \dfrac{4R_0S^3}{K_R^3} + \dfrac{R_0S^4}{K_R^4}\right) + \left(T_0 + \dfrac{4T_0S}{K_T} + \dfrac{6T_0S^2}{K_T^2} + \dfrac{4T_0S^3}{K_T^3} + \dfrac{T_0S^4}{K_T^4}\right)\right\}}$$

$$\bar{Y}_s = \frac{\dfrac{4R_0S}{K_R}\left(1 + \dfrac{3S}{K_R} + \dfrac{3S^2}{K_R^2} + \dfrac{S^3}{K_R^3}\right) + \dfrac{4T_0S}{K_T}\left(1 + \dfrac{3S}{K_T} + \dfrac{3S^2}{K_T^2} + \dfrac{S^3}{K_T^3}\right)}{4\left\{R_0\left(1 + \dfrac{4S}{K_R} + \dfrac{6S^2}{K_R^2} + \dfrac{4S^3}{K_R^3} + \dfrac{S^4}{K_R^4}\right) + T_0\left(1 + \dfrac{4S}{K_T} + \dfrac{6S^2}{K_T^2} + \dfrac{4S^3}{K_T^3} + \dfrac{S^4}{K_T^4}\right)\right\}}$$

Since

$$\left(1 + \frac{3S}{K_R} + \frac{3S^2}{K_R^2} + \frac{S^3}{K_R^3}\right) = \left(1 + \frac{S}{K_R}\right)^3$$

and

$$\left(1 + \frac{4S}{K_R} + \frac{6S^2}{K_R^2} + \frac{4S^3}{K_R^3} + \frac{S^4}{K_R^4}\right) = \left(1 + \frac{S}{K_R}\right)^4$$

the above expression simplifies to

$$\bar{Y}_s = \frac{\dfrac{4R_0S}{K_R}\left(1 + \dfrac{S}{K_R}\right)^3 + \dfrac{4T_0S}{K_T}\left(1 + \dfrac{S}{K_T}\right)^3}{4\left\{R_0\left(1 + \dfrac{S}{K_R}\right)^4 + T_0\left(1 + \dfrac{S}{K_T}\right)^4\right\}}$$

Since the allosteric constant $L = T_0/R_0$, T_0 can be replaced by LR_0 and the factor 4 can be cancelled.

$$\bar{Y}_s = \frac{\dfrac{R_0 S}{K_R}\left(1 + \dfrac{S}{K_R}\right)^3 + \dfrac{LR_0 S}{K_T}\left(1 + \dfrac{S}{K_T}\right)^3}{R_0\left(1 + \dfrac{S}{K_R}\right)^4 + LR_0\left(1 + \dfrac{S}{K_T}\right)^4}$$

$$\bar{Y}_s = \frac{\dfrac{S}{K_R}\left(1 + \dfrac{S}{K_R}\right)^3 + \dfrac{LS}{K_T}\left(1 + \dfrac{S}{K_T}\right)^3}{\left(1 + \dfrac{S}{K_R}\right)^4 + L\left(1 + \dfrac{S}{K_T}\right)^4} \tag{2.24}$$

If the number of binding sites on the protein is n, equation 2.24 can be expressed in the general form as follows.

$$\bar{Y}_s = \frac{\dfrac{S}{K_R}\left(1 + \dfrac{S}{K_R}\right)^{n-1} + L\dfrac{S}{K_T}\left(1 + \dfrac{S}{K_T}\right)^{n-1}}{\left(1 + \dfrac{S}{K_R}\right)^n + L\left(1 + \dfrac{S}{K_T}\right)^n} \tag{2.25}$$

If $S/K_R = \alpha$ and $K_R/K_T = c$ (so that $S/K_T = c\alpha$), equation 2.25 becomes

$$\bar{Y}_s = \frac{\alpha(1 + \alpha)^{n-1} + Lc\alpha(1 + c\alpha)^{n-1}}{(1 + \alpha)^n + L(1 + c\alpha)^n} \tag{2.26}$$

If the ligand S is assumed to bind only to the R state (exclusive binding) K_T will approach infinity and c will approach zero. Consequently, equation 2.26 can be further simplified.

$$\bar{Y}_s = \frac{\alpha(1 + \alpha)^{n-1}}{L + (1 + \alpha)^n} \tag{2.27}$$

(This is identical to equation 2.19 in Section D.2(b).)

There are several situations in which equation 2.26 reduces to that of a rectangular hyperbola:

(a) When the allosteric constant is either infinitely small (i.e. $L \to 0$) or infinitely large (i.e. $L \to \infty$). In these situations there is virtually only one state of the protein to be considered and obviously the source of sigmoidicity is removed.

If $L \to 0$, terms in L become negligible so that

$$\bar{Y}_s = \frac{\alpha(1 + \alpha)^{n-1} + Lc\alpha(1 + c\alpha)^{n-1}}{(1 + \alpha)^n + L(1 + c\alpha)^n}$$

simplifies to

$$\bar{Y}_s = \frac{\alpha(1 + \alpha)^{n-1}}{(1 + \alpha)^n}$$

$$= \frac{\alpha}{1 + \alpha}$$

If $L \to \infty$, all terms lacking L become negligible so that

$$\bar{Y}_s = \frac{Lc\alpha(1 + c\alpha)^{n-1}}{L(1 + c\alpha)^n}$$

$$= \frac{c\alpha(1 + c\alpha)^{n-1}}{(1 + c\alpha)^n}$$

$$= \frac{c\alpha}{1 + c\alpha}$$

(b) Hyperbolic curves result if there is only one binding site per protein molecule, i.e. $n = 1$

$$\bar{Y}_s = \frac{\alpha + Lc\alpha}{1 + \alpha + L + Lc\alpha}$$

$$= \frac{\alpha(1 + Lc)}{\alpha(1 + Lc) + (1 + L)}$$

$$= \frac{\alpha}{\alpha + \dfrac{(1 + L)}{(1 + Lc)}}$$

This equation has the form $\alpha/\alpha + B$ (where B is a constant) and it describes a hyperbola.

(c) If the affinity of the R state for the ligand is identical to that of the T state (i.e. $K_R = K_T$ and $c = 1$), hyperbolic curves result. In this situation the two states are identical (from the point of view of the ligand) and this removes the source of sigmoidicity

$$\bar{Y}_s = \frac{\alpha(1 + \alpha)^{n-1} + L\alpha(1 + \alpha)^{n-1}}{(1 + \alpha)^n + L(1 + \alpha)^n}$$

$$= \frac{\alpha(1 + L)(1 + \alpha)^{n-1}}{(1 + L)(1 + \alpha)^n}$$

$$= \frac{\alpha(1 + \alpha)^{n-1}}{(1 + \alpha)^n}$$

$$= \frac{\alpha}{1 + \alpha}$$

APPENDIX 2.2. DERIVATION OF THE FUNCTION OF STATE, $\bar{R}$, FOR THE MONOD–WYMAN–CHANGEUX MODEL

The function of state, $\bar{R}$, is defined as the fraction of the total protein in the R state. Thus, for a tetrameric protein,

$$\bar{R} = \frac{R_0 + R_1 + R_2 + R_3 + R_4}{(R_0 + R_1 + R_2 + R_3 + R_4) + (T_0 + T_1 + T_2 + T_3 + T_4)} \qquad (2.28)$$

Since R_1, R_2, etc., and T_1, T_2, etc., may all be expressed in terms of the free protein, R_0 and T_0, the ligand concentration, S, and the microscopic binding constants, K_R and K_T (for details see Appendix 2.1), equation 2.28 becomes

$$\bar{R} = \frac{\left(R_0 + \dfrac{4R_0S}{K_R} + \dfrac{6R_0S^2}{K_R^2} + \dfrac{4R_0S^3}{K_R^3} + \dfrac{R_0S^4}{K_R^4}\right)}{\left(R_0 + \dfrac{4R_0S}{K_R} + \dfrac{6R_0S^2}{K_R^2} + \dfrac{4R_0S^3}{K_R^3} + \dfrac{R_0S^4}{K_R^4}\right) + \left(T_0 + \dfrac{4T_0S}{K_T} + \dfrac{6T_0S^2}{K_T^2} + \dfrac{4T_0S^3}{K_T^3} + \dfrac{T_0S^4}{K_T^4}\right)}$$

$$= \frac{R_0\left(1 + \dfrac{4S}{K_R} + \dfrac{6S^2}{K_R^2} + \dfrac{4S^3}{K_R^3} + \dfrac{S^4}{K_R^4}\right)}{R_0\left(1 + \dfrac{4S}{K_R} + \dfrac{6S^2}{K_R^2} + \dfrac{4S^3}{K_R^3} + \dfrac{S^4}{K_R^4}\right) + T_0\left(1 + \dfrac{4S}{K_T} + \dfrac{6S^2}{K_T^2} + \dfrac{4S^3}{K_T^3} + \dfrac{S^4}{K_T^4}\right)}$$

$$= \frac{R_0\left(1 + \dfrac{S}{K_R}\right)^4}{R_0\left(1 + \dfrac{S}{K_R}\right)^4 + T_0\left(1 + \dfrac{S}{K_T}\right)^4}$$

Since $T_0 = L \cdot R_0$

$$\bar{R} = \frac{R_0\left(1 + \dfrac{S}{K_R}\right)^4}{R_0\left(1 + \dfrac{S}{K_R}\right)^4 + L \cdot R_0\left(1 + \dfrac{S}{K_T}\right)^4}$$

Cancelling R_0

$$\bar{R} = \frac{\left(1 + \dfrac{S}{K_R}\right)^4}{\left(1 + \dfrac{S}{K_R}\right)^4 + L\left(1 + \dfrac{S}{K_T}\right)^4} \qquad (2.29)$$

APPENDIX 2.3. DERIVATION OF EQUATIONS FOR HETEROTROPIC EFFECTS IN THE MONOD–WYMAN–CHANGEUX MODEL

(*i*) *Inhibition*

An inhibitor, I, is considered to bind preferentially to the T state of the enzyme and thus will shift the $R \rightleftarrows T$ equilibrium in favour of T (that is, the allosteric constant L is increased). As a result there is less protein in the R state to which the substrate may bind and inhibition results. Consider the case of a tetrameric protein in which the effect of the inhibitor I is to increase the allosteric constant L to L_I', the fractional saturation of enzyme with substrate is given by

$$\bar{Y}_s = \frac{\dfrac{S}{K_R}\left(1 + \dfrac{S}{K_R}\right)^3}{L_I' + \left(1 + \dfrac{S}{K_R}\right)^4} \tag{2.30}$$

where there is exclusive binding of substrate to the R state. L_I' may be expressed in terms of the concentration of inhibitor, I, and the microscopic dissociation constants, K_{I_R} and K_{I_T}, for the complexes of I with the R state and T state respectively. In the absence of inhibitor, the allosteric constant L is given by

$$L = \frac{T_0}{R_0}$$

In the presence of inhibitor, the new allosteric constant L_I' is given by

$$L_I' = \frac{T_0 + T_{1_I} + T_{2_I} + T_{3_I} + T_{4_I}}{R_0 + R_{1_I} + R_{2_I} + R_{3_I} + R_{4_I}} \tag{2.31}$$

The concentrations of T_{1_I}, T_{2_I}, etc., and R_{1_I}, R_{2_I}, etc., may be expressed in terms of free protein R_0 and T_0, concentration of inhibitor, I, and the microscopic dissociation constants K_{I_R} and K_{I_T} in exactly the same way as the concentrations of the enzyme–substrate complexes were derived (see Appendix 2.1), i.e.

$$T_{1_I} = \frac{4T_0I}{K_{I_T}} \qquad R_{1_I} = \frac{4R_0I}{K_{I_R}}$$

$$T_{2_I} = \frac{6T_0I^2}{K_{I_T}^2} \qquad R_{2_I} = \frac{6R_0I^2}{K_{I_R}^2}$$

$$T_{3_I} = \frac{4T_0I^3}{K_{I_T}^3} \qquad R_{3_I} = \frac{4R_0I^3}{K_{I_R}^3}$$

$$T_{4_I} = \frac{T_0I^4}{K_{I_T}^4} \qquad R_{4_I} = \frac{R_0I^4}{K_{I_R}^4}$$

Substituting these expressions in equation 2.31,

$$L_I' = \frac{T_0 + \dfrac{4T_0I}{K_{I_T}} + \dfrac{6T_0I^2}{K_{I_T}^2} + \dfrac{4T_0I^3}{K_{I_T}^3} + \dfrac{T_0I^4}{K_{I_T}^4}}{R_0 + \dfrac{4R_0I}{K_{I_R}} + \dfrac{6R_0I^2}{K_{I_R}^2} + \dfrac{4R_0I^3}{K_{I_R}^3} + \dfrac{R_0I^4}{K_{I_R}^4}}$$

$$= \frac{T_0\left(1 + \dfrac{4I}{K_{I_T}} + \dfrac{6I^2}{K_{I_T}^2} + \dfrac{4I^3}{K_{I_T}^3} + \dfrac{I^4}{K_{I_T}^4}\right)}{R_0\left(1 + \dfrac{4I}{K_{I_R}} + \dfrac{6I^2}{K_{I_R}^2} + \dfrac{4I^3}{K_{I_R}^3} + \dfrac{I^4}{K_{I_R}^4}\right)}$$

$$= \frac{T_0\left(1 + \dfrac{I}{K_{I_T}}\right)^4}{R_0\left(1 + \dfrac{I}{K_{I_R}}\right)^4}$$

Since $T_0/R_0 = L$ (the allosteric constant in absence of inhibitor)

$$L_I' = L\frac{\left(1 + \dfrac{I}{K_{I_T}}\right)^4}{\left(1 + \dfrac{I}{K_{I_R}}\right)^4} \tag{2.32}$$

Since I binds preferentially to the T state, $K_{I_T} < K_{I_R}$, $I/K_{I_T} > I/K_{I_R}$ and therefore $L_I' > L$, i.e. the allosteric constant is increased in the presence of inhibitor.

In the extreme case where I binds exclusively to the T state

$$L_I' = L\left(1 + \frac{I}{K_{I_T}}\right)^4$$

(ii) Activation

Activation is considered to arise in an analogous fashion to inhibition except that an activator is a compound which binds preferentially to the same state as that to which the substrate also binds (i.e. the R state). The microscopic dissociation constants for the R_A and T_A complexes are K_{A_R} and K_{A_T} respectively. If the same reasoning as in Section (i) above is applied, the allosteric constant, L, becomes L_A' in the presence of a fixed concentration of activator A, where L_A' is defined by

$$L_A' = L\frac{\left(1 + \dfrac{A}{K_{A_T}}\right)^4}{\left(1 + \dfrac{A}{K_{A_R}}\right)^4} \tag{2.33}$$

Since the activator binds preferentially to the R state, $K_{A_R} < K_{A_T}$ and $A/K_{A_R} > A/K_{A_T}$. Therefore $L'_A < L$. Thus, the activator causes a decrease in the allosteric constant—that is, it shifts the $R \rightleftarrows T$ equilibrium in favour of the R state. Therefore a greater proportion of the enzyme is present in the substrate-preferred conformation and sigmoidicity is decreased.

In the extreme case, the activator binds exclusively to the R state and

$$L'_A = \frac{L}{\left(1 + \dfrac{A}{K_{A_R}}\right)^4}$$

(iii) Inhibition and Activation

The variation of fractional saturation of an enzyme with varying substrate concentration, in the presence of a fixed inhibitor concentration I may be expressed in terms of the original allosteric constant, L, merely by substituting for L'_I in equation 2.30,

$$\bar{Y}_s = \frac{\dfrac{S}{K_R}\left(1 + \dfrac{S}{K_R}\right)^3}{L\dfrac{(1 + I/K_{I_T})^4}{(1 + I/K_{I_R})^4} + \left(1 + \dfrac{S}{K_R}\right)^4} \tag{2.34}$$

This equation applies when S binds exclusively to the R state. If I binds exclusively to the T state equation 2.34 simplifies to

$$\bar{Y}_s = \frac{\dfrac{S}{K_R}\left(1 + \dfrac{S}{K_R}\right)^3}{L\left(1 + \dfrac{I}{K_{I_T}}\right)^4 + \left(1 + \dfrac{S}{K_R}\right)^4} \tag{2.35}$$

Similarly, in the presence of a fixed concentration of activator A,

$$\bar{Y}_s = \frac{\dfrac{S}{K_R}\left(1 + \dfrac{S}{K_R}\right)^3}{L\dfrac{(1 + A/K_{A_T})^4}{(1 + A/K_{A_R})^4} + \left(1 + \dfrac{S}{K_R}\right)^4} \tag{2.36}$$

If A binds exclusively to the R state, equation 2.36 reduces to

$$\bar{Y}_s = \frac{\dfrac{S}{K_R}\left(1 + \dfrac{S}{K_R}\right)^3}{\dfrac{L}{(1 + A/K_{A_R})^4} + \left(1 + \dfrac{S}{K_R}\right)^4} \tag{2.37}$$

The simultaneous presence of both activator and inhibitor results in a new allosteric constant, L'', which is given by

$$L'' = L\frac{\left(1 + \dfrac{I}{K_{I_T}}\right)^4\left(1 + \dfrac{A}{K_{A_T}}\right)^4}{\left(1 + \dfrac{I}{K_{I_R}}\right)^4\left(1 + \dfrac{A}{K_{A_R}}\right)^4} \tag{2.38}$$

In the case of exclusive binding of both activator and inhibitor (to R and T states respectively)

$$L'' = L\frac{\left(1 + \dfrac{I}{K_{I_T}}\right)^4}{\left(1 + \dfrac{A}{K_{A_R}}\right)^4} \tag{2.39)*}$$

Thus the variation of fractional saturation, $\overline{Y}_s$, with substrate concentration, S, in the presence of both activator and inhibitor is given by substituting L'' for L in equation 2.30.

$$\overline{Y}_s = \frac{\dfrac{S}{K_R}\left(1 + \dfrac{S}{K_R}\right)^3}{\dfrac{L(1 + I/K_{I_T})^4(1 + A/K_{A_T})^4}{(1 + I/K_{I_R})^4(1 + I/K_{A_R})^4} + \left(1 + \dfrac{S}{K_R}\right)^4} \tag{2.40}$$

For the case of exclusive binding of both activator and inhibitor equation 2.40 may be simplified to

$$\overline{Y}_s = \frac{\dfrac{S}{K_R}\left(1 + \dfrac{S}{K_R}\right)^3}{L\dfrac{(1 + I/K_{I_T})^4}{(1 + A/K_{A_R})^4} + \left(1 + \dfrac{S}{K_R}\right)^4}$$

It may be extended to include preferential binding of the substrate, when

$$\overline{Y}_s = \frac{\dfrac{S}{K_R}\left(1 + \dfrac{S}{K_R}\right)^{n-1} + L\dfrac{(1 + I/K_{I_T})^n(1 + A/K_{A_T})^n}{(1 + I/K_{I_R})^n(1 + A/K_{A_R})^n} \cdot \dfrac{S}{K_T}\left(1 + \dfrac{S}{K_T}\right)^{n-1}}{\left(1 + \dfrac{S}{K_R}\right)^n + L\dfrac{(1 + I/K_{I_T})^n(1 + A/K_{A_T})^n}{(1 + I/K_{I_R})^n(1 + A/K_{A_R})^n}\left(1 + \dfrac{S}{K_T}\right)^n}$$

* N.B. Monod et al.[10] have replaced I/K_{I_T} and A/K_{A_R} by β and γ, so that

$$L'' = L\frac{(1 + \beta)^n}{(1 + \gamma)^n}$$

REFERENCES FOR CHAPTER 2

1. Roberts, R. B., Abelson, P. H., Cowie, D. B., Bolton, E. T. & Britten, R. J. (1955). In *Carnegie Institute of Washington Publication 607*, p. 196. Washington, D.C.
2. Umbarger, H. E. (1956). *Science*, **123**, 848.
3. Gerhart, J. C. & Pardee, A. B. (1962). *J. biol. Chem.* **237**, 891.
4. Monod, J., Changeux, J.-P. & Jacob, F. (1963). *J. molec. Biol.* **6**, 306.
5. Bohr, C., Hasselback, M. A. & Krogh, A. S. (1904). *Scand. Arch. Physiol.* **16**, 402.
6. Barcroft, J. & Hill, A. V. (1909). *J. Physiol.* **39**, 411.
7. Adair, G. S. (1923). *J. Physiol.* **58**, xxxix.
8. Adair, G. S. (1925). *J. biol. Chem.* **63**, 529.
9. Perutz, M. F., Rossman, M. G., Cullis, A. F., Muirhead, H., Will, G. & North, A. C. T. (1960). *Nature, Lond.* **185**, 416.
10. Monod, J., Wyman, J. & Changeux, J.-P. (1965). *J. molec. Biol.* **12**, 88.
11. Koshland, D. E., Némethy, G. & Filmer, P. (1966). *Biochemistry*, **5**, 365.
12. Koshland, D. E. (1958). *Proc. Nat. Acad. Sci. U.S.* **44**, 98.
13. Koshland, D. E. (1969). *Current Topics in Cellular Regulation*, **1**, 1. London & New York: Academic Press.
14. Scarano, E., Geraci, G. & Rossi, M. (1967). *Biochemistry*, **6**, 192 & 3645.
15. Wyman, J. (1964). *Adv. Prot. Chem.* **19**, 223.
16. Whitehead, E. P. (1970). *Prog. Biophys. molec. Biol.* **21**, 321.
17. Dalziel, K. & Engel, P. C. (1968). *FEBS Letters*, **1**, 349.
18. Conway, A. & Koshland, D. E. (1968). *Biochemistry*, **7**, 4011.
19. Engel, P. C. & Dalziel, K. (1969). *Biochem. J.* **115**, 621.
20. Kirschner, K., Eigen, M., Bittman, R. & Voigt, B. (1966). *Proc. Nat. Acad. Sci. U.S.* **56**, 1661.
21. Ogawa, S. & McConnell, H. (1967). *Proc. Nat. Acad. Sci. U.S.* **58**, 19.
22. Gerhart, J. C. & Schachman, H. K. (1968). *Biochemistry*, **7**, 538.
23. Changeux, J.-P. & Rubin, M. M. (1968). *Biochemistry*, **7**, 553.
24. Rabin, B. R. (1967). *Biochem. J.* **102**, 22C.
25. Dalziel, K. (1957). *Acta Chem. Scand.* **11**, 1706.
26. Ferdinand, W. (1966). *Biochem. J.* **98**, 278.
27. Holzer, H. (1969). *Adv. Enzymol.* **32**, 297.
28. Gerhart, J. C. & Schachman, H. K. (1965). *Biochemistry*, **4**, 1054.
29. Newsholme, E. A. & Start, C. (1972). In *Handbook of Physiology and Endocrinology*, 1, Ed. D. F. Steiner & N. Freinkel. Washington, D.C.: American Physiological Society.

CHAPTER 3

REGULATION OF CARBOHYDRATE METABOLISM IN MUSCLE

A. INTRODUCTION

1. The glycolytic pathway

The degradation of the simple sugar, glucose, into the 3-carbon compound, pyruvate, by the sequence of enzyme-catalysed reactions shown in Figure 3.1 appears to be a universal system for liberation of energy, some of which is

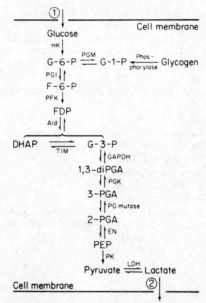

Figure 3.1. The glycolytic pathway in muscle. (1) Entry of glucose into muscle by a specific transport process. (2) Exit of lactate from the muscle by diffusion across cell membrane. HK, hexokinase; PGM, phosphoglucomutase; PGI, phosphoglucoisomerase; PFK, phosphofructokinase; Ald, aldolase; TIM, triose phosphate isomerase; GAPDH, glyceraldehyde-3-phosphate dehydrogenase; PGK, phosphoglycerate kinase; PGmutase, phosphoglycerate mutase; EN, enolase; PK, pyruvate kinase; LDH, lactate dehydrogenase

conserved in the chemical bonds of ATP. The pathway is sometimes known as the Embden–Meyerhof–Parnas pathway after the three investigators who elucidated most of the individual reactions. Although the reactions involved in the conversion of glucose to pyruvate are very similar in all organisms, the fate of the pyruvate depends upon the organism and its environment. The pathway is presumed to have arisen early in the course of evolution since it provides a mechanism for the generation of ATP under anaerobic conditions.

The initial reaction is the transport of glucose across the cell membrane and this involves a specific carrier mechanism. The first intracellular reaction is the conversion of glucose to glucose-6-phosphate (involving ATP conversion to ADP) and is catalysed by the enzyme hexokinase

$$\text{Glucose} + \text{ATP} \rightarrow \text{Glucose-6-phosphate} + \text{ADP}$$

This reaction ensures that the intermediates of glycolysis are phosphorylated and this may be important in restricting these compounds to the cytoplasmic compartment (where the glycolytic enzymes are located) since both the cell membrane and the mitochondrial membrane are generally impermeable to phosphorylated compounds. In the glycolytic pathway glucose-6-phosphate is converted to fructose-6-phosphate which is further phosphorylated by ATP to form fructose-1,6-diphosphate. The conversion of glucose to fructose ensures that the C=O group is adjacent to the third C atom in the molecule.

The bond between the third and fourth C atoms is split by an aldol cleavage to produce two triose phosphate molecules which are maintained in equilibrium by the enzyme triose phosphate isomerase.

$$
\begin{array}{ccc}
CH_2O\textcircled{P} & & CH_2O\textcircled{P} \\
| & & | \\
C=O & & C=O \\
| & & | \\
CHOH & \xrightarrow{\text{Aldolase}} & CH_2OH \\
----+-- & \rightleftharpoons & + \\
CHOH & & CHO \\
| & & | \\
CHOH & & CHOH \\
| & & | \\
CH_2O\textcircled{P} & & CH_2O\textcircled{P}
\end{array}
$$

Glyceraldehyde-3-phosphate is oxidized to phosphoglycerate. During this oxidation NAD^+ is converted to NADH and inorganic phosphate (P_i) is taken up and converted into the 'energy rich' mixed anhydride bond

$$
\begin{array}{c}
O \\
\diagup\!\!\diagup \\
C \\
\diagdown \\
O\textcircled{P}
\end{array}
$$

$$
\begin{array}{ccc}
CHO & & COOP\textcircled{P} \\
| & & | \\
CHOH + NAD^+ + P_i & \rightarrow & CHOH + NADH \\
| & & | \\
CH_2O\textcircled{P} & & CH_2O\textcircled{P}
\end{array}
$$

In this form the phosphate group is transferred by phosphoglycerate kinase onto ADP to form ATP and 3-phosphoglycerate. The combination of the glyceraldehyde-3-phosphate dehydrogenase and 3-phosphoglycerate kinase reactions provides an oxidative reaction in which some of the energy released by the oxidation is conserved in the ATP molecule. The other important aspect of this reaction is the conversion of NAD^+ to NADH which must be continually reoxidized to NAD^+ in order to maintain glycolytic flux (see below).

The 3-phosphoglycerate is converted to phosphoenolpyruvate by mutase and enolase reactions. Finally the phosphate from this compound is transferred to ADP with the formation of ATP and pyruvate. Presumably the initial product of the pyruvate kinase reaction is enol-pyruvate, but this is rapidly converted to the more stable keto-form.

$$
\text{ADP} + \begin{array}{c} CH_2 \\ \| \\ C-O\!\!\!\!P \\ | \\ COOH \end{array} \rightarrow \begin{array}{c} CH_2 \\ \| \\ C-OH \\ | \\ COOH \end{array} + \text{ATP}
$$

$$
\updownarrow
$$

$$
\begin{array}{c} CH_3 \\ | \\ C=O \\ | \\ COOH \end{array}
$$

2. Regeneration of NAD^+ for glycolysis

The reduction of NAD^+ in the glyceraldehyde-3-phosphate dehydrogenase reaction requires that the NADH which is produced must be reoxidized at the same rate as glycolysis. In most types of muscle under anaerobic conditions this is accomplished by the lactate dehydrogenase reaction:

$$CH_3COCOOH + NADH \rightarrow NAD^+ + CH_3CHOHCOOH$$

Thus, anaerobic glycolysis is a self-sufficient process. White anaerobic vertebrate skeletal muscles (such as rabbit leg and pheasant pectoral muscle) obtain almost all of their energy for contraction from anaerobic glycolysis: they have little aerobic capacity for pyruvate oxidation, a poor blood supply, a low activity of hexokinase and a high activity of phosphorylase[1] (Table 3.1). Consequently the conversion of pyruvate to lactate is more important in these muscles than in the more aerobic red vertebrate muscles and insect flight muscles which have highly active enzymes of the TCA cycle and the mitochondrial electron transport chain.

In red muscles the conversion of pyruvate to lactate is only important when the demand for energy is greater than the availability of oxygen. Under

Table 3.1. Activities of hexokinase, phosphorylase, phosphofructokinase, mitochondrial and cytoplasmic glycerol 1-phosphate dehydrogenase and lactate dehydrogenase in various muscles[1]

Animal	Muscle	Enzyme activities (μmol/min per g fresh weight at 25 °C)					
		Hexokinase	Phosphorylase	Phospho-fructokinase	Glycerol-1-phosphate dehydrogenase		Lactate dehydrogenase
					Mitochondrial	Cytoplasmic	
Insecta							
Locust (*Schistocerca gregaria*)	Flight	11·5	7·5	17·0	43·0	141·0	2·9
Wasp (*Vespa vulgaris*)	Flight	77·0	3·0	74·0	120·0	—	—
Honey-bee (*Apis mellifera*)	Flight	29·0	4·0	20·0	44·0	257·0	1·5
Blowfly (*Phormia terranova*)	Flight	14·0	54·0	46·0	110·0	300·0	1·7
Pisces							
Trout (*Salmo gairdneri*)	Red	2·6	14·0	12·2	0·1	9·0	23·0
	White	1·6	48·0	58·3	0·1	18·0	—
Amphibia							
Frog (*Rana temporaria*)	Sartorius (white)	1·3	29·0	22·0	0·4	24·0	398·0
Aves							
Domestic pigeon (*Columba livia*)	Pectoral (red)	3·0	18·0	24·0	1·2	33·0	314·0
Mallard (*Anas platyrhynchos*)	Pectoral (red)	3·8	50·0	41·0	1·9	35·0	276·0

Table 3.1. Continued

Animal	Muscle	Enzyme activities (μmol/min per g fresh weight at 25 °C)					
		Hexokinase	Phosphorylase	Phospho-fructokinase	Glycerol-1-phosphate dehydrogenase		Lactate dehydrogenase
					Mitochondrial	Cytoplasmic	
Domestic fowl (*Gallus gallus*)	Pectoral (white)	1·1	83·0	105·0	0·6	76·0	870·0
Pheasant (*Phasianus colchicas*)	Pectoral (white)	2·3	120·0	143·0	2·8	103·0	542·0
Mammalia Rabbit (*Oryctolagus cuniculus*)	Semitendinosus (red)	1·9	8·0	8·0	0·2	4·6	60·0
	Adductor longus (white)	0·3	30·0	26·0	0·8	55·0	3772·0
Laboratory rat (Wistar strain)	Heart (red)	6·1	12·0	10·0	0·3	6·0	311·0
	Quadriceps femoris (white)	1·9	50·0	47·0	1·2	48·0	448·0

aerobic conditions pyruvate is oxidized within the mitochondria and therefore it is unavailable for the oxidation of glycolytic NADH. Another pathway for the oxidation of this NADH must be present in these muscles.

In aerobic muscle the mitochondrial electron-transport chain provides the obvious means of oxidation of glycolytic NADH, but a problem arises from the impermeability of the inner mitochondrial membrane to pyridine nucleotides. Indirect means must be employed for the transport of reducing equivalents from the cytoplasm to the mitochondria. In insect flight muscle this is achieved by a process known as the glycerol-1-phosphate cycle[2]: in the cytoplasm the enzyme glycerol-1-phosphate dehydrogenase catalyses the conversion of dihydroxyacetone phosphate (formed along with glyceraldehyde-3-phosphate in glycolysis) and NADH to glycerol-1-phosphate and NAD$^+$. The glycerol-1-phosphate enters the mitochondria where it is oxidized to dihydroxyacetone phosphate by the mitochondrial glycerol-1-phosphate dehydrogenase (a flavoprotein enzyme). The dihydroxyacetone phosphate returns from the mitochondrion to the cytoplasm to complete the cycle (Figure 3.2). An obvious question arises as to why the NADH cannot

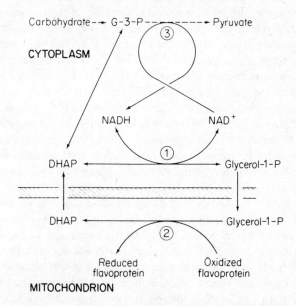

Figure 3.2. The glycerol-1-phosphate cycle. (1) Cytoplasmic glycerol-1-phosphate dehydrogenase. (2) Mitochondrial glycerol-1-phosphate dehydrogenase. (3) Glyceraldehyde-3-phosphate dehydrogenase. G-3-P is glyceraldehyde 3-phosphate. DHAP is dihydroxyacetone phosphate

enter the mitochondria directly and avoid the necessity for such a complex cycle. The answer is that the mitochondrial membrane is impermeable to pyridine nucleotides and as a result the redox state (i.e. $NAD^+/NADH$ ratio) in the cytoplasm can be maintained at a more oxidized level than that in the mitochondria. The pyridine nucleotide system in the cytoplasm has to be maintained in a relatively highly oxidized state ($NAD^+/NADH$ is about 10^3) in order to ensure that the equilibrium of the reaction catalysed by glyceraldehyde-3-phosphate dehydrogenase lies in favour of glycolysis: a more reduced ratio would favour the conversion of 1:3-diphosphoglycerate to glyceraldehyde-3-phosphate (i.e. gluconeogenesis). However, the mitochondrion must maintain its pyridine nucleotides much more reduced ($[NAD^+]/[NADH]$ is about 10) in order to provide sufficient driving force for the electron-transport chain and oxidative phosphorylation.

The glycerol-1-phosphate cycle must be irreversible in order to prevent the two pools of pyridine nucleotides equilibrating by means of the cycle. Irreversibility is achieved through the mitochondrial glycerol-1-phosphate dehydrogenase reaction which is non-equilibrium. It is interesting that although glycerol-1-phosphate is produced in the cytoplasm by the NADH-linked reduction of dihydroxyacetone phosphate, in the mitochondrion the oxidation of glycerol phosphate involves a flavin-linked reduction in the electron-transport chain, so that the resultant P/O ratio is 2 (instead of 3). This extra energy is not conserved in ATP but is lost as heat, in order to ensure the non-equilibrium character of the mitochondrial dehydrogenase reaction and of the cycle as a whole (Chapter 1, Section B).

The glycerol-1-phosphate cycle does not appear to play such an important quantitative role in NADH oxidation in vertebrate aerobic muscle, in which the activity of the mitochondrial glycerol-1-phosphate dehydrogenase is very low[1] (Table 3.1). In these muscles the malate-oxaloacetate shuttle may perform a similar function to the glycerol-1-phosphate cycle in insect flight muscle.[3] In this case oxaloacetate is reduced to malate (and NADH is oxidized to NAD^+) in the cytoplasm by malate dehydrogenase and malate traverses the mitochondrial membrane and is then oxidized to oxaloacetate by the mitochondrial dehydrogenase. Two problems complicate the system: first, oxaloacetate does not traverse the mitochondrial membrane very readily and therefore it has been proposed that it leaves as aspartate which requires transaminase reactions on both sides of the mitochondrial membrane (see Figure 3.3); second, the malate dehydrogenases function on both sides of the membrane as NAD^+-linked enzymes which would produce a reversible cycle and result in equilibration of mitochondrial and cytoplasmic pools of pyridine nucleotides. Therefore at least one of the reactions in the cycle must be irreversible. This is possibly the transport of malate into the mitochondria or the transport of aspartate out of the mitochondria.

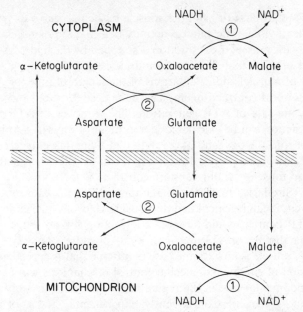

Figure 3.3. The malate-oxaloacetate cycle. (1) Malate dehydrogenase. (2) Glutamate-oxaloacetate transaminase

3. Energy relationship between glycolysis and the TCA cycle

When glycolysis functions anaerobically, the net energy gain is 2 ATP molecules per glucose molecule. However, in most anaerobic situations that occur physiologically in muscle, endogenous glycogen is the substrate for glycolysis and this produces 3 ATP molecules per glucose residue. In aerobic muscles the complete oxidation of glucose produces 34 ATP molecules per glucose molecule (or 38 if the mitochondrial oxidation of glycolytic NADH is taken into account). Therefore aerobic metabolism is at least 10-fold more efficient in terms of energy production per glucose residue.

4. The need for control of glycolysis

The control of glycolysis is necessary to ensure that carbohydrate is degraded only as rapidly as energy is required by the cell. The requirement for energy will vary from organism to organism and from tissue to tissue. In the case of microorganisms, the synthetic processes involved in growth and replication will largely determine the need for ATP synthesis and the rates of these processes must be adapted to the nature of the environment or medium in which the microorganism is growing. At the other extreme of biological complexity, the cells of vertebrate tissues are subservient to the needs of the organism as a whole. This may place demands upon a particular tissue such that extremely sudden and drastic changes in the rate of ATP synthesis are required. For example, muscle tissue may have to switch from rest to a state of violent mechanical activity in a fraction of a second.

The energy for muscular contraction is supplied by the hydrolysis of ATP. The amount of ATP that is found in muscle is not very large (5–7 μmol/g fresh weight of muscle) and calculations of the length of time for which this ATP could support contraction emphasize the need for rapid and controlled variation in the rate of ATP generation. The turnover of ATP in muscle during contraction can be calculated in a number of ways (see Appendix 3.1 for details). From the oxygen uptake data of a flying insect (such as *Lucilia sericata*), or an isolated perfused rat heart, it can be calculated that the total ATP in these muscles would support contraction for about 0·1 s and 5 s, respectively. Similarly, from the maximum glycolytic capacity of white skeletal muscle, it can be calculated that during vigorous mechanical activity the total ATP content could support contraction for no longer than one second in the absence of ATP regeneration (Appendix 3.1).

Obviously, muscle is an extreme case of a tissue that is specialized for the rapid provision of energy and specific control mechanisms will be expected to play a fundamental role in the regulation of the utilization of fuels (such as glucose and glycogen). Consequently, experimental studies of glycolytic control mechanisms have centred upon muscle tissue and provide the basis for the discussion in this chapter. It is now becoming clear that other glycolysing cells including microorganisms (such as *E. coli* and yeast) and other mammalian tissues (such as brain and red blood cells) may utilize similar control mechanisms. At the present state of the investigations, differences between tissues or between organisms appear to be merely quantitative: it cannot be easily assessed whether they reflect variations of an experimental nature or whether they can provide a basis for important differences in control mechanisms.

B. IDENTIFICATION OF NON-EQUILIBRIUM REACTIONS OF GLYCOLYSIS

The study of the control of glycolysis provides a good example of the application of the approach outlined in Chapter 1 for the identification of regulatory enzymes and the development of an acceptable theory of metabolic control. The first stage of the investigation is the identification of non-equilibrium reactions by measurements of mass-action ratios and maximal enzyme activities.

1. Mass-action ratios and equilibrium constants for the glycolytic reactions

Mass-action ratios for the reactions of glycolysis from a variety of tissues are collated in Table 3.2 together with the apparent equilibrium constants. Several points emerge from a consideration of the data in this table.

Table 3.2. A comparison of apparent equilibrium constants with mass-action ratios for the reactions of glycolysis[16,17,65,66,67]

Reactions catalysed by:	Apparent equilibrium constant (K')	Mass-action ratios (Γ)				Units of K' and Γ*
		Brain	Heart	Erythrocytes	Ascites tumour	
Hexokinase	$3 \cdot 9$–$5 \cdot 5 \times 10^{3}$	$0 \cdot 04$	$0 \cdot 08$	$7 \cdot 6 \times 10^{-4}$	$2 \cdot 6 \times 10^{-2}$	
Phosphoglucoisomerase	$0 \cdot 36$–$0 \cdot 47$	$0 \cdot 22$	$0 \cdot 24$	$0 \cdot 41$	$0 \cdot 23$	
Phosphofructokinase	$0 \cdot 9$–$1 \cdot 2 \times 10^{3}$	$0 \cdot 13$	$0 \cdot 03$	$4 \cdot 4 \times 10^{-2}$	$0 \cdot 63$	
Aldolase	$6 \cdot 8$–$13 \cdot 0 \times 10^{-5}$	$2 \cdot 4 \times 10^{-6}$	9×10^{-6}	$1 \cdot 4 \times 10^{-5}$	$2 \cdot 9 \times 10^{-5}$	M
Triosephosphate isomerase	$3 \cdot 6$–$4 \cdot 5 \times 10^{-2}$	—	$0 \cdot 24$	$0 \cdot 35$	$1 \cdot 5$	
Glyceraldehyde-3-phosphate dehydrogenase plus phosphoglycerate kinase	$0 \cdot 2$–$1 \cdot 5 \times 10^{3}$	53	9	124	$17 \cdot 8$	M^{-1}
Phosphoglycerate mutase	$0 \cdot 1$–$0 \cdot 2$	$0 \cdot 1$	$0 \cdot 12$	$0 \cdot 15$	$0 \cdot 43$	
Enolase	$2 \cdot 8$–$4 \cdot 6$	$3 \cdot 6$	$1 \cdot 4$	$1 \cdot 7$	$1 \cdot 6$	
Pyruvate kinase	2–20×10^{3}	$5 \cdot 4$	40	51	$2 \cdot 8$	

* Unless otherwise stated, K' and Γ are dimensionless

(a) The mass-action ratios for each reaction are fairly similar in all the tissues studied. This facilitates the assessment of the data and emphasizes the basic similarity of different tissues.

(b) Apparently the reactions catalysed by phosphoglucoisomerase, phosphoglycerate mutase and enolase are close to equilibrium, whereas those catalysed by hexokinase, phosphofructokinase and pyruvate kinase are removed far from equilibrium.

(c) The aldolase/triose phosphate isomerase system and the glyceraldehyde-3-phosphate dehydrogenase/phosphoglycerate kinase system are more difficult to assess. However, it is concluded for the purpose of this discussion that both these enzyme systems catalyse reactions close to equilibrium. Therefore they do not enter into any further consideration of the control of glycolysis by feedback mechanisms. The experimental problems concerning calculation of mass-action ratio data for these reactions are discussed in Appendices 3.2 and 3.3.

2. Maximum catalytic activities of the enzymes of glycolysis

In general, enzymes that catalyse non-equilibrium reactions possess low catalytic activities in comparison to those catalysing near-equilibrium reactions. The maximum activities of the glycolytic enzymes from a variety of tissues (measured *in vitro* under optimal conditions) are presented in Table 3.3. Despite the variation in total activities there is an overall pattern,

Table 3.3. Maximal activities of glycolytic enzymes in different tissues. The enzyme activities are expressed as μmol of substrate transformed/min/g fresh tissue[68,69,70]

| | Enzyme activities | | | |
Reactions catalysed by:	Brain	Heart	Skeletal muscle	Erythrocytes
Hexokinase	17	7	1·5	0·3
Phosphoglucoisomerase	80	65	176	5·6
Phosphofructokinase	24	14	56	1·8
Aldolase	15	24	78	0·7
Triosephosphate isomerase	415	580	2,650	97
Glyceraldehyde-3-phosphate dehydrogenase	105	135	440	17·1
Phosphoglycerate kinase	610	74	169	25·6
Phosphoglycerate mutase	122	27	100	8·6
Enolase	47	15	158	1·6
Pyruvate kinase	164	145	387	4·6
Lactate dehydrogenase	100	386	366	20·4

which is similar in all tissues. This pattern becomes clear upon consideration of the *relative* activities of the enzymes as calculated in Table 3.4 in which the activity of hexokinase has arbitrarily been assigned as unity. The enzymes, hexokinase, phosphofructokinase, aldolase and (in most cases) enolase have low activities in comparison with the remainder of the glycolytic enzymes.

Table 3.4. The relative activities of glycolytic enzymes

| Reactions catalysed by: | Enzyme activities (based on a value of 1 μmol/min/g for hexokinase) | | | |
	Brain	Heart	Skeletal muscle	Erythrocytes
Hexokinase	1	1	1	1
Phosphoglucoisomerase	5	9	117	19
Phosphofructokinase	2	2	37	6
Aldolase	1	4	52	2·5
Triosephosphate isomerase	28	83	1,768	323
Glyceraldehyde-3-phosphate dehydrogenase	7	19	295	57
Phosphoglycerate kinase	41	10	113	85
Phosphoglycerate mutase	8	3	67	28
Enolase	3	2	105	5
Pyruvate kinase	11	21	258	15
Lactate dehydrogenase	7	55	244	67

Thus, from the criterion of maximal enzyme activity, these enzymes should be classified as catalysing non-equilibrium reactions. However, if these activities are taken in conjunction with mass-action ratios, only hexokinase and phosphofructokinase can be definitely classified as 'non-equilibrium' enzymes. This suggests that there may be problems associated with the measurement of the maximum activities of aldolase and enolase *in vitro*, so that the assays underestimate the total catalytic capacity that is available in the intact tissue. These problems remain unresolved at present. Another problem enzyme is pyruvate kinase: the mass-action ratio strongly indicates that it catalyses a non-equilibrium reaction whereas the maximal catalytic activity suggests otherwise. It is assumed for this discussion that the mass-action ratio data provide a better criterion and that pyruvate kinase catalyses a non-equilibrium reaction.

C. IDENTIFICATION OF REGULATORY ENZYMES

1. Introduction

The identification of non-equilibrium reactions indicates those enzymes whose activities limit the flux through the pathway. How can the activity of such an enzyme be controlled? One possible mechanism is by variation of the substrate concentration. However, if control is effected by compounds other than the substrate, the enzyme would be a regulatory enzyme according to the more restricted definition presented in Chapter 1 (Section C.2). An enzyme can be shown to be regulatory (according to the latter definition) if the concentration of the pathway substrate (that is, the pathway intermediate which is the substrate for the enzyme under consideration) changes in the opposite direction to the change in flux. The rationale for this type of experiment has been discussed in detail in Chapter 1 (Section C.2). There has been a great deal of experimental work on variations of glycolytic flux and the changes in glycolytic intermediates. For the sake of clarity each of the possible non-equilibrium reactions of glycolysis is considered in turn and selected evidence which positively identifies regulatory reactions is presented.

2. Glucose transport into the cell

Although there is very little known about the molecular details of the transport process, there is every indication that a specific carrier within the membrane is responsible for the entry of glucose (see Appendix 3.4). In order to establish that this transport process is regulatory, it is necessary first to show that it is removed from equilibrium. It is not possible to measure the activity of this process *in vitro* and therefore conclusions must be based solely on mass-action ratio data (that is, the ratio of the concentration of intracellular glucose to the concentration of extracellular glucose). A mass-action ratio approaching unity indicates that transport is an equilibrium process (providing that glucose equilibrates completely within the intracellular water). Unfortunately, there is a major experimental problem in the precise measurement of the concentration of intracellular glucose. Any measurement of the tissue content of glucose includes that which is external to the cell membrane as well as that which is intracellular. This problem may be surmounted by the measurement of the extracellular fluid volume using a compound (such as sorbitol) that cannot traverse the cell membrane (see Figure 3.4). Since the concentration of glucose in the extracellular water is the same as that in the medium, the intracellular concentration may be calculated (for an example, see Appendix 3.5).

A large difference between the total tissue content and the extracellular content of glucose enables the intracellular content to be estimated with

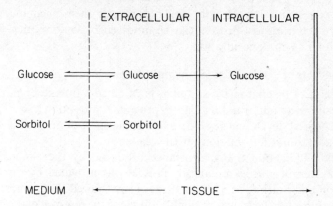

Figure 3.4. Use of sorbitol to measure extracellular fluid volume

reasonable precision. This is not possible when there is only a small difference between these contents. Nevertheless, if the concentration of the intracellular glucose is very small (i.e. non-detectable) and the extracellular concentration is high, the concentration ratio of intracellular glucose to extracellular glucose will be very large and will indicate that transport is a non-equilibrium process. This is found to be the case in many experimental preparations of muscle (for example, isolated rat diaphragm and isolated perfused rat heart). Thus, it can be concluded that under many conditions the rate of glycolysis from extracellular glucose is limited by the transport process at the muscle cell membrane.

It can also be demonstrated that the glucose transport process in muscle is regulatory since it is modified by factors other than the concentration of extracellular glucose. The rate of glucose uptake by the isolated rat diaphragm and the perfused rat heart can be increased under conditions in which the transport process is non-equilibrium (for example by anaerobiosis or the presence of respiratory poisons or uncoupling agents). The flux is increased and the substrate concentration (extracellular glucose) is decreased in comparison to the control condition. Therefore the transport process must have been increased by factors other than concentration of extracellular glucose.[4,5] This conclusion can be confirmed by experiments in which the transport of non-utilizable sugars (such as xylose and arabinose) is studied. Apparently these sugars enter the cell by the same carrier-mediated process as glucose (see Appendix 3.4) so their accumulation can be used as a direct measure of the rate of the transport process. Anaerobiosis, respiratory poisons, uncoupling agents and insulin all increase the rate of accumulation of these sugars by the isolated rat diaphragm and perfused rat heart, whereas the oxidation of fatty acids decreases their accumulation.[4,5,6] Therefore the transport process can be modified by factors other than the extracellular sugar concentration.

(a) The effects of insulin on glucose uptake by muscle

The effect of insulin on the stimulation of glucose uptake by muscle and other tissues is an important regulatory process. At this point a short account of the historical development of ideas about the effect of insulin will provide useful background information for the reader.

The first indication that a substance produced by the pancreas could affect the rate of glucose uptake by muscle was provided by the work of Knowlton and Starling as early as 1912.[7] They showed that glucose uptake by the perfused dog heart was negligible following the removal of the pancreas but was restored to normal by the addition of a boiled extract of pancreas to the medium. In 1922, Banting and Best isolated the hormone, insulin, from the pancreas[8] and there followed a number of experiments that showed that insulin was responsible for the stimulation of glucose uptake in muscle tissue, but a controversy arose over which reaction in the pathway of glucose utilization was stimulated by insulin. Two major theories were proposed to explain the effect of insulin on glucose metabolism; the hexokinase theory and cell membrane transport theory. Since hexokinase catalyses an early reaction in the utilization of glucose it was considered to be a potential regulatory enzyme. Hexokinase activity of muscle extracts was found to be inhibited by anterior pituitary and adrenal cortical extracts supplied either in vitro or in vivo and this inhibition could be removed by insulin.[9] At the time it seemed possible that the activity of hexokinase was regulated by a critical balance of hormones and that insulin exerted its effect on glucose uptake in muscle by removing the inhibition of hexokinase. Although the observations of hexokinase inhibition by pituitary extracts may have some validity, this stimulatory effect of insulin could not be repeated.[10]

However, a paper had been published as early as 1939 which presented good evidence that the effect of insulin was due to accelerated membrane transport:[11] glucose uptake of the musculature of the eviscerated cat obeyed saturation kinetics and, even at saturation, no significant intracellular accumulation of glucose was observed. This indicated a specific process for the transport of glucose. Furthermore, in the perfused hind-limb preparation, insulin increased glucose uptake three-fold but the intracellular glucose concentration remained very low. Since the glucose concentration gradient across the cell membrane did not change, insulin must have stimulated the transport process.

It is usual to credit Levine and colleagues[12] with the first evidence for the action of insulin on membrane transport in muscle. They found that in eviscerated-nephrectomized dogs the volume of distribution of D-galactose was approximately extracellular in the absence of insulin but was increased to greater than the extracellular volume (that is, extra- plus intracellular) when insulin was administered. Since galactose is not metabolized to any great extent in this preparation, these workers concluded that insulin had specifically accelerated a membrane transport process. Accordingly, they proposed that the hormone would exert a similar effect on glucose transport. Since these experiments, a substantial body of evidence has accumulated in support of this theory.[13,14]

3. The hexokinase reaction

Hexokinase can be shown to be a regulatory enzyme if the rate of glucose phosphorylation can be changed in the opposite direction to the concentration of substrate (intracellular glucose). The practical demonstration is hindered by the problems involved in the accurate measurement of the intracellular glucose concentration. The presence of insulin and a high concentration of glucose (5–10 mM) in the perfusion medium activates glucose transport in the perfused rat heart so that the activity of hexokinase limits glucose uptake and there is an accumulation of intracellular glucose. Therefore the latter can be measured with reasonable precision. If glycolysis is increased (and therefore glucose phosphorylation is increased) by addition of respiratory poisons, uncoupling agents or by anaerobiosis, the intracellular glucose content is markedly reduced (in comparison to the control situation).[5] On the other hand, the oxidation of an alternative substrate to glucose (such as fatty acids, ketone bodies or pyruvate) decreases the rate of glycolysis and the content of intracellular glucose is increased.[6] Therefore in this tissue, under certain conditions, hexokinase can be shown to be a regulatory enzyme. In skeletal muscle, intracellular glucose is not experimentally detectable (even in the presence of insulin) and it is not possible to conclude that hexokinase is a regulatory enzyme (according to the second definition).

4. The phosphofructokinase reaction

Phosphofructokinase can be shown to be regulatory if the rate of fructose-6-phosphate phosphorylation is increased under conditions where the concentration of fructose-6-phosphate is decreased, or vice versa. In the perfused heart and isolated rat diaphragm preparations (and in brain) the stimulation of glycolysis by respiratory poisons or by anoxia is accompanied by a fall in the fructose-6-phosphate content of the tissue.[14] Conversely, the oxidation of a substrate other than glucose (such as fatty acids, ketone bodies or pyruvate) in perfused-heart and diaphragm preparations decreases the rate of glycolysis (and therefore of fructose-6-phosphate phosphorylation) and the content of fructose-6-phosphate is increased.[14] In experiments with the blowfly, the initiation of flight stimulates glycolysis in the flight muscles about 100-fold and the content of fructose-6-phosphate decreases.[15] Thus, there is ample evidence to support the view that PFK is a regulatory enzyme for glycolysis in muscle. This is also the case for other tissues (see references 16 and 17 for brain tissue).

In experiments in which glycolysis in a skeletal muscle preparation (such as frog sartorius) is increased by electrical stimulation, there is an increase in the content of fructose-6-phosphate as well as the other hexose mono-phosphates.[18] The probable reason for this is that phosphorylase is activated by electrical stimulation to a greater extent than PFK. But it cannot be concluded that PFK is regulatory, because the increase in fructose-6-phosphate concentration could be responsible for the increase in PFK activity. However, it has been shown that treatment of this muscle preparation with adrenaline, which increases phosphorylase activity (see Chapter 4) and raises the content of fructose-6-phosphate to a level higher than that obtained with electrical stimulation, produces a smaller increase in glycolytic flux (as measured by lactate formation).[19] Thus in the electrical stimulation experiments the activity of PFK must have been increased by factors other than the fructose-6-phosphate concentration.

5. The pyruvate kinase reaction

Although it appears that pyruvate kinase catalyses a non-equilibrium reaction in muscle and other tissues, it has not been possible to show that it is a regulatory enzyme, except in the case of cerebral cortex slices. (The stimulation of glycolysis by several agents—cyanide, glutamate, K^+ ions—results in a decrease in the tissue content of phosphoenolpyruvate.[17]) In experiments with the blowfly, initiation of flight results in a very marked stimulation of glycolysis (about 100-fold) but there is very little change in the concentration of phosphoenolpyruvate.[15] It would require a large increase in the concentration of this substrate to increase the activity of pyruvate kinase by 100-fold and, since large increases in content of substrate are not observed, this suggests that the enzyme is regulated by other factors.

6. Summary

A summary of the possible regulatory reactions in glycolysis in muscle is presented in Figure 3.5.

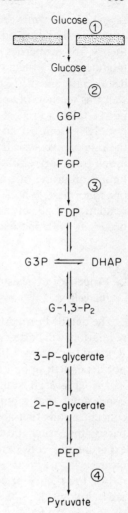

Figure 3.5. The regulatory reactions of glycolysis in muscle. (1) Glucose transport. (2) Hexokinase. (3) Phosphofructokinase. (4) Pyruvate kinase

D. PROPERTIES OF REGULATORY ENZYMES AND THEORIES OF METABOLIC REGULATION

1. Introduction

Once the regulatory enzymes have been identified, the next step in the general approach is to identify the controlling factors. These factors may be elucidated during a systematic *in vitro* study of the properties of the proposed regulatory enzymes. A theory based upon these properties may then be constructed and tested. If the results of such a test do not comply with the theory, the properties of the enzymes must be rę-examined and the theory modified and tested once more. The following discussion centres upon hexokinase and PFK in muscle simply because they illustrate particularly well this method of approach. The emphasis upon these two enzymes must not be taken to reflect their overriding importance in control of the rate of glycolysis from extracellular glucose or glycogen. The major limitation in the rate of glycolysis from glucose in muscle may occur at the level of membrane transport, about which little is known. On the other hand, the major limitation in the rate of glycolysis from glycogen may occur at the level of phosphorylase, whose regulation is described in Chapter 4. However, the regulation of glycolysis from intracellular glucose and glucose-6-phosphate occurs at hexokinase and PFK, respectively.

2. Properties of phosphofructokinase and control by the 'energy status' of the cell

The detailed properties of PFK, which appear to be relevant to metabolic regulation, will be described as the story of the regulatory mechanism unfolds. It should be stressed that the physiological theory of control of glycolysis is not dependent upon knowledge of the mechanism of control of PFK at the *molecular level*; it is sufficient for the physiological theory that the metabolic compounds that modify the activity do so in a reversible manner and at concentrations that are reasonably physiological. Whether or not a theory based upon such properties is acceptable depends upon theoretical and experimental considerations of a physiological rather than a molecular nature.

For the theory of control of glycolysis the essential properties of PFK are as follows: it is inhibited by ATP above a certain optimum concentration (Figure 3.6a) and this inhibition is relieved by AMP, P_i, fructose diphosphate or fructose-6-phosphate (see Figure 3.6 and references 20, 21). If the activity is plotted against the fructose-6-phosphate concentration at an inhibitory concentration of ATP, the resultant plot is sigmoid (Figure 3.6b). These properties can be explained by a kinetic mechanism similar to that proposed by Ferdinand, or by a mechanism based on equilibrium binding of ATP to various conformational states of the protein (see Chapter 2). At present there is not sufficient information to distinguish between these possibilities. Nonetheless, from desensitization experiments, it can be concluded that PFK possesses one catalytic site for ATP and at least one regulatory site.[22]

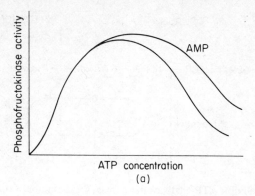

ATP concentration
(a)

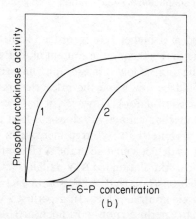

F-6-P concentration
(b)

Figure 3.6. (a) Plot of phosphofructokinase activity against ATP concentration in the presence and absence of AMP. (b) Plot of phosphofructokinase activity against fructose-6-phosphate concentration at a non-inhibitory level (1) and an inhibitory level (2) of ATP

(a) The problems associated with control of phosphofructokinase by ATP

A simple theory of glycolytic control can be proposed which is based solely upon the inhibition of PFK by ATP. The theory is that ATP controls its own rate of formation (from glycolysis and the TCA cycle) by feedback inhibition of PFK. Such a simple closed-loop system would function as follows: when the ATP-utilizing reactions are stimulated (for example, by increased contractile activity) the level of ATP would fall and this would lead to stimulation of PFK (Figure 3.7). Glycolysis would be stimulated and ATP

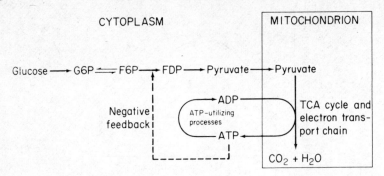

Figure 3.7. Simple ATP-feedback mechanism for the inhibition of glycolysis in muscle. For simplicity, ATP generation from glycolysis is omitted

would be synthesized at a higher rate in order to satisfy the increased requirement. According to this theory, the content of ATP should be high when the rate of ATP utilization is low (for example, in resting muscle) and the content of ATP should be low when the rate of energy utilization is high (for example, during contraction). However, it has been known for many years that increased mechanical activity does *not* lead to large decreases in the content of ATP despite the very large increase in energy expenditure. (Indeed, the inability to detect a change in the ATP content in muscles made to contract by electrical stimulation led A. V. Hill in 1950 to issue a challenge to biochemists to demonstrate that ATP was in fact the primary energy intermediate for muscle contraction.)[23] In a perfused working isolated rat heart (in comparison to a perfused non-working heart) the rate of contraction, the coronary flow, the oxygen uptake and glucose utilization are all increased.[24] When the heart is made to work, the flux through PFK is increased about four-fold, whereas the content of ATP is decreased by only 16% (Table 3.5). Similarly when the blowfly is forced to fly, the rate of flux through glycolysis (and therefore through PFK) is increased by about 100-fold, whereas the ATP content is decreased by only 10% (Table 3.5).[25] The question is, could such a small change in ATP content lead to sufficient stimulation of PFK activity? This question could be answered by reference to the experimental response curve of PFK activity to ATP concentration, but it is always possible that changes in the assay conditions will result in an increase in sensitivity to ATP and the number of possible changes in assay conditions are almost infinite. If PFK interacts with ATP at the regulatory site by a process of equilibrium binding, the response can be described either by a hyperbolic or by a sigmoid curve, depending upon whether or not the ATP binding sites are independent. It may be calculated from the Monod–Wyman–Changeux model that a change in enzyme activity from 10% to 90% requires a change in regulator concentration of at least four-fold (for

Table 3.5. Effects of mechanical activity and anaerobiosis on the glycolytic rate and contents of adenine nucleotides in muscle[24,25,26]

Tissue preparation	Physiological condition	Glycolytic flux (μmol of glucose equiv./g/30 min)	Muscle contents (μmol/g)				
			ATP	ADP	AMP	P_i	ATP/AMP
Perfused isolated rat heart	Non-working	14·7	5·3	1·1	0·09	3·9	49
	Working	59·4	4·5	1·3	0·17	5·9	27
Perfused isolated rat heart	Aerobic	20·0	4·2	0·8	0·06	1·5	70
	Anaerobic	180·0	3·4	1·2	0·2	5·2	17
Insect flight muscles	Rest	1·0*	7·0	1·6	0·12	6·8	58
	Flight	100·0*	6·3	1·9	0·26	7·6	24

* These are proportional rates as the precise rates of glycolytic flux under conditions of rest and flight in the living insect are not known. The 100-fold increase is calculated from oxygen consumption data (see reference 1 for details of calculation).

assumptions see Table 2.1). It is therefore exceedingly unlikely that the small changes in ATP content observed in the above experiments could explain the large increases in activity of PFK.

It is possible, of course, to suggest that changes in concentration of ATP in the local environment of PFK may be decreased four-fold, and that this is not detected in the total tissue measurements. The role of ATP as the fundamental energy-transfer compound would suggest otherwise. Any change in the concentration of ATP would produce a change in the opposite direction in ADP, and large changes would seriously modify the amount of energy released during ATP hydrolysis (see Table 3.6). Variations in the

Table 3.6. The effect of changes in the ATP/ADP concentration ratio on the free energy of hydrolysis of ATP

	Concentration (mM)			ΔG for ATP hydrolysis (calories)
	ATP	ADP	P_i	
A	4·95	0·05	8·0	12,834
	3·90	1·0	8·0	10,849
	2·20	2·0	8·0	10,047
	1·42	2·15	8·0	9,734
B	11·0	1·0	8·0	11,475
	10·0	2·0	8·0	10,986
	6·0	6·0	8·0	9,990
	2·0	10·0	8·0	8,993

The change in free energy was calculated from $\Delta G = \Delta G° + RT \ln ADP.P_i/ATP$; $\Delta G°$ was taken to be $-7,000$ cal; by convention the concentration of water was taken to be unity. In section A the changes in the concentrations of ATP and ADP are in accord with an adenylate kinase equilibrium and a total nucleotide concentration of 5 mM (see Table 3.7). In section B the changes in concentrations of ATP and ADP are not related to adenylate kinase and the total nucleotide concentration is 12 mM. In both A and B the concentration of inorganic phosphate has been kept constant to simplify the calculation of the change in free energy.

The table shows that a small change in the ATP concentration results in a considerable decrease in the quantity of energy released from the hydrolysis of ATP. The normal contents of adenine nucleotides in muscle are approximately those shown in the top line of section A in this table and suggest that the amount of energy released from the hydrolysis of 1 mole of ATP is between 11,000–13,000 calories. A decrease in ATP content of four-fold causes a 30% decrease in the free energy released. At this level the hydrolysis of ATP may not provide sufficient energy for many of the energy-requiring processes in muscle.[27]

amount of energy transferred would produce inefficiency in energy conversions generally.[27] All unidirectional reactions must release some energy as heat but a proportion of the total available energy is used for 'useful work' (such as the concentration of ions or mechanical activity). If the energy available from the hydrolysis of ATP varied, then, in order to maintain the same amount of chemical work and 'unidirectionality' (i.e. heat loss) when the concentration of ATP was low (i.e. low energy level), more heat would have to be lost when the ATP concentration was high (i.e. high energy level,

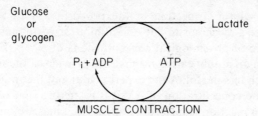

Figure 3.8. Generation of energy for mechanical activity. Hydrolysis of the terminal phosphate bond of ATP to form ADP and P_i provides the universal means by which energy is transferred in living systems. However, this is a means for *transference* of energy rather than *storage*. Energy is released, for example, in the conversion of glucose or glycogen to lactate and this energy is used by the living organism to carry out all the energy-requiring processes of life (for example, muscle contraction, ion transport, biosynthesis). The energy released from the process of glycolysis is not used directly but is transferred initially into the chemical bonds of ATP which donates the energy for processes such as muscle contraction, etc. Hence, when the rate of the energy-consuming processes is increased, the rate of utilization *and regeneration* of ATP must also increase. Thus, the energy for the contraction process is ultimately obtained from the conversion of glucose to lactate and *not* from the hydrolysis of ATP. This hydrolysis only acts as the *energy link* between the process that releases the energy (glycolysis) and the process that uses the energy (muscle contraction). Consequently, the concentrations of ATP and ADP should not change to any appreciable extent during contraction[71]

see Figure 3.8). The advantages that stem from a stable energy currency in the cell are not unlike those that stem from a stable international currency. Transactions or transformations involving biological energy can thus be performed at any time with supreme confidence that the free energy available from the reaction will be relatively constant.

(b) *AMP as an amplification system for changes in ATP*

Despite the biochemical problems associated with ATP as a feedback inhibitor for control of its own formation, the system has the essential simplicity of a satisfactory feedback mechanism. Since large changes in the concentration of ATP are precluded on the basis of energy-transfer efficiency, a mechanism that can detect and magnify small changes in ATP concentration is required. A closer inspection of the properties of PFK indicates the existence of such a mechanism. The ATP inhibition of this enzyme is relieved by the presence of physiological concentrations of AMP (Figure 3.6). The role of AMP in an amplification mechanism provides a theory of control of glycolysis which has the following experimental and theoretical basis.

In the cell the concentration of AMP is related to that of ATP through the equilibrium reaction catalysed by adenylate kinase (often referred to as 'myokinase' in muscle tissue),

$$2ADP \rightleftarrows ATP + AMP$$

There are two essential properties of this reaction in the living cell which provide amplification: the ATP concentration is maintained very much higher than that of AMP and the reaction is always close to equilibrium. The equilibrium nature of the reaction is indicated by the extremely high activity of adenylate kinase and by the mass-action ratio which is very similar to the equilibrium constant. If the concentration of any one of the

Table 3.7. Variations in adenine nucleotide concentrations based on the equilibrium of the reaction catalysed by adenylate kinase

Concentration (mM)				$\dfrac{\% \text{ change in [AMP]}}{\% \text{ change in [ATP]}}$
ADP	ATP	AMP	[ATP]/[ADP]	
0·1	4·899	0·001	49·0	–
0·2	4·796	0·004	24·0	190
0·3	4·691	0·009	15·6	102
0·5	4·48	0·02	8·9	49
1·0	3·89	0·11	3·9	42
1·5	3·19	0·31	2·1	16
2·0	2·2	0·80	1·1	9

The concentrations are calculated from the equilibrium constant for the adenylate kinase reaction,

$$K = \frac{[AMP][ATP]}{[ADP]^2} = 0.44,$$

assuming a constant total nucleotide concentration of 5 mM. The algebraic equation for the calculation is

$$x = + \sqrt{\left\{\left(\frac{c-a}{2}\right)^2 - 0.44a^2\right\}} + \frac{c-a}{2},$$

where c is the total nucleotide concentration, a is the ADP concentration, and x is the AMP concentration. In the computation of the values in this table the restriction that $[ATP] \gg [AMP]$ has been applied.

This table shows that a small percentage change in ATP concentration results in a larger percentage change in the concentration of AMP. The magnitude of the change in concentration of AMP is dependent upon the initial [ATP]/[ADP] ratio and is always constant for any given ratio.[27]

three nucleotides changes, compensatory changes in the others will auto-matically result and, since [ATP] is about 50-fold higher than [AMP], a small decrease in [ATP] must cause a much larger fractional increase in [AMP]. The data in Table 3.7 show the results of theoretical calculations of concentrations of adenine nucleotides as dictated by the equilibrium characteristics of the adenylate kinase reaction. Clearly, the extent of the amplification that can be achieved depends upon the [ATP]/[ADP] ratio and must remain constant for any given value of this ratio. For example, a 10 % change in ATP con-centration can produce a four-fold change in that of AMP. Two points should be emphasized here : first, it is the *fractional* change in the concentra-tion of ATP or AMP which is important for the response of the enzyme and not the *absolute* concentration (even the minimum concentration of AMP in the muscle is probably 100-fold higher than that of PFK); second, this role of AMP is based upon the properties of an isolated enzyme (PFK), and upon theoretical calculations of changes in concentrations of adenine nucleotides assuming equilibrium of the adenylate kinase reaction.

(c) Primary evidence for the amplification theory of control of phospho-fructokinase

This theory has been tested experimentally using intact tissue preparations. Glycolysis can be increased in the perfused isolated rat heart by approxi-mately nine-fold under anaerobic conditions (or in the presence of respiratory poisons) when the concentration of ATP changes only 19 % but [AMP] is increased about four-fold (Table 3.5). One of the difficulties of investigating metabolic control is that in order to detect statistically significant changes in the contents of important metabolites, the metabolic system has to be considerably perturbed. It is often necessary to employ unphysiological conditions (such as anaerobiosis) in order to ensure sufficiently large changes in the concentrations of metabolic regulators. However, the rate of glycolysis in the perfused heart can be modified by such physiological conditions as increased work or provision of alternative substrates to glucose (see later). In insects, the process of flight requires such a large expenditure of energy that, upon the transition from rest to flight, there is a very large increase in the rate of metabolism. In experiments with blowfly (*Phormia regina*) Sacktor and colleagues have shown that glycolysis is stimulated about 100-fold, that the concentration of ATP is decreased only 10 % but that of AMP is increased about 250 % (Table 3.5).[25]

Inorganic phosphate also relieves the ATP inhibition of PFK and in the experiments described above (see Table 3.5) the inorganic phosphate content was increased when glycolysis was stimulated. Therefore it should reinforce the effects of changes in the AMP concentration. The increase in inorganic phosphate may result from the hydrolysis of creatine phosphate (or arginine phosphate in invertebrate muscle). Creatine phosphate is broken down during muscular activity and could give rise to phosphate via the following reactions

$$\text{Creatine-P} + \text{ADP} \xrightleftharpoons[\text{phosphokinase}]{\text{creatine}} \text{ATP} + \text{creatine}$$

$$\text{ATP} \xrightarrow{\text{Actomyosin ATPase}} \text{ADP} + \text{P}_\text{i}$$

Net reaction

$$\text{creatine-P} \xrightarrow{\hspace{2cm}} \text{creatine} + \text{P}_\text{i}$$

The net result of the breakdown of creatine phosphate is an increase in creatine and inorganic phosphate while the levels of ATP and ADP remain fairly constant. Hence, under these conditions, creatine phosphate may act, not only as an energy donor for the synthesis of ATP, but also as a reservoir of inorganic phosphate for the stimulation of glycolysis.

Fructose diphosphate decreases the ATP inhibition of PFK. This property provides the basis for yet another amplification mechanism. A stimulation of the PFK reaction may increase the concentration of fructose diphosphate which would result in a further stimulation of PFK. The process is to some extent autocatalytic, although it cannot produce unlimited stimulation of PFK since it only relieves ATP inhibition. Evidence for this role of fructose diphosphate is obtained from studies with intact tissues in which it can be shown that the concentration of this compound increases under conditions in which PFK is stimulated.[14,26]

(d) *Secondary evidence for the amplification theory of the control of phospho-fructokinase*

The evidence described in the previous section supports the proposed theory for the control of glycolysis. However, it is indirect evidence: it does not *prove* that the theory is correct; it is merely consistent with it. Evidence of a more direct nature would be obtained if the concentration of the regulator could be measured in the immediate environment of PFK in the cell or if the properties of this enzyme could be studied under more physiological conditions (for example, at a concentration of 1 mg/ml). Such investigations are at present technically impossible. It is interesting that perhaps the strongest support for the above theory is obtained from what may be described as secondary evidence, which is, in fact, even more indirect than the primary evidence described above.

(i) *Oscillations in glycolysis.* This phenomenon was first detected in studies on the reduction and oxidation of pyridine nucleotides in intact yeast cells. It was observed that when a certain concentration of glucose was administered to the yeast cells under anaerobic conditions, damped oscillations in the state of reduction of the pyridine nucleotides occurred.[28]

Computer-aided calculations of the kinetics of various types of model systems[29] indicate that at certain substrate and product concentrations a system of the type,

$$
\begin{array}{ccc}
 & \text{Positive} & \\
 & \overset{\frown}{} & \\
\longrightarrow \text{F6P} & \longrightarrow & \text{FDP} \\
 & & \\
\text{ATP} & & \text{ADP}
\end{array}
$$

should oscillate—that is, the concentrations of reactants should increase to a maximum as the products decline to a minimum and then spontaneously the reactants should decline and the products accumulate. This cycle of events is spontaneously repeated and oscillations are induced in the products which are 180° out of phase with the oscillations in the reactants. The activation of PFK by the product is essential in order for spontaneous oscillations to occur. In extracts of yeast or beef heart, sustained oscillations in the redox state of the pyridine nucleotides can be induced by the supply of a glycolytic substrate (glucose) and by addition of either hexokinase, PFK or an ATPase to the system. Oscillations of the same frequency as those of the pyridine nucleotides (4–10 cycles/hour) are seen in the adenine nucleotides and the glycolytic intermediates. An analysis of the phase relationships indicates that the PFK reaction is the source of the oscillations that is, fructose 6-phosphate and fructose diphosphate oscillate 180° out of phase. Moreover, in yeast the oscillations may be initiated by the addition of glucose, fructose, glucose-6-phosphate or fructose-6-phosphate but not by addition of fructose diphosphate or any other glycolytic intermediate that occurs after the PFK reaction.[30,31] In beef-heart extracts the oscillations are modified by factors that affect the activity of PFK.[30] All this evidence supports the suggestion that the PFK reaction is the oscillatory source. Since calculations based upon the *in vitro* properties of PFK predicted the occurrence of oscillations, the fact that oscillations in glycolysis do in fact occur in intact cells strongly supports the theory of control of PFK based on its *in vitro* properties.

It is not known if these oscillations have any biological significance, although it is tempting to speculate that oscillations propagated in this way might provide a molecular basis for circadian (and other) rhythms. Obviously the frequency of glycolytic oscillations is much too high to be directly involved in such rhythms, but a basic rhythm could be easily reduced in frequency. In this respect it is interesting that the most important tissue for generating rhythmicity in higher animals, the brain, has a continual requirement for glucose (see Chapter 6). It remains to be seen whether this requirement stems from an abnormal need for energy derived solely from the catabolism of carbohydrate or whether glycolysis plays a more subtle role in brain metabolism such as rhythm generation.

(*ii*) *Role for adenylate kinase.* The amplification theory described above provides a specific and possibly unique role for the enzymatic reaction catalysed by adenylate kinase (that is, amplification of small changes in ATP concentration). However, the adenylate kinase reaction has been known for many years, whereas this theory for the control of glycolysis is relatively recent. Previously, the postulated role for this enzyme was the conversion of ADP into ATP whenever the ATP level was critically reduced. Under these extreme conditions adenylate kinase would catalyse the conversion of ADP into ATP according to the reaction:

$$2ADP \rightarrow ATP + AMP$$

Since AMP is produced in this reaction, the ADP could be used only once and, since the total nucleotide concentration is low, this mechanism could provide energy for only a very short period of time. For example, in the perfused heart the total content of ATP turns over once every 7 seconds, so that at most adenylate kinase could supply ATP for about 3 seconds. In muscles with a higher turnover of ATP it could supply energy for a much shorter period. Such a process would have little 'survival' value.

Another possible role for the enzyme is the phosphorylation of AMP that is produced in the reactions that 'activate' amino acids and fatty acids (amino acyl-t-RNA synthetase and fatty acid thiokinase, respectively). However the activities of these activating enzymes in muscle are very low (< 3 μmol/min/g fresh wt) whereas the activity of adenylate kinase is extremely high (approximately 100 μmol/min/g fresh weight). Furthermore adenylate kinase has a higher activity in white skeletal muscle than in red skeletal muscle (and heart) whereas fatty acid oxidation occurs almost exclusively in the red muscle.

Thus, the amplification role for adenylate kinase appears to be the only plausible one at the present time, and as such it provides indirect evidence for the theory of control of glycolysis by changes in the concentrations of adenine nucleotides.

(*e*) *Reason for a direct effect of ATP on phosphofructokinase*

The inhibition of PFK by ATP would appear to be something of an enigma if changes in the concentration of ATP are not significant in regard to changes in the activity of the enzyme. In view of the suggested role of AMP, it might have been expected that phosphofructokinase would be directly activated by AMP. The evolutionary development of the control mechanisms of PFK could explain the indirect effect of AMP. The most primitive form of feedback control of this enzyme may have been the ATP-inhibition mechanism, but this suffers from the disadvantage of inefficiency in energy transfer as discussed above. However, it is a general biological axiom that Nature, when evolving new mechanisms, simply adapts or modifies mechanisms already in existence. Therefore ATP inhibition represents an evolutionary primitive control mechanism and the enzyme has adapted by providing the de-inhibitory response to AMP, which now appears to play the major role in regulation of activity of phosphofructokinase in many organisms.

3. Properties of hexokinase and the control of glucose phosphorylation

Since hexokinase (HK) catalyses a non-equilibrium reaction, the regulation of PFK activity need not necessarily control glucose uptake. Inhibition of PFK without simultaneous control of hexokinase (or membrane transport) would cause an enormous accumulation of hexose monophosphates. The properties of isolated hexokinase provide a basis for a theory of control which links both this enzyme and PFK in a concerted control mechanism. The properties of this control system are consistent with the known character-istics of the reactions involved in glycogen synthesis and breakdown and with the effects of insulin upon glucose transport and UDPG-glucosyl transferase. These metabolic interrelationships provide further indirect evidence for the control of the early stages of glycolysis by adenine nucleo-tides.

(a) *Properties of hexokinase and theory of control*

Hexokinases from a variety of tissues are inhibited by the reaction product, glucose-6-phosphate. This inhibition is non-competitive with respect to the substrate, glucose. This property alone provides the basis for a control theory: inhibition of PFK results in an increase in the concentrations of fructose-6-phosphate and glucose-6-phosphate and therefore the phosphorylation of glucose is inhibited. Conversely, stimulation of PFK results in a decrease in glucose-6-phosphate concentration and stimulation of phosphorylation. The changes in glucose-6-phosphate content in muscle are consistent with this theory (for example, in the perfused isolated rat heart the content of glucose-6-phosphate is increased when the glycolytic rate is depressed, and vice versa[6,14,26]); a simple diagram of the concerted mechanism of control of HK and PFK is given in Figure 3.9.

(b) *Indirect evidence for the theory of control of hexokinase and phospho-fructokinase*

The non-competitive nature of the glucose-6-phosphate inhibition of hexokinase is of fundamental importance in this concerted control mechan-ism. If an increase in the concentration of intracellular glucose could stimulate HK and lead to an increase in the concentration of hexose monophosphate, this would effectively overcome the control of PFK by the adenine nucleotide system (fructose-6-phosphate counteracts ATP inhibition; Figure 3.6b). In

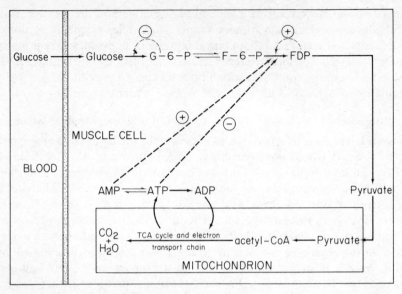

Figure 3.9. Control of glycolysis in muscle at the hexokinase and phosphofructokinase reactions

other words, glycolytic flux could vary in response to variations in the
concentration of intracellular glucose. However, the inhibition of HK by
glucose-6-phosphate is non-competitive and therefore cannot be overcome
by excess glucose.* This is an example of a concerted control system involving
two enzymes both of whose properties are designed to provide efficient
control of the pathway as a whole and neither of which would be effective
alone.

At first sight, a much simpler control mechanism could be expected from
non-competitive adenine nucleotide control of hexokinase. Such a mechanism would reduce the complexity of control at the PFK reaction, but hexokinase would be inhibited when the muscle was at rest and glycogen synthesis
would be prevented. The separation of glycolytic control between PFK and
HK permits glucose residues to be converted to glycogen even though
glycolysis is severely inhibited at the level of PFK. The dual effect of insulin
in stimulating both glucose transport (see Section C.2(a)) and the activity of
the enzyme UDPG-glucosyltransferase (see Chapter 4, Section E.5) supports
this theory (Figure 3.10).

---

* In liver a specific bypass of the glucose-6-phosphate control of hexokinase exists. This
tissue possesses the enzyme, glucokinase, which is *not* inhibited by glucose-6-phosphate and
which has a high K_m for glucose (10 mM). Therefore it is able to respond to changes in blood
glucose (via the intracellular glucose) without any restriction by the hepatic concentration of
glucose-6-phosphate. This mechanism is discussed in detail in Chapter 6, Section B.1.

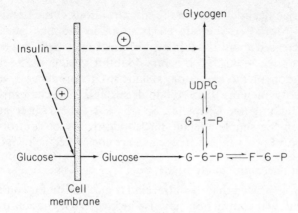

Figure 3.10. Stimulation of glucose transport and UDPG-glucosyltransferase by insulin. The stimulation of glucosyltransferase by insulin may not be brought about directly, but via a secondary messenger

An effect of insulin solely on transport would raise the intracellular levels of glucose and glucose-6-phosphate. The latter would restrict the flux through the hexokinase reaction and minimize the rate of glycogen synthesis. The additional stimulation of glucosyltransferase activity by insulin ensures that the steady-state concentrations of the intermediates between glucose and glycogen (particularly glucose-6-phosphate) remain fairly constant and therefore the conversion of glucose-6-phosphate to glycogen is optimized.

The HK-PFK concerted control system provides a flexible mechanism of control of glycolysis, permitting glycogen synthesis when glycolysis is inhibited, and enabling the specific hormonal and nervous control of phosphorylase to modify PFK activity through the fructose-6-phosphate concentration.

4. An extension of the adenine nucleotide theory of control of phosphofructokinase in muscle

(a) Problems of the adenine nucleotide theory

The evidence in support of the theory of control of phosphofructokinase by the concentration changes in adenine nucleotides is reasonably substantial. However, in some experiments it has not been possible to detect any changes in the concentrations of the adenine nucleotides despite large increases in the rate of muscle glycolysis. Thus, electrical stimulation of the isolated frog sartorius muscle and the *in situ* hind-limb preparation of a cat causes contraction and increases the rate of glycolysis, but there are no statistically-significant changes in the concentrations of the adenine nucleo-tides.[18,19,32] Moreover, the rate of glycolysis in the flight muscle of the blowfly is increased about 100-fold by the initiation of flight, but the increase in [AMP] is only 2·5-fold.[15,25] It is very doubtful whether a 2·5-fold increase in concentration of the regulator is sufficient to produce an increase in enzyme activity of more than 100-fold through a mechanism based on equilibrium binding (see Chapter 2, Section F.2). These observations have cast doubt on the simple adenine nucleotide theory of control and have led to alternative proposals, two of which are considered below.

(b) Ca^{2+} and the control of glycolysis

It has been suggested that the intracellular mechanism for controlling the process of muscular contraction may also be involved in the control of glyco-lysis at the enzymatic levels of PFK, phosphorylase and possibly HK. The control of glycolysis by adenine nucleotides may be generally described as 'control in series', whereas this alternative mechanism may be termed 'control in parallel' (see Figure 3.11). The sarcoplasmic concentration of Ca^{2+}

1. CONTROL IN SERIES

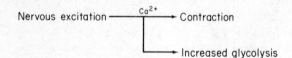

2. CONTROL IN PARALLEL

Figure 3.11. Control of glycolysis in muscle

provides the link between nervous excitation (electrical stimulation) and contraction: excitation promotes a release of Ca^{2+} from the sarcoplasmic reticulum and the concentration of Ca^{2+} in the sarcoplasm increases over the approximate range 10^{-8}–10^{-6} M. This is sufficient to activate the myofibrillar ATPase and initiate contraction. Relaxation is brought about by the uptake of Ca^{2+} by the sarcoplasmic reticulum so that its concentration in the sarcoplasm is reduced to about 10^{-8} M. Thus for the 'control in parallel' mechanism to operate, the activities of hexokinase, PFK and phosphorylase should be modified by Ca^{2+} in the concentration range 10^{-8}–10^{-6} M.

In fact, the activity of phosphorylase *is* stimulated by Ca^{2+} in this con-centration range, although it is an indirect stimulation operating through an enzymatic interconversion. (Details of this mechanism are given in the next chapter where the regulation of Ca^{2+} distribution within the muscle is discussed.) However, Ca^{2+} in the concentration range $10^{-9}–10^{-5}$ M has no effect upon HK and PFK activities nor upon their regulatory properties.[33] Therefore it is unlikely that physiological changes in Ca^{2+} concentration can influence the activities of these enzymes *in situ*. Higher concentrations of Ca^{2+} (10^{-3} M) have been found to inhibit PFK and HK and this observation has led to the suggestion that these enzymes might be localized within the sarcoplasmic reticulum where the concentration of Ca^{2+} would be about 10^{-3} M at rest. During contraction when the concentration of reticulum Ca^{2+} must fall, HK and PFK would be activated.[34] The only evidence in support of this theory of the localization of PFK is that during centrifugation of frog skeletal muscle extracts some of the PFK sediments with the sarcoplasmic reticulum. Such experiments do not prove that PFK is localized within the reticulum in the intact muscle: an alternative explanation is that PFK in crude muscle extracts polymerizes to produce large aggregates which co-sediment with the reticulum fraction. Furthermore, in a comparative study it has been shown that, although the Ca^{2+} inhibition of these enzymes is common to all types of muscle tested, the distribution of the enzymes between mitochondria, reticulum and sarcoplasm is variable.[33] The hypothesis that these enzymes are located in the reticulum so that they can be regulated by high concentrations of Ca^{2+} would predict a fairly constant pattern of intracellular distribution of the enzymes in different muscles.

(c) *Substrate cycling at the level of phosphofructokinase and fructose diphosphatase*

The enzyme, fructose-1,6-diphosphatase (FDPase) catalyses the following reaction,

$$\text{Fructose-1,6-diphosphate} \rightarrow \text{Fructose-6-phosphate} + P_i$$

This enzyme has long been known to be present in liver where its function in the gluconeogenic pathway is to bypass the energy barrier of the PFK reaction (see Chapter 6). However, FDPase is also present in muscle, where there is no indication that quantitatively significant rates of gluconeogenesis can occur. Significant activities of FDPase are found in white skeletal muscle of vertebrates and in certain insect flight muscles. However, they are not detectable in heart muscle, smooth muscle, some vertebrate red muscles and some insect flight muscles.

The properties of FDPase which are relevant to its proposed role in regulation are as follows: it has a low K_m for its substrate, FDP (about 1 μM); it is inhibited by AMP; and, when the enzyme is detected in muscle, it has a maximal activity between 2 and 10 % of that of the maximal activity of PFK.[35]

These properties provide a basis for an extension of the theory of control of PFK by adenine nucleotides. It is proposed that, when the muscle is at rest and the rate of glycolysis is low, PFK is not maximally inhibited but retains a considerable residual activity which is 'opposed' by the activity of FDPase. Both enzymes are considered to be simultaneously active (in resting muscle) so that a *substrate cycle* between fructose-6-phosphate and fructose-1,6-diphosphate is catalysed, with the continual hydrolysis of ATP (Figure 3.12).

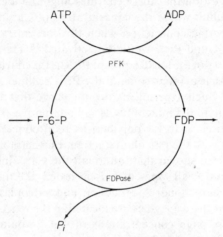

Figure 3.12. The PFK/FDPase substrate cycle. F-6-P represents fructose 6-phosphate; FDP represents fructose diphosphate

In this case the advantage of such a cycle is that it provides a threshold response of fructose-6-phosphate phosphorylation to changes in the AMP concentration, in addition to an increase in the sensitivity of the response of fructose-6-phosphate phosphorylation to changes in [AMP] (see Table 3.8 and Figure 3.13). Such a cycle is necessary in these muscles in order to improve the response between the rate of fructose-6-phosphate phosphorylation and changes in the concentration of AMP. Such an increase in efficiency of regulation is necessary in some muscles for at least two reasons. First, the adenine nucleotide control theory proposes that small changes in the concentration of ATP cause larger percentage changes in the concentration of AMP, through the adenylate kinase reaction. Although amplification is produced, it is pre-set and cannot be increased (see Section D.2(b)). This amplification mechanism is different from the type that occurs in electronic circuitry, in which the degree of amplification can be increased with the 'gain control'. The amplification provided by adenylate kinase is analogous to a 'lever system', in which a small change near the fulcrum is magnified progressively as the distance from the fulcrum is increased. Second, vertebrate white

Table 3.8. Theoretical effects of changes in the AMP concentration on the activities of PFK and FDPase, and on the net rate of fructose-6-phosphate phosphorylation (assuming that PFK and FDPase catalyse a substrate cycle)

Concentration of AMP (arbitrary units)	Fractional saturation of enzyme with AMP	PFK activity (max = 100)	FDPase activity (max = 10)	Net F-6-P phosphoryla-tion (i.e. PFK-FDPase)
0·0	0·000	0·0	10·0	0·0
1·0	0·010	1·0	9·9	0·0
2·0	0·050	5·0	9·5	0·0
2·5	0·093	9·3	9·1	0·2
3·0	0·150	15·0	8·5	6·5
4·0	0·310	31·0	6·9	24·1
5·0	0·470	47·0	5·3	41·7
6·0	0·600	60·0	4·0	56·0
8·0	0·770	77·0	2·3	74·7
12·0	0·890	89·0	1·1	87·9
18·0	0·940	94·0	0·6	93·4
20·0	0·950	95·0	0·5	94·5

PFK activity is increased and that of FDPase is decreased by AMP. It is assumed that the maximum activity of PFK is 100 units whereas that of FDPase is 10 units. Also, at an AMP concentration approaching zero, PFK is completely inhibited and FDPase is maximally active. The fractional saturation of the enzyme with AMP is calculated from the model of Monod, Wyman and Changeux (see Table 2.1).

In the absence of a substrate cycle, the activity of PFK is reduced to a level approaching zero only when the AMP concentration approaches zero. However, in the presence of a substrate cycle the rate of fructose-6-phosphate phosphorylation can be reduced to zero at a concentration of AMP that is slightly lower than 2·5 arbitrary units. Under these conditions the rate of fructose-6-phosphate phosphorylation can be increased from 0·2% to almost 90% of the maximum (about 440-fold increase) by only a five-fold increase in AMP (2·5 to 12·0 units).[35]

skeletal muscles and insect flight muscles may remain inactive for long periods while the animal is at rest, but occasionally the muscles will be maximally active. The rate of energy utilization will vary widely between these two extremes. Consequently the rate of fructose-6-phosphate phosphorylation cannot be regulated adequately by changes in AMP concentration without the amplification provided by a substrate cycle.

At present there is no direct evidence to support the theory of cycling at the PFK-FDPase level. However, this is the only plausible theory which explains the presence of FDPase in muscle. Furthermore, it explains the surprising fact that this enzyme is found in extremely anaerobic muscles (such as the pectoral muscles of game-birds) and in extremely aerobic muscles (such as insect flight muscles). It also accounts for the absence of FDPase in smooth and tonic muscles which are always mechanically active (for example heart) and in which variations in energy demand are never very large.

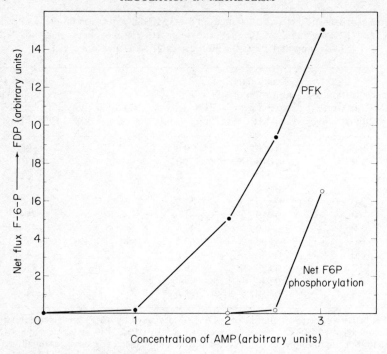

Figure 3.13. Effect of AMP on the activity of phosphofructokinase and on the net rate of fructose-6-phosphate phosphorylation assuming the existence of a substrate cycle between fructose-6-phosphate and fructose diphosphate

Finally, this cycling hypothesis may explain why changes in AMP content have not been observed in skeletal muscle upon electrical stimulation.[19,32] The cycle provides a regulatory enzyme system which is extremely sensitive to changes in the concentration of AMP. The present techniques for assaying AMP are so imprecise that experimental variations (as well as biological variations) could be greater than the actual changes in AMP concentration that influence this regulatory system (see Table 3.8).

5. The regulation of glycolysis by the oxidation of pyruvate, ketone bodies or fatty acids

The rate of glucose uptake and glycolysis in the perfused isolated rat heart and in the isolated rat diaphragm are markedly decreased by the presence of pyruvate, ketone bodies or fatty acids in the perfusion (or incubation) medium (Table 3.9).[6,14,36] There is now extremely strong evidence to indicate that the inhibition of glycolysis is dependent upon the oxidation of these compounds by the muscle. The decreased rate of glycolysis is associated with an increase in the levels of glucose-6-phosphate and fructose-6-phosphate, and in the perfused heart (when insulin is present) the intracellular

Table 3.9. The effects of fatty acids, ketone bodies, alloxan diabetes, starvation and fluoroacetate on glycolytic flux and the contents of citrate and other intermediates in the isolated perfused rat heart

Conditions of animals	Additions to perfusion medium	Glycolytic flux (μmol/g/hr)	Content in perfused heart (nmol/g fresh wt.)					Ratio Acetyl-CoA/ CoA
			Glucose-6-phosphate	Fructose-6-phosphate	Citrate	Acetyl-CoA	CoA	
Normal	None	74	290	63	220	1·0	67	0·01
	Palmitate (0·75 mM)	46	390	70	700	5·0	29	0·19
	Butyrate (4 mM)	32	470	91	490	21·0	28	0·74
	β-Hydroxybutyrate (5·5 mM)	20	560	87	620	20·0	30	0·67
Alloxan-diabetic	None	50	380	83	530	9·0	68	0·13
Alloxan-diabetic treated with insulin	None	74	240	70	130	—	—	—
Starved for 40 hours	None	61	380	83	340	—	—	—
Normal	Fluoroacetate (0·22 mM)	33	800	200	2,000	—	—	—

Hearts were perfused for 15 or 30 minutes in the presence of glucose and insulin. The condition of the animals from which the hearts were removed is indicated in the table. All additions indicated in the table were made to the perfusion medium. Alloxan-diabetic animals were injected with the insulin 24 hours before the experiments. [6,14,36,37,40]

content of glucose is also increased (Table 3.9). These experimental findings indicate that HK and PFK are regulated by the oxidation of fatty acids or ketone bodies. There is also evidence that the membrane transport of glucose can be inhibited by the oxidation of these compounds. However, inhibition of glucose transport can be completely overcome by the presence of a high concentration of insulin[6] whereas the inhibition of HK and PFK cannot.[14] Nothing is known about the molecular mechanism of transport or its regulation. Therefore this process cannot enter into the following discussion, despite the fact that the regulation of glucose transport is physiologically important.

In the experiments with the perfused rat heart and isolated diaphragm preparations, the simultaneous provision of glucose and an alternative fuel (such as fatty acids) did not lead to any changes in the contents of the adenine nucleotides. Therefore, a re-investigation of the properties of PFK was necessary in order to try to explain the inhibition of the enzyme under these conditions. Accordingly, it was found that physiological concentrations of citrate caused specific inhibition of PFK *in vitro* provided that the enzyme was already inhibited by ATP—that is, citrate potentiates the inhibition by ATP (Figure 3.14). This is a very specific effect of citrate which is not observed with comparable concentrations of other TCA cycle intermediates, or the citrate analogue, tricarballylic acid.

$$CH_2COOH \qquad\qquad CH_2COOH$$
$$|\qquad\qquad\qquad\qquad\qquad |$$
$$CHCOOH \qquad\qquad HOC \cdot COOH$$
$$|\qquad\qquad\qquad\qquad\qquad |$$
$$CH_2COOH \qquad\qquad CH_2COOH$$

Tricarballylic acid   Citric acid

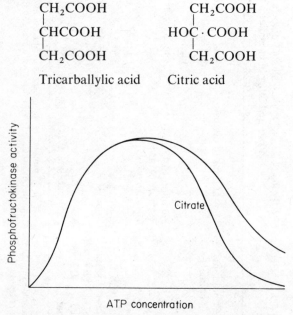

Figure 3.14. Effect of ATP on the activity of phosphofructokinase in the presence and absence of citrate

On the basis of this finding, a theory was proposed that the oxidation of pyruvate, ketone bodies or fatty acids elevates the concentration of citrate in the muscle and that this causes inhibition of PFK. The resultant increase in the concentration of glucose-6-phosphate inhibits HK (Figure 3.15).

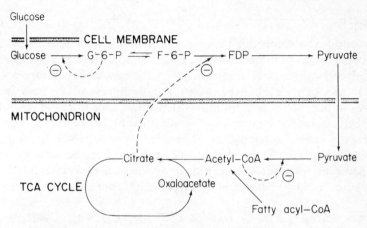

Figure 3.15. Control of glycolysis and pyruvate oxidation in muscle by citrate and acetyl-CoA

This theory was tested by measuring the content of citrate in the muscle:[37] in the perfused heart, it was elevated about four-fold by the oxidation of these compounds (Table 3.9). However, the results of such experiments are only consistent with the theory and do not prove it. One specific problem is that citrate is produced within the mitochondrion and must traverse the mitochondrial membrane in order to inhibit PFK. The translocation of ionic compounds (including citrate) across the mitochondrial membrane has been clearly demonstrated in liver mitochondria[3,38] and a specific transportation system for citrate has also been identified in heart muscle mitochondria.[39]

There is a substantial amount of indirect evidence which supports the theory of the control of PFK by citrate.

(a) The effects of fatty acids on glycolysis are not observed if the process of electron transport is inhibited by respiratory poisons (such as cyanide). Under these conditions the rates of glucose uptake and glycolysis and the contents of hexose phosphates are unaffected by the presence of fatty acids, etc.[6,14] This suggests that the mere presence of fatty acids *per se* does not cause inhibition of PFK.

(b) Perfusion of the isolated rat heart with fluoroacetate causes inhibition of glucose uptake, decreased glycolysis and an accumulation of hexose monophosphates.[40] These effects may all be explained by the increase in content of citrate that occurs in the perfused heart upon the administration of fluoroacetate. Upon entering the cells, fluoroacetate is activated to fluoroacetyl-CoA and then converted to fluorocitrate by the enzyme, citrate synthase.

$$\text{F-acetate} \xrightarrow[\text{thiokinase}]{\text{CoA} \cdot \text{ATP} \quad \text{AMP}} \text{F-acetyl-CoA} \xrightarrow[\text{citrate synthase}]{\text{oxaloacetate}} \text{F-citrate}$$

Fluorocitrate is a competitive inhibitor of aconitase and therefore it causes an accumulation of citrate. Thus, the effects of fluoroacetate administration upon glycolysis and PFK are predicted by the citrate control theory.

(c) In a series of elegant experiments, Randle and coworkers have studied changes in metabolite concentrations that occur after the system has been perturbed but before the new steady-state situation has been attained: such changes are known as 'transients'. The contents of acetyl-CoA, citrate and glucose-6-phosphate in the perfused heart were measured after switching from perfusion with glucose to perfusion with glucose plus either β-hydroxybutyrate or acetate. Although the acetyl-CoA content reached the new

Table 3.10. Changes in the contents of ATP, acetyl-CoA, citrate and glucose-6-phosphate and in the rate of glucose phosphorylation in the perfused heart after switching from glucose to glucose plus acetate in the perfusion medium

Time after switching to acetate + glucose perfusion (minutes)	Contents of intermediates in perfused heart (nmol/g fresh wt.)				Rate of glucose phosphorylation (nmol/min/g fresh wt.)
	ATP	Acetyl-CoA	Citrate	Glucose-6-phosphate	
0·0	5,250	5	12	325	1,625
0·5	—	67	25	—	—
1·0	5,000	65	30	380	—
2·0	4,500	45	42	387	1,325
4·0	5,000	47	55	432	—
6·0	5,250	—	77	412	1,075
8·0	—	40	70	420	950

Hearts were perfused for 5 minutes with a medium containing glucose alone and then switched to a perfusion medium containing glucose plus acetate (5 mM). For assay of metabolic intermediates the hearts were freeze-clamped at various times after switching to glucose plus acetate perfusion. Glucose phosphorylation was measured as glucose disappearance from the medium minus any accumulation of intracellular glucose. The content of ATP decreases slightly after 2 minutes of perfusion and then remains constant. The content of acetyl-CoA increases to a maximum within 30 seconds of switching to acetate, whereas the changes in contents of citrate and glucose-6-phosphate and the decrease in glucose phosphorylation attain maximal or minimal levels in about 8 minutes.[41,42]

steady-state level in about 1 minute, citrate required approximately 10 minutes[41] (Table 3.10). There was a similar delay in the maximum accumulation of glucose-6-phosphate and in the reduction of the rate of glucose phosphorylation.[42] Thus, there is the same temporal response between the concentration changes of citrate and glucose-6-phosphate and the rate of phosphorylation of glucose.

(d) A perfused heart from an alloxan-diabetic rat* has a severely depressed rate of glucose uptake and glycolysis even in the presence of high perfusate concentrations of glucose and insulin. This can be attributed to inhibition of PFK by citrate. The citrate content is increased by the oxidation of fatty acid derived from endogenous triglyceride. The compound α-bromostearate is known to inhibit fatty acid oxidation, and addition of this compound to the perfusion medium of hearts from diabetic rats causes glucose uptake and glycolysis to increase to the rates observed in perfused hearts from normal rats.[43] Furthermore, the contents of intracellular glucose, hexose monophosphates, fructose-1,6-diphosphate and citrate are all returned to the normal range (Table 3.11). Since the contents of the adenine nucleotides

Table 3.11. Effect of bromostearate on the glycolytic rate and contents of metabolic intermediates in the isolated perfused rat heart from alloxan-diabetic animals

Measured parameter	Hearts from alloxan-diabetic rats		Hearts from normal control animals
	No addition	1·0 mM-bromostearate	
Rates in μmol/g fresh weight of ventricle/hour			
glucose uptake	35	81	79
glycolysis	35	81	79
glucose oxidation	13	48	56
Contents of metabolic intermediates			
intracellular glucose (mM)	1·61	1·11	0·87
glucose-6-phosphate (nmol/g fresh wt of ventricle)	762	420	415
fructose-6-phosphate	232	152	—
citrate	712	180	245
ATP	4,525	4,800	4,775
ADP	850	825	—
AMP	225	200	—

Animals were made alloxan-diabetic as described in the text. Hearts were pre-perfused for 10 minutes with medium containing either 2% albumin (controls) or 2% albumin plus 1 mM 2-bromostearate (together with glucose and insulin) and they were perfused for a further 10 or 20 minutes with medium containing glucose and insulin alone.[43]

* The β-cells of the pancreas are damaged by alloxan injection and within 48 hours the animal becomes severely diabetic.

remain unchanged, the effects of α-bromostearate are not those of a general respiratory inhibitor. However, they are precisely those effects which are predicted by the theory of the regulation of glycolysis by citrate.

Physiological importance of the control of glycolysis in muscle by fatty acids

Experiments performed *in vitro* on the isolated perfused heart and diaphragm preparations have demonstrated that fatty acid oxidation can cause inhibition of glycolysis. A detailed biochemical mechanism of the control of this process has been established (see above). Is this effect of fatty acids likely to be of any physiological importance to the animal?

The importance of plasma fatty acids as a fuel of respiration in various physiological conditions, the evidence for their concentration-dependent oxidation and the mechanism of release of fatty acids by adipose tissue is discussed in detail in Chapter 5. On the basis of *in vitro* effects of fatty acids on the perfused heart and diaphragm preparations, there is no doubt that the oxidation of the available plasma fatty acids during conditions such as starvation could cause a substantial inhibition of glycolysis in muscle. The physiological importance of this inhibition is explained by the observation that even during prolonged starvation the concentration of blood glucose is decreased by only 20–25 %. Therefore both glucose and fatty acids are present in the blood simultaneously during starvation. The blood glucose level must not fall unduly since tissues such as the brain, nervous system and red blood cells have almost a continual requirement for glucose for energy production. In the fed animal the fatty acid concentration is low and the main fuel for oxidation is glucose but with the onset of starvation the fatty acid concentration gradually increases so that both fuels become available. Under these conditions fatty acids are oxidized by muscle and their oxidation restricts glucose utilization by this tissue. Consequently glucose is conserved for the brain, etc. If these tissues did not require a constant supply of glucose, the concentration in the blood could fall to very low levels in starvation, and the inhibition of glycolysis by fatty acids would be unnecessary.

6. Properties and regulation of pyruvate kinase

The mass-action ratio data for pyruvate kinase indicate that this enzyme catalyses a reaction which is removed far from equilibrium. However, there have been very few detailed studies in which the content of the substrate, phosphoenolpyruvate, has been measured when the glycolytic flux is changed. In the blowfly the onset of flight, which increases glycolytic flux in the flight muscle about 100-fold, does not cause any marked change in the content of phosphoenolpyruvate.[15] A further problem is that the maximum activity of pyruvate kinase *in vitro* is very high in comparison to that of PFK (see Table 3.3), so that the enzyme must be severely inhibited, particularly when the muscle is at rest.

Investigations into the properties of pyruvate kinase *in vitro* have so far not provided any illuminating information about a possible control mechanism. The only interesting property of the mammalian muscle enzyme is that it is inhibited by ATP with a K_i of approximately 3·5 mM.[44] Such inhibition may be partially responsible for reduction of the enzyme activity *in situ*. The low level of phosphoenolpyruvate in the muscle (10–20 μM) in comparison to the K_m value for this substrate (100 μM) may also play a role in reduction of the activity *in situ*. However, changes in the concentrations of both ATP and phosphoenolpyruvate during mechanical activity are rather small and therefore they cannot be responsible for the marked increase in activity of this enzyme under these conditions. At the present time, details of the mechanism of control of pyruvate kinase are unknown and much more intensive work on this enzyme (and this particular area of metabolism) is necessary in order to provide information upon which a satisfactory control theory could be based. It must be emphasized that control of pyruvate kinase cannot regulate glucose uptake: inhibition of this enzyme could lead only to accumulation of the glycolytic intermediates between fructose diphosphate and phosphoenolpyruvate.

7. Properties and theory of regulation of the pyruvate dehydrogenase complex

Experiments with the isolated perfused rat heart and the isolated diaphragm preparation have shown that pyruvate oxidation is inhibited by the oxidation of fatty acids or ketone bodies.[45] The first enzyme involved in the utilization of pyruvate is the pyruvate dehydrogenase enzyme complex which converts pyruvate into acetyl-CoA with the involvement of thiamine pyrophosphate, lipoic acid and the enzyme lipoate dehydrogenase. The activity of pyruvate dehydrogenase is inhibited by acetyl-CoA (competitively with CoA).[46] This property provides the basis for a theory of control of pyruvate dehydrogenase by fatty acids and ketone bodies: oxidation of these compounds increases the concentration ratio of acetyl-CoA to CoA. Evidence for this theory has been obtained from experiments with the isolated rat heart perfused with fatty acids or ketone bodies in which a marked increase in the ratio [acetyl-CoA]/[CoA] is observed (Table 3.9). Furthermore, the ratio is increased in hearts from alloxan diabetic animals which also show inhibited pyruvate oxidation upon perfusion.[45]

Fatty acid oxidation raises the contents of acetyl-CoA and citrate and decreases the content of CoA. These changes regulate the enzymes PFK and pyruvate dehydrogenase: the regulation of PFK leads to changes in the concentration of glucose-6-phosphate which in turn regulates HK. Thus, with the exception of pyruvate kinase the enzymes that catalyse non-equilibrium reactions between glucose and its entry into the TCA cycle are regulated by fatty acid oxidation. This obviously represents a concerted mechanism of control not only of the glycolytic flux but also of the steady-state concentrations of the glycolytic intermediates. The maintenance of the concentrations of these intermediates is important because they are often precursors for other reactions (for example, glycerol-1-phosphate for the glycerol phosphate cycle or for triglyceride synthesis). Also some glycolytic intermediates are reactants in a number of equilibria that involve important cofactors (for example, ADP and ATP at the phosphoglycerate kinase reaction; NAD^+ and NADH at the lactate dehydrogenase reaction).

Recent work has shown that pyruvate dehydrogenase may exist in two enzymatically interconvertible forms, one of which is catalytically active and the other inactive.[47] The interconverting enzymes appear to be a phosphokinase and a phosphatase, although they have not been purified. Phosphorylation of pyruvate dehydrogenase leads to inactivation, whereas dephosphorylation produces the active form. The interconversions are somewhat similar to those of UDPG-glucosyltransferase, which are discussed in detail in Chapter 4. Although the control mechanisms of these interconverting enzymes are not yet known, one possibility is that phosphorylation of pyruvate dehydrogenase is stimulated by a high-energy state of the mitochondria, so that when the [ATP]/[ADP] ratio reaches a certain level, the rate of acetyl-CoA formation from pyruvate is severely inhibited. Enzymatic interconversions provide increased sensitivity in a control system over that provided by equilibrium-binding of a regulator to an enzyme (see Chapter 2, Section F.2.a(ii)). A sensitive control mechanism might be required for pyruvate dehydrogenase because it depends upon feedback information of the [ATP]/[ADP] ratio within the mitochondria and variations in this ratio are severely restricted because of the need to maintain the efficiency of energy transfer.

Thus, there appear to be at least two quite distinct methods of regulation of pyruvate dehydrogenase; enzymatically interconvertible forms and the equilibrium binding of acetyl-CoA. At the present time it is not known if these two mechanisms are related. It is tempting to speculate that the phosphorylated form (inactive) is very sensitive to the [acetyl-CoA]/[CoA] ratio, so that it is active only if CoA is high and acetyl-CoA is low: the non-phosphorylated form would be much less sensitive to this ratio. This combined mechanism would provide a simple cellular control of enzyme activity based on changes in the concentrations of acetyl-CoA and CoA, and a more sophisticated and sensitive control dependent upon changes in the energy status of the mitochondrion. Such a mechanism would provide another example of flexibility in biological control.

E. CONTROL OF THE TRICARBOXYLIC ACID CYCLE

1. Identification of regulatory enzymes

One of the major problems in the formulation of control theories for the TCA cycle is the identification of regulatory enzymes. It is even difficult to ascertain which reactions are non-equilibrium. It is possible to calculate mass-action ratios for many of the reactions but the interpretation of such data is difficult. Most of the intermediates of the cycle are present both inside and outside the mitochondria and the mass-action ratio data includes both compartments. However, the reactions of the TCA cycle occur within the mitochondria so that only the mitochondrial concentrations should be considered. Since the proportional distribution of metabolites (for example, citrate, acetyl-CoA, CoA, oxaloacetate) between the mitochondria and cytoplasm is not known, meaningful mass-action ratios cannot be calculated. Since the initial reactions of the TCA cycle are involved in the control of the citrate concentration, and since little is known about the control of the later stages, this discussion will centre upon the regulation of the activities of citrate synthase and isocitrate dehydrogenase. (It is generally assumed that aconitase catalyses a reaction which is close to equilibrium, despite the problems associated with the interpretation of mass-action ratio data.) There are two enzymes which catalyse the oxidative decarboxylation of isocitrate, NAD^+-linked isocitrate dehydrogenase (NAD^+-ICDH) and $NADP^+$-linked isocitrate dehydrogenase ($NADP^+$-ICDH), and their presence also complicates the interpretation of experimental data.

Somewhat surprisingly, little work has been done on the measurement of maximal activities of the TCA cycle enzymes. A comparative study of the activities of citrate synthase, NAD^+-ICDH and $NADP^+$-ICDH in muscle has recently been carried out and some of the results are included in Table 3.12.[50] In most cases the activity of citrate synthase is about five times greater than that of NAD^+-ICDH. In insect flight muscle the activity of the NAD^+-ICDH is usually much greater than that of the $NADP^+$-linked enzyme so that even the combined activities of ICDH are much less than that of citrate synthase. Moreover an estimate of the maximum capacity of the TCA cycle in some insect flight muscles can be obtained from the oxygen uptake measured during flight and it is clear from these data that the activity of NAD^+-ICDH is only slightly greater than that predicted from the maximum oxygen uptake (see Table 3.12). This suggests that, at least in insect flight muscles, isocitrate dehydrogenase catalyses a non-equilibrium reaction whereas citrate synthase catalyses an equilibrium reaction. In vertebrates, the situation is complicated by the fact that in any given muscle the activity of $NADP^+$-ICDH is usually much higher than that of the NAD^+-linked enzyme and the combined activities of the two enzymes may be similar to that of citrate synthase. Furthermore, previous work had indicated that only the NAD^+-linked isocitrate dehydrogenase was involved in the TCA cycle whereas the recent comparative study suggests that both ICDH enzymes are involved. Thus the NAD^+-ICDH activity alone is not sufficient to account for the flux through the TCA cycle as estimated from the oxygen-consumption data in the flying pigeon and the swimming trout (see Table 3.12). If the $NADP^+$-ICDH is involved in the

Table 3.12. The activities of citrate synthase, NAD+-ICDH and NADP+-ICDH and the maximal TCA cycle activities (calculated from oxygen uptake data) in insect and vertebrate muscles

Animal	Muscle	Maximum TCA cycle activity calculated from oxygen uptake (μmol/min/g muscle at 25 °C)	Experimentally determined enzyme activities (μmol/min/g muscle at 25 °C)		
			Citrate synthase	NAD+-linked isocitrate dehydrogenase	NADP+-linked isocitrate dehydrogenase
Insecta					
Locust (*Schistocerca gregaria*)	Flight	28	242	54	4·0
Cockroach (*Periplaneta americana*)	Flight	30	185	74	2·5
Honey bee (*Apis mellifera*)	Flight	64	345	94	4·0
Peacock butterfly (*Vanessa io*)	Flight	40	379	120	8·5
Silver-Y moth (*Plusia gamma*)	Flight	25	351	117	10·9
Pisces					
Trout (*Salmo gairdneri*)	Red muscle	2·0	50	0·3	125
Dogfish (*Scylliorhinus canicula*)	Red muscle	—	35	0·4	31
	Heart	—	46	0·3	53
Aves					
Pigeon	Pectoral	4·8	114	3·6	63
	Heart	—	137	11·7	62
Mammalia					
Rat	Heart	2·7	96	5·0	71

The enzyme activity data are taken from reference 50. The oxygen uptake data for the locust, cockroach, honey bee, peacock butterfly and silver-Y moth are the maximal rates of oxygen consumption during flight and are collated from references 58, 59, 60 and 61 respectively. The oxygen uptake has been measured in the swimming trout (and it is assumed that only the red muscle is involved in normal continual swimming).[62] The oxygen uptake has also been measured for the flying pigeon (for this calculation is is assumed that the pectoral muscles use most of the oxygen)[63] and in the isolated, perfused, working heart preparation.[64]

operation of the TCA cycle in these muscles, the total activity (NAD^+-ICDH + $NADP^+$-ICDH), which is greater than the predicted TCA cycle flux, would imply that the reaction is close to equilibrium. If this is so, there remains the question of why the vertebrate muscle requires both enzymes, or indeed why the vertebrate and insect muscles should be so different.

An alternative approach to the identification of non-equilibrium reactions in the TCA cycle has been adopted by Randle and colleagues.[52] These workers administered pulses of ^{14}C-acetate to isolated perfused rat hearts and at various times after the pulse-addition the hearts were freeze-clamped. Acetyl-CoA, citrate and other TCA-cycle intermediates were isolated and their specific radioactivities measured. It was found that even 60 minutes after the administration of the pulses of ^{14}C-acetate, the specific activity of the citrate remained below that of the acetyl-CoA. Since the two pools had obviously not equilibrated, it was concluded that citrate synthase in the rat heart catalyses a reaction which is far from equilibrium. Perfusions were also performed with ^{14}C-HCO_3^- and the incorporation of the label into isocitrate was followed. The results confirmed those of the ^{14}C-acetate experiment and also indicated that the reverse reaction of isocitrate dehydrogenase (reductive carboxylation of α-ketoglutarate) occurred at 46 % of the rate of the forward reaction (oxidative decarboxylation of isocitrate). In other words, the isocitrate dehydrogenase reaction is close to equilibrium in rat heart. This conclusion rests upon the assumption, implicit in the computer calculations of Randle et al., that there is one single pool of citrate and isocitrate in the cell (that is, they assumed that mitochondrial citrate and isocitrate readily exchange with cytoplasmic citrate and isocitrate, or that the cytoplasmic pools are negligible). If this conclusion is valid, the question is, do both of the isocitrate dehydrogenases catalyse reversible reactions? Certainly the $NADP^+$-ICDH readily catalyses a reversible reaction in vitro. However, all attempts to demonstrate reversibility of the NAD^+-linked enzyme have failed.[51] This failure may be due to an inadequacy of the in vitro system. For example, if the K_m of the NAD^+-ICDH for CO_2 is much higher than that of the $NADP^+$-linked enzyme, the concentration of dissolved CO_2 in the reaction mixture may be well below the K_m: the reverse reaction would be limited simply by substrate availability.

In summary, the evidence from the perfused rat heart suggests that citrate synthase catalyses a non-equilibrium reaction and that the isocitrate dehydrogenase reaction is close to equilibrium. In contrast, enzyme activity data from insect flight muscle suggests that, in this tissue, citrate synthase catalyses a reaction close to equilibrium, whereas the isocitrate dehydrogenase reaction is non-equilibrium.

There have been few studies in which changes in the contents of TCA cycle intermediates have been followed when the flux rate through the cycle is changed. Only the perfused rat heart has been used in this type of study and in this case the results did not indicate any regulatory enzymes (according to the second definition given in Chapter 1).[51,53] In other words it is not possible to conclude from these experiments that the TCA cycle is controlled by anything other than the concentration of acetyl-CoA.

2. Properties of citrate synthase and isocitrate dehydrogenase and theory of control

Any regulatory properties of citrate synthase and NAD^+-ICDH will only be of physiological relevance if these enzymes catalyse non-equilibrium reactions. The difficulties in the identification of 'non-equilibrium' enzymes and the possible species variations have been outlined above.

Citrate synthase is inhibited by ATP *in vitro* and this property might suggest that the TCA cycle is controlled by the energy status of the mitochondrion. However, in muscle tissue the variation in ATP content is very small and this casts doubt upon the physiological importance of the ATP inhibition. Citrate synthase is located within the mitochondrion and, if the total mitochondrial content of adenine nucleotides is low in comparison with the cytoplasm, large changes in the mitochondrial concentrations of ATP and ADP may occur without producing any marked changes in their total cellular content. This difficulty may only be resolved when the mitochondrial and cytoplasmic contents of metabolites can be measured independently.

The work of Randle and colleagues[51] has indicated that the activity of heart muscle citrate synthase may be regulated by the concentration of its pathway substrate, acetyl-CoA. The available data on the content of this substrate imply that it is present at well below saturating concentrations for citrate synthase. Furthermore, when the flux through the TCA cycle is increased by acetate perfusion (a 67% increase in flux rate), the contents of acetyl-CoA, citrate, isocitrate and α-ketoglutarate are all increased considerably. Therefore the activation of the acetate by acetate thiokinase could be responsible for the increased content of acetyl-CoA and hence for the stimulation of citrate synthase by increased substrate availability.* If it is assumed that ICDH catalyses a reversible reaction in the heart, the increase in concentration of its pathway substrate, isocitrate, automatically results in increased oxidation to α-ketoglutarate.

The properties of the NAD^+-linked ICDH provided the basis for earlier theories on the control of the TCA cycle. Thus, *in vitro* experiments show that ADP is a specific activator of this enzyme.[55] A simple theory of control would be that changes in the intra-mitochondrial ADP concentration modify the activity of NAD^+-ICDH (for example, increased activity of the

---

* A similar mechanism could be responsible for the increased contents of acetyl-CoA and, citrate when substrates such as fatty acids and ketone bodies are oxidized by the heart, and such increases are important because they cause inhibition of pyruvate dehydrogenase and PFK.

myofibrillar ATPase during muscle contraction might be expected to increase the concentration of ADP). This theory has similar problems to that of the ATP control of citrate synthase described above.

It has been shown comparatively recently that calcium ions inhibit NAD^+-ICDH but that the inhibition is removed when the concentration of Ca^{2+} is decreased below 10^{-7} M.[56] Mitochondria are capable of concentrating Ca^{2+} ions to sufficiently high levels to inhibit NAD^+-ICDH. It has been suggested that the mitochondria release Ca^{2+} ions during muscle contraction and in this respect supplement the role of the sarcoplasmic reticulum.[57] However, nothing is known of the control of the release of Ca^{2+} by the mitochondria, neither is it known whether the intramitochondrial concentration of Ca^{2+} falls sufficiently (i.e. $<10^{-7}$ M) to de-inhibit NAD^+-ICDH. Nonetheless, the facts that the enzyme activity can be modified by such low concentrations of Ca^{2+}, that the effects of Ca^{2+} and ADP on the enzyme are independent and that the $NADP^+$-linked ICDH is not affected by either Ca^{2+} or ADP suggest that these properties might be significant in the regulation of the TCA cycle.

Obviously it is not possible at present to propose a simple theory of regulation of the early stages of the TCA cycle that is consistent with the experimental data and that is physiologically satisfactory. A problem of investigating the TCA cycle is that it occurs at what may be described as the centre of metabolism. Therefore perturbation of the cycle is difficult to achieve and changes in the contents of intermediates are difficult to interpret. The authors consider that the most fruitful investigations into the control of the TCA cycle will be those upon insect flight muscle. Initiation of flight in the insect will increase the turnover rate of the TCA cycle enormously and changes in the contents of intermediates of the cycle and related pathways may provide an experimental basis for testing the various theories.

APPENDIX TO CHAPTER 3

APPENDIX 3.1   CALCULATION OF ATP TURNOVER
IN MUSCLE

(a) Insect flight muscle

In order to satisfy the large demand for energy required for insect flight, the rate of oxidative metabolism must be increased very markedly upon the transition from rest to flight. Since the ATP production in the flight muscles arises exclusively from aerobic metabolism, the increase in metabolic rate can be estimated from the change in oxygen consumption. The energy demands for other tissues are so small in comparison to the requirements of the flight muscle that they can be ignored. The maximum rate of oxygen uptake by the fly, *Lucilia sericata*, is 187 ml O_2/hr/g fly,[48] or approximately 3,000 μl O_2/min/g. If it is assumed that the weight of the flight muscles is about 20% of the body weight of the fly, this value becomes 670 μmol O_2/min/g muscle (assuming 1 μmol occupies 22·4 μl). Assuming a P/O ratio of 3 (that is, for every atom of oxygen utilized by the electron transport chain, 3 molecules of ADP will be phosphorylated to ATP), 670 μmol O_2 is equivalent to 4,020 μmol of ATP produced every minute per gram of muscle, or approximately 66 μmol/s/g muscle. Since the concentration of ATP in the muscle remains constant during flight, 66 μmol must be hydrolized and rephosphorylated every second and the total amount of ATP in the muscle (approximately 7 μmol/g) would support contraction for about 0·1 s (in the absence of any mechanism for the rephosphorylation of ADP).

(b) Perfused isolated rat heart

In the rat heart perfused aerobically, more than 90% of the energy is obtained from mitochondrial oxidative phosphorylation. In this tissue the uptake of oxygen is 10 μmol/min/g fresh weight, which is equivalent to 0·17 μmol/s/g or 1 μmol ATP used per second per gram of muscle (assuming a P/O ratio of 3). The total ATP in the muscle (5 μmol/g) would sustain contractions for no more than 5 seconds.

(c) White vertebrate muscle

In white vertebrate muscle (such as rabbit leg or pheasant pectoral muscle) the energy for contraction is supplied almost exclusively from anaerobic glycolysis, the main substrate being endogenous glycogen. The maximal capacity for glycolysis in these muscles is assumed to be equivalent to the maximal activity of phosphorylase.[1] In rabbit leg muscle the activity of this enzyme is about 100 μmol/min/g muscle (at 37 °C) and, since 3 ATP molecules are produced (from ADP) for every glucose residue which is degraded anaerobically, this represents a maximum ATP turnover of 300 μmol/min/g or 5 μmol/s/g muscle. Thus the total ATP in the muscle would support contraction for about 1 second.

APPENDIX 3.2   MASS-ACTION RATIO FOR THE ALDOLASE/TRIOSE PHOSPHATE ISOMERASE REACTION

The equilibrium constant for the aldolase reaction is obtained from the concentration ratio [GAP] × [DHAP]/[FDP], where the concentrations of the GAP and DHAP are equal. However, in the cell the action of triose phosphate isomerase disturbs this situation so that the concentrations of these two triose phosphates are not identical. Furthermore, the equilibrium position of this reaction is 22:1 in favour of DHAP, and the intracellular content of GAP is too small to measure accurately. Therefore the mass-action ratio for the aldolase reaction has been calculated assuming that triose phosphate isomerase catalyses an equilibrium (see reference 17). The mass-action ratio is obtained as follows

$$\Gamma = \frac{[\text{triose phosphate}]^2 \times 22}{[\text{fructose diphosphate}] \times 23^2}$$

This is derived, from the assumption that triose phosphate isomerase catalyses on equilibrium, as follows.

$$[\text{DHAP}] = [\text{triose phosphate}] \times 22/23$$

$$[\text{GAP}] = [\text{triose phosphate}] \times 1/23$$

$$[\text{Aldolase}] = \frac{[\text{DHAP}] \times [\text{GAP}]}{[\text{fructose diphosphate}]}$$

Therefore

$$\Gamma = \frac{[\text{triose phosphate}]^2 \times 22}{[\text{fructose diphosphate}] \times 23^2}$$

APPENDIX 3.3   MASS-ACTION RATIOS AND APPARENT EQUILIBRIUM CONSTANTS FOR THE GLYCERALDEHYDE-3-PHOSPHATE DEHYDROGENASE/PHOSPHOGLYCERATE KINASE REACTION

Experimentally the determination of the content of 1,3-diphospho-glycerate in tissues is difficult because it is present only in very low concentrations. Therefore it is convenient to combine the reactions producing and utilizing this compound (glyceraldehyde-3-phosphate dehydrogenase (GAPDH) and phosphoglycerate kinase (PGK)). The two apparent equilibrium constants are given by

$$K'_{GAPDH} = \frac{[\text{1,3-diphosphoglycerate}^{4-}] \times [\text{NADH}] \times [\text{H}^+]}{[\text{glyceraldehyde-3-phosphate}^{2-}] \times [\text{HPO}_4^{2-}] \times [\text{NAD}^+]}$$

$$K'_{PGK} = \frac{[\text{3-phosphoglycerate}^{2-}] \times [\text{ATP}^{4-}]}{[\text{1,3-diphosphoglycerate}^{4-}] \times [\text{ADP}^{3-}] \times [\text{H}^+]}$$

The combination of these two constants eliminates the 1,3-diphospho-glycerate:

$$K'_{GAPDH} \times K'_{PGK}$$

$$= \frac{[\text{3-phosphoglycerate}^{2-}] \times [\text{NADH}] \times [\text{ATP}^{4-}]}{[\text{glyceraldehyde-3-phosphate}^{2-}] \times [\text{NAD}^+] \times [\text{HPO}_4^{2-}] \times [\text{ADP}^{3-}]}$$

Although this overcomes the problem of measurement of 1,3-diphospho-glycerate the measurement of the combined mass-action ratio is still fraught with difficulties. The total P_i content is unlikely to represent the free concentration of P_i in the region of the enzymes, since much of the P_i may be bound in the cell. The determination of total NADH and NAD^+ contents is similarly misleading, since some of the pyridine nucleotides are both bound to protein and localized within the mitochondria. However, it is possible to estimate the cytoplasmic $[NADH]/[NAD^+]$ ratio indirectly by assuming that lactate dehydrogenase, which is located exclusively in the cytoplasm, catalyses a reaction close to equilibrium. If this is the case, the ratio, $[\text{pyruvate}] \times [\text{NADH}]/[\text{lactate}] \times [\text{NAD}^+]$ will approximate to the measured equilibrium constant K'_{LDH}, i.e. $1 \cdot 11 \times 10^{-11}$ (see reference 49).

$$K'_{LDH} = \frac{[\text{pyruvate}] \times [\text{NADH}] \times [\text{H}^+]}{[\text{lactate}] \times [\text{NAD}^+]} = 1 \cdot 11 \times 10^{-11}$$

However, at pH 7·0 the H^+ can be removed from consideration by dividing K'_{LDH} by 10^{-7}, that is

$$K'_{LDH} = \frac{[\text{pyruvate}] \times [\text{NADH}]}{[\text{lactate}] \times [\text{NAD}^+]} = 1 \cdot 11 \times 10^{-4} \text{M}$$

If the contents of lactate and pyruvate are measured, $[NAD^+]/[NADH]$ in the cytoplasm can be calculated from

$$\frac{[NAD^+]}{[NADH]} = \frac{[pyruvate]}{[lactate]} \times \frac{1}{K'_{LDH}}$$

Therefore the mass-action ratio for the combined GAPDH and PGK reaction is

$$\frac{23 \times [\text{3-phosphoglycerate}] \times [ATP] \times [\text{lactate}] \times 1 \cdot 11 \times 10^{-4}}{[\text{triose phosphate}] \times [P_i] \times [ADP] \times [\text{pyruvate}]} M^{-1}$$

A further problem is the large error involved in the measurement of the extremely small amounts of G3P and 3PGA in the tissue. Obviously the measured mass-action ratio may not reflect the situation within the cell. There are also discrepancies in the calculated values for the equilibrium constants for each of the two reactions so that the product $K'_{GAPD} \times K'_{PGK}$ may be anything from 180 to 1,500. Consequently, it is impossible to conclude whether or not the reactions catalysed by the GAPDH and PGK system are non-equilibrium and therefore a possible control point. Even if this question were answered, there would remain the problem of which of the two enzymes were non-equilibrium especially since the situation may vary from tissue to tissue.

APPENDIX 3.4   GLUCOSE TRANSPORT IN MUSCLE

There are at least two mechanisms by which glucose could enter a cell; by simple diffusion or by combination with a specific carrier localized within the membrane. Such a carrier may transport glucose along a concentration gradient by a process which is sometimes referred to as *facilitated diffusion*. If the carrier transported glucose against a concentration gradient, energy would be required and the process would be described as *active transport*. The available evidence indicates that glucose is transported across the membrane of many types of cells by a process of carrier-mediated diffusion which does not require energy, although active transport of glucose occurs from the lumen of the gut and during reabsorption into the kidney tubules. The evidence is summarized below (see also reference 13).

(a) At low extracellular concentrations of glucose, the rate of transport is directly proportional to the concentration, but at high concentrations it approaches a maximum asymptotically. This type of saturation kinetics is predicted by a carrier-mediated mechanism.

(b) The rate of entry of glucose is decreased by the presence of other transportable sugars (such as arabinose).

(c) There are large differences in the transportation rates of structurally similar sugars. In the extreme case, the D forms of hexoses and pentoses are transported, whereas the L forms are not. Such specificity is not exhibited by simple diffusion.

(d) The transport process has a high Q_{10}, i.e. the increase in the rate of entry with a 10 °C rise in temperature is much higher than would be expected for simple diffusion but is of the same order as the Q_{10} of enzymic catalysis.

(e) In certain experimental situations it is possible to demonstrate the movement of a sugar against a concentration gradient (although ATP hydrolysis is not involved). This phenomenon can be explained on the basis of a carrier-mediated transport process. If an isolated heart is perfused with a medium containing a high concentration of arabinose, the concentration of arabinose inside the cell slowly increases. (Arabinose is not metabolized by the heart.) If glucose is then added to the perfusion medium, it is taken up by the heart and the intracellular concentration of arabinose progressively decreases: presumably it is being transported out of the cells against a concentration gradient. This can be explained on the basis of competition between the sugars for the carrier in the cell membrane: glucose competes with arabinose on the outside of the cell membrane but, since glucose is metabolized within the cell, the intracellular glucose concentration is much lower than the extracellular concentration. Therefore competition is less on the inner side of the membrane and there is net movement of arabinose out of the cell against a concentration gradient. This is sometimes termed 'counter current' transport because it is dependent upon the movement of sugars in opposite directions.

APPENDIX 3.5   THE MEASUREMENT OF THE CONCENTRATION OF INTRACELLULAR GLUCOSE

A piece of tissue is incubated in a medium containing sorbitol and glucose. After a period of time (which is sufficient for extracellular equilibration of the sugars) the tissue is frozen and rapidly extracted with a deproteinization agent (such as $HClO_4$). The concentrations of glucose and sorbitol are measured in both the tissue extract and the incubation medium. These values and the details of the calculation of the intracellular glucose concentration are given below.

Experimental measurements

Sorbitol concentration in the incubation medium   0·05 g/ml
Sorbitol concentration in the tissue   0·015 g/g tissue
Glucose concentration in the incubation medium   0·05 g/ml
Glucose concentration in the tissue   0·02 g/g tissue.

Calculations

The tissue space is defined as the volume of the tissue in which the sugar is present at the same concentration as that in the medium, that is

$$\text{Tissue space (ml/100 g)} = \frac{\text{muscle content (g/100 g fresh weight)}}{\text{medium concentration (g/ml)}}$$

Therefore

$$\text{Sorbitol space} = \frac{0.015}{0.050} \times 100 \text{ (ml/100 g tissue)}$$

$$= 30 \text{ ml/100 g tissue}$$

$$\text{Glucose space} = \frac{0.02}{0.05} \times 100$$

$$= 40 \text{ ml/100 g tissue.}$$

$$\text{Intracellular glucose space} = \text{Total glucose space} -$$
$$\text{extracellular (i.e. sorbitol) space}$$

$$= 40 - 30$$

$$= 10 \text{ ml/100 g tissue}$$

This value is the volume of intracellular water in 100 g of tissue that contains glucose at the same concentration as in the medium. The advantage of this method of expressing the intracellular concentration is that the calculation is a simple ratio of medium/tissue concentrations, so that the actual measurements of the concentration (for example, optical density units or counts per minute) can be used directly in the calculation.

An estimate of the actual intracellular concentration (mg/ml) is obtained as follows.

Intracellular concentration

$$= \frac{\text{Intracellular glucose space (ml/100 g)} \times \text{medium glucose concentration (g/ml)}}{\text{Total tissue water} - \text{extracellular space (ml/100 g)}}$$

$$\left(\text{The total tissue water (ml/100 g)} = \frac{(\text{wet weight} - \text{dry weight}) \times 100}{\text{wet weight}} \right)$$

If the total tissue water is assumed to be 80 ml/100 g, the intracellular glucose in the above example is calculated as follows:

$$\text{Intracellular glucose concentration} = \frac{10 \times 0.05}{80 - 30}$$

$$= 0.01 \text{ g/ml of intracellular water}$$

$$= 55 \text{ mM}$$

Thus the concentration of glucose in the intracellular water is 55 mM (assuming complete distribution) whereas the extracellular concentration is approximately 280 mM. Thus the mass-action ratio would be 55/280 = approximately 0·2. Under these conditions transport is approaching equilibrium. The above values are fictitious.

REFERENCES FOR CHAPTER 3

1. Crabtree, B. & Newsholme, E. A. (1972). *Biochem. J.* **126,** 49.
2. Sacktor, B. (1961). *Ann. Rev. Ent.* **6,** 103.
3. Chappell, J. B. (1968). *Brit. Med. Bull.* **24,** 150.
4. Randle, P. J. & Smith, G. H. (1958). *Biochem. J.* **70,** 490.
5. Morgan, H. E., Randle, P. J. & Regen, D. M. (1959). *Biochem. J.* **73,** 573.
6. Randle, P. J., Newsholme, E. A. & Garland, P. B. (1964). *Biochem. J.* **93,** 652.
7. Knowlton, F. P. & Starling, E. H. (1912). *J. Physiol.* **45,** 146.
8. Banting, F. G. & Best, C. H. (1922). *J. Lab. Clin. Med.* **7,** 251.
9. Colowick, S. P., Cori, G. T. & Stein, M. W. (1947). *J. biol. Chem.* **168,** 583.
10. Stadie, W. C., Haugaard, N. & Hills, A. G. (1950). *J. biol. Chem.* **184,** 617.
11. Lundsgaard, E. (1939). *Uppsala Läkarefören. Förh.* **45,** 143.
12. Levine, R., Goldstein, M. S., Huddlestun, B. & Klein, S. P. (1950). *Amer. J. Physiol.* **163,** 70.
13. Randle, P. J. & Morgan, H. E. (1962). *Vitamins & Hormones,* **20,** 199.
14. Newsholme, E. A. & Randle, P. J. (1964). *Biochem. J.* **93,** 641.
15. Sacktor, B. & Wormser-Shavit, E. (1966). *J. biol. Chem.* **241,** 624.
16. Lowry, O. H., Passonneau, J. V., Hasselberger, F. X. & Schulz, D. W. (1964). *J. biol. Chem.* **239,** 18.
17. Rolleston, F. S. & Newsholme, E. A. (1967). *Biochem. J.* **104,** 524.
18. Karpatkin, S., Helmreich, E. & Cori, C. F. (1964). *J. biol. Chem.* **239,** 3139.
19. Helmreich, E., Danforth, W. H., Karpatkin, S. & Cori, C. F. (1965). In *Control of Energy Metabolism,* p. 299. Ed. B. Chance, R. W. Estabrook & J. R. Williamson. New York: Academic Press.
20. Passonneau, J. V. & Lowry, O. H. (1962). *Biochem. biophys. Res. Commun.* **7,** 10.
21. Mansour, T. E. (1963). *J. biol. Chem.* **238,** 2285.
22. Ahlfors, C. E. & Mansour, T. E. (1969). *J. biol. Chem.* **244,** 1247.
23. Hill, A. V. (1950). *Biochim. biophys. Acta,* **4,** 4.
24. Opie, L. H., Mansford, K. R. L. & Owen, P. (1971). *Biochem. J.* **124,** 475.
25. Sacktor, B. & Hurlbut, E. C. (1966). *J. biol. Chem.* **241,** 632.
26. Regen, D. M., Davis, W. W., Morgan, H. E. & Park, C. R. (1964). *J. biol. Chem.* **239,** 43.
27. Newsholme, E. A. (1970). In *Essays in Cell Metabolism,* p. 189. Ed. W. Bartley, H. L. Kornberg & J. R. Quayle. London: Wiley-Interscience.
28. Chance, B., Estabrook, R. W. & Ghosh, A. (1964). *Proc. Nat. Acad. Sci. U.S.* **51,** 1244.
29. Higgins, J. (1967). *Industrial & Engineering Chem.* **59,** no. 5, 18.
30. Frenkel, R. (1968). *Arch. Biochem. Biophys.* **125,** 151 & 157.
31. Hess, B. & Boiteux, A. (1968). In *Regulatory Functions of Biological Membranes,* p. 148. Ed. J. Järnefelt. Amsterdam: Elsevier.
32. Wilson, J. E., Sacktor, B. & Tiekert, C. G. (1967). *Arch. Biochem. Biophys.* **120,** 542.
33. Vaughan, H., Thornton, S. D. & Newsholme, E. A. (1973). *Biochem. J.* (In press).
34. Margreth, A., Cantani, C. & Schiaffino, S. (1967). *Biochem. J.* **102,** 35C.

35. Newsholme, E. A. & Crabtree, B. (1970). *FEBS Letters*, **7**, 195.
36. Randle, P. J., Garland, P. B., Hales, C. N., Newsholme, E. A., Denton, R. M. & Pogson, C. I. (1966). *Rec. Progr. Horm. Res.* **22**, 1.
37. Garland, P. B. & Randle, P. J. (1964). *Biochem. J.* **93**, 678.
38. Chappell, J. B. & Robinson, B. H. (1968). In *Metabolic Roles of Citrate*, p. 123. Ed. T. W. Goodwin. London & New York: Academic Press.
39. England, P. J. & Robinson, B. H. (1969). *Biochem. J.* **112**, 8P.
40. Bowman, R. H. (1964). *Biochem. J.* **93**, 13C.
41. Randle, P. J., Denton, R. M. & England, P. J. (1968). In *Metabolic Roles of Citrate*, p. 87. Ed. T. W. Goodwin. London & New York: Academic Press.
42. England, P. J. & Randle, P. J. (1967). *Biochem. J.* **105**, 907.
43. Randle, P. J. (1969). *Nature, Lond.* **221**, 777.
44. Tanaka, K., Harano, Y., Sue, F. & Morimura, H. (1967). *J. Biochem. (Tokyo)*, **62**, 71.
45. Garland, P. B., Newsholme, E. A. & Randle, P. J. (1964). *Biochem. J.* **93**, 665.
46. Garland, P. B. & Randle, P. J. (1964). *Biochem. J.* **91**, 6C.
47. Reed, L. J. (1969). *Current Topics in Cellular Regulation*, **1**, 233. London & New York: Academic Press.
48. Davis, R. A. & Fraenkel, G. (1940). *J. exp. Biol.* **17**, 402.
49. Williamson, D. H., Lund, P. & Krebs, H. A. (1967). *Biochem. J.* **103**, 514.
50. Alp, P. & Newsholme, E. A. (1973). *Biochem. J.* (In press).
51. Goebell, H. & Klingenberg, M. (1964). *Biochem. Z.* **340**, 441.
52. Randle, P. J., England, P. J. & Denton, R. M. (1970). *Biochem. J.* **117**, 677.
53. Bowman, R. H. (1966). *J. biol. Chem.* **241**, 3041.
54. Moriyama, T. & Srere, P. A. (1971). *J. biol. Chem.* **246**, 3217.
55. Chen, R. F. & Plaut, G. W. E. (1963). *Biochemistry*, **2**, 1023.
56. Vaughan, H. & Newsholme, E. A. (1969). *FEBS Letters*, **5**, 124.
57. Patriarca, P. & Carafoli, E. (1969). *Experientia*, **25**, 598.
58. Krogh, A. & Weis-Fogh, T. (1951). *J. exp. Biol.* **28**, 344.
59. Polacek, L. & Kubista, V. (1960). *Physiol. Bohemoslov.* **9**, 228.
60. Jongbloed, J. & Wiermsa, C. A. G. (1934). *Z. vergl. Physiol.* **21**, 519.
61. Zebe, E. C. (1954). *Z. vergl. Physiol.* **36**, 290.
62. Webb, P. W. (1971). *J. exp. Biol.* **55**, 521.
63. Tucker, V. A. (1968). *J. exp. Biol.* **48**, 67.
64. Neely, J. R., Liebermeister, H., Battersby, E. J. & Morgan, H. E. (1967). *Amer. J. Physiol.* **212**, 804.
65. Williamson, J. R. (1965). *J. biol. Chem.* **240**, 2308.
66. Hess, B. (1962). In *Funktionelle und morphologische organisation der zelle*, p. 163. Ed. P. Karlson. Berlin: Springer Verlag.
67. Minakami, S. & Yoshikawa, H. (1966). *J. Biochem. (Tokyo)*, **59**, 139.
68. Shonk, C. E., Koven, B. J., Majima, H. & Boxer, G. E. (1964). *Cancer Res.* **24**, 722.
69. Lowry, O. H. & Passonneau, J. V. (1964). *J. biol. Chem.* **239**, 33.
70. Chapman, R. G., Hennessey, M. A., Wattersdorph, A. M., Haennekens, F. M. & Gabrio, B. W. (1962). *J. clin. Invest.* **41**, 1249.
71. Banks, B. E. C. & Vernon, C. A. (1970). *J. theor. Biol.* **29**, 301.

CHAPTER 4

REGULATION OF GLYCOGEN METABOLISM

A. INTRODUCTION

1. Pathways of synthesis and degradation

Glycogen is a highly branched polysaccharide made up of D-glucose residues linked by α-1,4-glycosidic bonds to form long chains which are branched by the formation of 1,6-linkages: there are about 12 to 18 residues between branch points (Figure 4.1). Glycogen is similar to most polymers of this

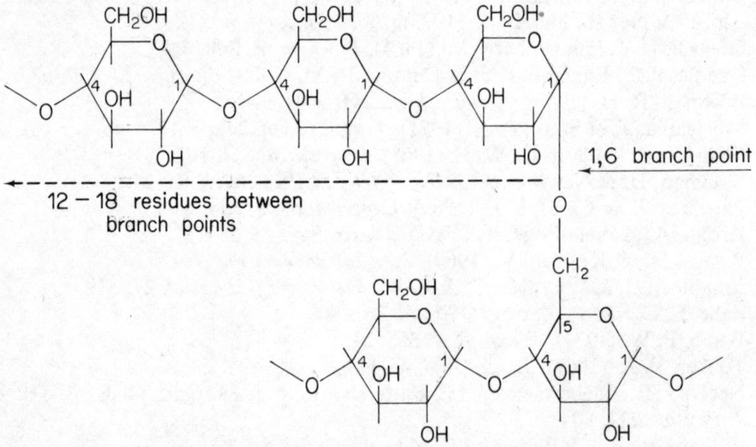

Figure 4.1. Diagram of the structure of glycogen

type in that it has no unique molecular structure in terms of the number of glucose residues and their relative position within the molecule. The molecular weights of these molecules range from about 10^6 to 10^8.

The synthesis of glycogen in the muscle cell begins with the phosphorylation of glucose to form glucose-6-phosphate. The phosphate group is transferred (by the action of phosphoglucomutase) to carbon-1 and the glucose-1-phosphate formed is reacted with UTP to form uridine diphosphate-glucose (UDPG). The glucose residue is then transferred from the nucleotide onto the end of an uncompleted chain in the glycogen molecule (sometimes known as the glycogen primer) to increase the length of this chain by one glucose residue: this reaction is catalysed by the enzyme **UDPG**-glucosyltransferase (or glycogen synthetase). The cleavage of the sugar-phosphate bond provides the driving force for the synthesis of the α-1,4-glycosidic bond. The pathway of glycogen synthesis from glucose is shown in Figure 4.2.

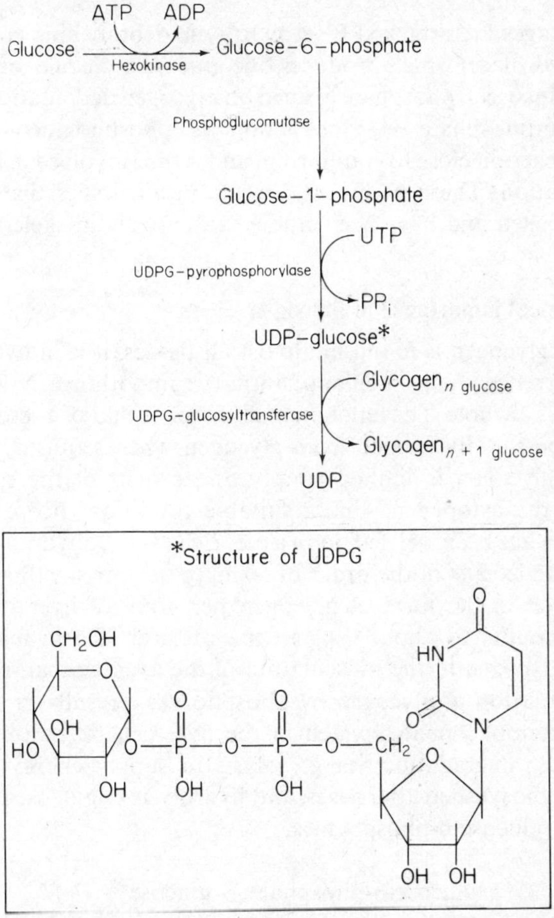

Figure 4.2. The pathway of glycogen synthesis

As the chain length of the polymer is increased to between 12 and 18 residues, the branching enzyme (α-1,4-glucan:α-1,4-glucan 6-glycosyl transferase) is activated (possibly by substrate availability, that is, chains of 12 to 18 residues linked by 1,4-glycosidic bonds) and a glycosyl residue is transferred from the 1,4 to the 1,6-linkage.

The degradation of glycogen proceeds by an entirely separate pathway. Glycogen phosphorylase (or simply 'phosphorylase') catalyses the phosphorolytic cleavage of the 1,4-glycosidic bonds to give glucose-1-phosphate.

$$\text{glycogen}_{(n\,\text{glucose})} + P_i \xrightarrow{\text{phosphorylase}} \text{glucose-1-phosphate} + \text{glycogen}_{(n-1\,\text{glucose})}$$

The 1,6-linkages are attacked by a hydrolytic debranching enzyme (dextrin 6-glucanohydrolase) which produces one glucose molecule for every branch point. The glucose-1-phosphate formed on glycogen degradation is converted to glucose-6-phosphate via the action of phosphoglucomutase, which catalyses a reaction close to equilibrium and is thus involved in both synthesis and degradation. These pathways operate in all tissues that are found to contain glycogen and have been studied extensively in skeletal muscle and in liver.

2. Physiological importance of glycogen

Although glycogen is found in almost all tissues, it is in liver and muscle that its occurrence is of particular quantitative importance in the metabolism of the body as a whole. The function of glycogen is that of a reserve of glucose which can be rapidly formed from glycogen when required. The capacity for storing glycogen is limited simply on account of the space which it occupies in the cytoplasm. Under suitable conditions (for example, in an animal which has been well fed upon a diet rich in carbohydrate) the glycogen content of the liver is of the order of 50 mg/g fresh tissue (that is, 250 μmol glucose stored in the form of glycogen per gram of liver: the total liver glycogen amounts to about 0·4 g in the rat and 70 g in man). The total amount of glycogen in the musculature of the average man is about 120 g.

The degradation of glycogen by phosphorylase results in the formation of hexose monophosphates which in the liver can be utilized for at least two purposes; degradation via glycolysis to supply energy and/or intermediates for biosynthetic purposes, and hydrolysis to glucose in the reaction catalysed by glucose-6-phosphatase,

$$\text{glucose-6-phosphate} \rightarrow \text{glucose} + P_i$$

Hydrolysis of glucose-6-phosphate is of particular importance since it means that the hepatic glycogen stores can be utilized for the maintenance of blood glucose levels in conditions where a serious fall in glucose level would have otherwise occurred (for example, excessive insulin secretion, starvation or carbohydrate deprivation). However, there is not sufficient glycogen stored in the liver to maintain the blood glucose level during a period of prolonged starvation (liver glycogen lasts for about 12–24 hours of starvation in man and rat) and glucose must be synthesized from non-carbohydrate sources (gluconeogenesis—see Chapter 6). Hepatic glycogen is probably partially utilized between meals and to a greater extent during the diurnal fast.[1] Physical exercise also increases the breakdown of glycogen in the liver.[2]

In muscle, glycogen functions solely as a fuel reserve for ATP generation during contraction. In accordance with this function, skeletal muscle lacks the enzyme glucose-6-phosphatase, and consequently is unable to convert glucose-6-phosphate to glucose. The activity of phosphorylase in muscle is generally very high, and necessarily so, since glycogen must be degraded rapidly in order to produce energy at a sufficient rate for muscle contraction. Skeletal muscle may be subdivided into at least two types, namely red (aerobic) and white (anaerobic) (Figure 4.3) which differ in both appearance and metabolism. Red muscle has a good blood supply and contains many mitochondria. It possesses a high capacity for aerobic oxidation of either glucose or fatty acids (i.e. enzymes of fat oxidation, TCA cycle and electron transport are present in high activity, see Table 4.1). The supply of these fuels via the blood should be sufficient to provide energy rapidly enough for moderate mechanical activity. If the energy requirement for contraction exceeds the rate of energy production from glucose and/or fatty acids, glycogen may be oxidized to provide additional energy for a comparatively long period. However, if the energy demands of contraction exceed the aerobic capacity of the muscle (that is, the supply of oxygen is limiting), glycogen can be degraded anaerobically to lactate and extra ATP obtained from glycolysis. In this situation the rate of glycogenolysis must be high since the anaerobic rate of ATP production is less than 10 % of the aerobic rate. However, the glycogen reserve is soon depleted and the extra ATP generation may only be maintained for a short time. White muscle contracts violently for short periods (for example, during escape of an animal from a predator) and its metabolism is well adapted to such a role: it has a poor blood supply, very few mitochondria and a low activity of the TCA cycle, but it has a high capacity for glycogen degradation via glycolysis (see Table 4.1). The glycogen stores are somewhat greater in white muscle than in red: domestic fowl pectoral muscle (white) and rat heart (red) contain respectively 20 and 12 μmol glucose residues as glycogen per gram of fresh muscle (approximately). In white muscle the phosphorylase activity is about 100 μmol/min/g compared with about 20 μmol/min/g in red muscle. Therefore glycogen degradation can occur extremely rapidly in white muscle whereas its poor blood supply and low-activity hexokinase (about 2 μmol/min/g) indicate that anaerobic glycolysis from glucose would not supply sufficient energy for contraction. The pectoral muscles of game birds and domestic fowls are good examples of white muscles: they are used solely for escape from predators or for flying to a high perch to roost in the evening (see Figure 4.4).

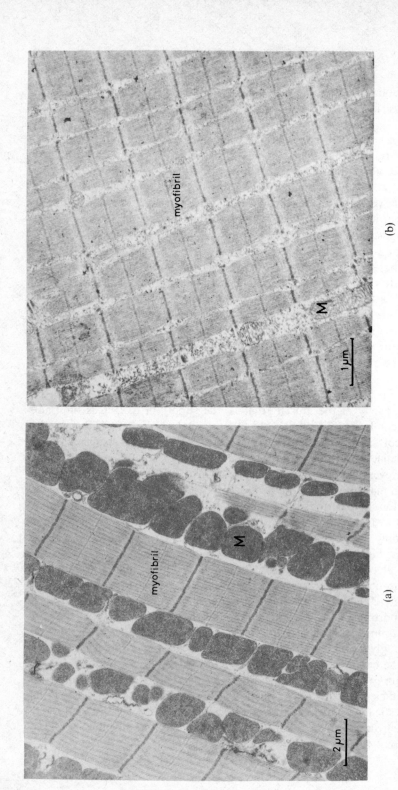

(a)

(b)

Figure 4.3. Electron micrographs of aerobic and anaerobic muscle. (a) Aerobic muscle (in this case insect flight muscle). L.S. dorso-longitudinal muscle (flight muscle) of the bumble-bee showing the high frequency of mitochondria (M). (b) Anaerobic muscle. L.S. pectoral muscle (white muscle) of the pheasant showing the low frequency of mitochondria (M). The electron micrographs were kindly supplied by Dr M. Cullen and Mrs B. Luke of the A.R.C. Unit, Zoology Dept, Oxford

Table 4.1. The activities of hexokinase, phosphorylase, phosphofructokinase, citrate synthase, triglyceride (or diglyceride) lipase and carnitine palmitoyltransferase in various muscles

Species	Muscle	Enzyme activities (μmol/min/g fresh weight at 25 °C)					
		Hexokinase	Phosphorylase	Phosphofructokinase	Citrate synthase	Triglyceride lipase	Carnitine palmitoyltransferase
Locust (*Schistocerca gregaria*)	Flight	8·0	8·0	13·0	230	0·6*	3·6
Bumble-bee (*Bombus hortorum*)	Flight	114·0	8·0	33·0	350	0·2*	0·7
Peacock butterfly (*Vanessa io*)	Flight	—	—	—	—	0·9*	1·7
Blowfly (*Phormia terranova*)	Flight	14·0	54·0	46·0	300	0·2*	0·2
Trout (*Salmo gairdneri*)	Red	2·6	14·0	12·2	30	0·02	0·2
Pigeon (*Columba livia*)	Pectoral (red)	3·0	18·0	24·0	100	0·07	3·2
Pheasant (*Phasianus colchicas*)	Pectoral (white)	2·3	120·0	143·0	15	0·01	0·03
Rabbit (*Oryctolagus cuniculus*)	Semitendinosus (red)	1·9	8·0	8·0	—	0·03	0·51
	Adductor longus (white)	0·3	30·0	26·0	—	0·01	0·06
Rat (Wistar strain)	Heart	6·1	12·0	10·0	95	0·06	2·2

Some of the information in this table is taken from references 58 and 60: the remainder is the unpublished work of B. Crabtree and of P. R. Alp of the Department of Zoology, Oxford.
* Diglyceride lipase.

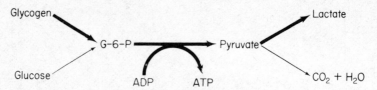

Figure 4.4. Emphasis upon glycogen conversion to lactate for energy production in anaerobic muscle

The inefficient production of ATP in anaerobic muscles is offset by their high glycolytic capacity. The limitation that is imposed by the rapid depletion of the glycogen stores is illustrated by the fact that mechanical activity can be maintained for only short periods (if phosphorylase in these muscles were fully activated all the glycogen would be used in about 10 seconds). It has been known for many centuries that game birds are very easily fatigued. In his *Anabasis*, Xenophon wrote in about 400 BC, 'The bustards on the other hand, can be caught if one is quick in starting them up, for they fly only a short distance, like partridges and soon tire; and their flesh was delicious.'[3]

3. Identification of the regulatory enzymes of glycogen metabolism

The pathways of glycogen degradation and synthesis consist of comparatively few reactions and therefore identification of regulatory enzymes is fairly straightforward. There is good evidence that phosphorylase catalyses a non-equilibrium reaction in the cell.

(*a*) The maximum activity of phosphorylase is low in comparison to that of some other enzymes of glycolysis: its activity is similar to that of the 'non-equilibrium' enzyme phosphofructokinase (Table 4.1).

(*b*) The mass-action ratio for the phosphorylase reaction should be given by [glucose-1-phosphate] $\times$ [glycogen$_{n-1}$]/[P_i] $\times$ [glycogen$_n$], where n refers to the number of glucose residues in the glycogen. Since glycogen consists of molecules of different sizes, it is impossible to determine the ratio [glycogen$_{n-1}$]/[glycogen$_n$]. It seems very likely that this ratio is approximately unity and in this case the mass-action ratio reduces to [glucose-1-phosphate]/[P_i]. This ratio is found to be about 0·003 in muscle, whereas at equilibrium the ratio [glucose-1-phosphate]/[P_i] is about 0·3. Therefore the mass-action ratio is much lower than the ratio at equilibrium, so that phosphorylase catalyses the unidirectional degradation of glycogen in the cell. The mass-action ratio for this reaction is low because the cell maintains the level of inorganic phosphate at about 10 mM and the level of hexose monophosphate at about 0·6 mM. Moreover, the equilibrium position of phosphoglucomutase, which catalyses the interconversion of the two glucose phosphates, is about 95% in favour of glucose-6-phosphate.

It is possible to demonstrate that phosphorylase is a regulatory enzyme according to the more restricted definition given in Chapter 1. When glycogenolysis is stimulated (for example, by adrenaline or muscle contraction), the catalytic activity of phosphorylase must have increased, whereas the content of its substrate, glycogen, is obviously decreased. Thus the activity of phosphorylase is controlled by factors other than the concentration of its pathway substrate.

The evidence that glucosyltransferase is non-equilibrium for glycogen synthesis is based on enzyme activity measurements: its activity is much less than the activities of UDPG—pyrophosphorylase and phosphoglucomutase and it is similar to or less than the activities of hexokinase and phosphofructokinase (Table 4.2). In liver tissue it has been demonstrated that, under some conditions when glycogen synthesis is increased, the hepatic content of UDPG is decreased. This positively identifies the enzyme as regulatory.[4]

The properties of phosphorylase and glucosyltransferase are relevant to any theory of control of glycogenolysis and glycogen synthesis. Since these properties are exceedingly complex and the theories of control exceptionally involved, their description is presented in several separate sections in this chapter. This must not imply that there is any segregation of control in the living cell: segregation is necessary in the present context merely to aid the understanding of highly complex and well-integrated control systems for both glycogenolysis and glycogen synthesis.

B. EARLY STUDIES OF THE PROPERTIES
OF PHOSPHORYLASE

Some knowledge of the early studies of phosphorylase is helpful in an appreciation of present theories of its control (for review see reference 5). The fascinating new control theory for phosphorylase (probably the most thoroughly understood metabolic control system in higher animals) is based upon a large amount of experimental data which began to accumulate with the early pioneering work on the enzyme by G. T. Cori and C. F. Cori. More recently the enzymology of the interconversions has been studied in great detail by Fischer, Krebs and coworkers (for early review, see reference 6) and the involvement of cyclic AMP in the control of phosphorylase has been elucidated by the brilliant work of Sutherland and his colleagues (for an early review see reference 7).

Studies on phosphorylase have been complicated by the fact that the enzyme exists in two distinct forms which have different properties. In the early 1940s it proved possible to isolate the enzyme in either an active form (phosphorylase *a*) or an inactive form (phosphorylase *b*). The inactive phosphorylase could be activated by AMP.[8] Following the crystallization

Table 4.2. The maximal activities of hexokinase, phosphofructokinase, UDPG-glucosyltransferase, UDPG-pyrophosphorylase, and phosphoglucomutase in tissues of the rat

Tissue	Enzyme activities (μmol/min/g fresh weight at 25 °C)				
	Hexokinase	Phosphofructokinase	UDPG-glucosyltransferase	UDPG-pyrophosphorylase	Phosphoglucomutase
Skeletal muscle	2·0	47·0	3·7	10·7	111·0
Heart	6·1	10·0	2·8	3·8	10·0
Liver	2·5*	2·5	3·1	59·0	37·0
Brain	14·0	18·0	0·5	1·5	3·6
Kidney	2·8	2·8	0·5	3·4	8·4

Some of the data are from references 44, 58 and 59 and some are the unpublished work of P. H. Sugden and E. A. Newsholme.
* This value includes the activity of glucokinase (see Chapter 6).

of phosphorylase *a* from muscle tissue, an enzyme was demonstrated in muscle extracts that catalysed the conversion of the *a* form into the *b* form. Crystals of phosphorylase *b* could be isolated after exposing phosphorylase *a* to the action of the interconverting enzyme, which at that time was called the 'prosthetic group removing enzyme' (PR enzyme). It was thought that, since phosphorylase *b* became active in the presence of AMP, the PR enzyme might be removing bound AMP. The discovery that the molecular weight of phosphorylase *a* was twice that of phosphorylase *b* led to the interconverting enzyme being renamed the 'phosphorylase-rupturing enzyme' (still 'PR' enzyme).

In 1955 Fischer and Krebs found an enzyme which catalysed the conversion of phosphorylase *b* to phosphorylase *a*.[9] This reaction required Mg^{2+} and involved the hydrolysis of ATP to ADP. Thus it appeared to bring about phosphorylation of phosphorylase *b* by ATP. The activating enzyme, phosphorylase *b* kinase, was partially purified and the stoichiometry of the interconversion *in vitro* was established as:

$$2 \text{ phosphorylase } b + 4\text{ATP} \xrightarrow{Mg^{2+}} \text{phosphorylase } a + 4\text{ADP}$$

The demonstration that the activation of phosphorylase involved a phosphorylation reaction and a kinase enzyme with the probable transfer of a phosphate group to the phosphorylase protein, suggested that the inactivating enzyme was a phosphatase (that is, a phosphate-releasing or PR enzyme). This enzyme was partially purified and shown to catalyse the following phosphatase-type reaction.

$$\text{Phosphorylase } a + 4\text{H}_2\text{O} \rightarrow 2 \text{ phosphorylase } b + 4\text{P}_i$$

The existence of two forms of phosphorylase with different catalytic activities which were capable of being enzymatically interconverted suggested that the two forms might be involved in metabolic control of glycogenolysis in muscle tissue. However, in the early studies, whenever phosphorylase was assayed in extracts of muscle it was always found to be in the *a* form. This was the case even in extracts prepared from resting muscle, in which it is known that glycogen is not degraded.

Fischer and Krebs realized that if the distribution of the two forms of phosphorylase in muscle was to be accurately assessed, it was vital to inhibit the interconverting enzymes during extraction of the muscle tissue. Knowledge of the properties of these enzymes indicated suitable inhibitors: the phosphatase was inhibited by fluoride ions and the kinase was inhibited by EDTA, which chelated the essential Mg^{2+}. Under these conditions extracts of many muscles were found to contain proportions of phosphorylase *b* which accounted for more than 90% of the total activity.[9]

The theory developed that phosphorylase *b* was always the inactive species of the enzyme and that whenever glycogenolysis was necessary, phosphorylase b had to be converted to phosphorylase a.[6] Although this theory explained many of the known facts, some modification was necessary in the early 1960s to take into account new experimental data. These experiments and the modification of the control theory are described in the following section, while discussion of the further developments in the enzymology of the interconverting enzymes is deferred until Section D.

C. CONTROL OF THE ACTIVITY OF PHOSPHORYLASE b IN MUSCLE

The simple theory of control of phosphorylase activity, based upon the interconversions between the two forms, required the fundamental assumption that phosphorylase b was inactive under all conditions, although in their review article in 1962 Krebs and Fischer[6] voiced some reservations on this assumption. The early work of the Coris had shown that phosphorylase b could be activated by AMP (50% activation was obtained at about 10^{-5} M) and prior to about 1960 it was considered that the level of AMP in muscle was always lower than 10^{-5} M.[9] Therefore it appeared that the effect of AMP was unphysiological and that phosphorylase b was inactive in muscle. This theory had to be modified since experiments of three different kinds suggested that phosphorylase b could indeed be active in muscle.

(a) The development of rapid-freezing techniques and enzymatic assay methods for the determination of tissue metabolite levels in the late 1950s permitted an experimental reappraisal of the AMP content of muscle.[10] It was found that the content of AMP in skeletal muscle was about 0.1 μmol/g fresh tissue (or 10^{-4} M). Since 50% of the maximal activity of phosphorylase b was obtained at 10^{-5} M AMP, this form of the enzyme should be always active even in resting muscle. This theory is obviously untenable since little if any glycogen degradation occurs in resting muscle.

(b) A strain of mice (I-strain) was discovered in which the muscles specifically lack the enzyme phosphorylase b kinase, so that in these muscles the conversion of phosphorylase b to phosphorylase a is impossible. Therefore, according to the theory, glycogen should not be degraded. However, enforced physical exercise in these mice (swimming in a bucket of water),[11] or electrical stimulation of the muscles in vitro,[12] caused glycogen depletion.

(c) In perfused heart experiments it was shown very convincingly that under certain conditions phosphorylase b must be active. In the isolated rat heart perfused with glucose, no glycogenolysis could be detected and, consistent with this, it was shown that 98% of the phosphorylase was in the b form (see Table 4.3). The addition of the hormone, glucagon, which stimulates glycogen breakdown, caused 44% of the phosphorylase b to be converted to the a form. However, the effect of anaerobiosis on the rate of glycogenolysis

Table 4.3. The effects of glucagon and anaerobiosis on the content of glycogen and the percentage of phosphorylase a in the perfused isolated rat heart[13]

Substances measured	Aerobic conditions		Anaerobic conditions
	Control	Glucagon	
Glycogen content (mg/g dry weight)	13·5	8·0	3·5
Phosphorylase content (percentage a)	2	44	16

The hearts were perfused for 12 minutes and the control values represent the glycogen content and percentage phosphorylase a at 12 minutes. Glucagon was added to the perfusate, or hearts were made anaerobic, at 12 minutes, and then perfusions were continued for two minutes before freeze-clamping the heart. The content of glycogen and the activity of phosphorylase were measured. Thus, in two minutes 5·5 mg of glycogen was degraded as a result of glucagon addition and 10·0 mg was degraded as a result of anaerobiosis.

was much greater than the effect of glucagon, despite the fact that only a slight conversion (16 %) of phosphorylase b to phosphorylase a had occurred.[13] The obvious conclusion was that phosphorylase b had been activated by the anaerobic conditions so that both phosphorylase a and b were active.

At this stage Morgan and Parmeggiani reinvestigated the properties of phosphorylase b from skeletal muscle. They found that phosphorylase b was activated not only by AMP but also by inorganic phosphate. The activation caused by these compounds was decreased in the presence of ATP and glucose-6-phosphate. In contrast, phosphorylase a was much less sensitive to these compounds.[14] The discovery of these properties provided the answer to the problems cited above. In resting muscle the concentration of AMP is not sufficient to activate phosphorylase b because the levels of ATP and glucose-6-phosphate are inhibitory, but conditions which cause an increase in the concentrations of AMP and P_i and a decrease in those of ATP and/or glucose-6-phosphate (for example, exercise in the I-strain of mice; anaerobiosis in the perfused heart) result in an increase in phosphorylase b activity. Therefore glycogenolysis proceeds without the need for the conversion of phosphorylase b to phosphorylase a.

The discovery that both forms of phosphorylase can be catalytically active in muscle (and when both are fully active the catalytic activities are similar) immediately poses a question: why has Nature gone to the trouble to provide a dual mechanism of control of this enzyme? The control of phosphorylase b by changes in the concentrations of adenine nucleotides and/or glucose-6-phosphate can be considered as a basic cellular mechanism of control which is not unlike the regulation of phosphofructokinase (Chapter 3, Section D.2). Thus, in any situation in which the energy level of the cell is decreased, or in which the glucose-6-phosphate level is decreased, phosphorylase b will be activated and glycogenolysis will result. The ability of the cell to activate phosphorylase by conversion of the b form to the a form can be considered as a more sophisticated mechanism of control that has been grafted onto the basic control mechanism during evolutionary development. The advantage of this mechanism is that it permits glycogenolysis to proceed despite normal (i.e. high) levels of ATP and glucose-6-phosphate (see Figure 4.5). The physiological advantage of this is that in stressful

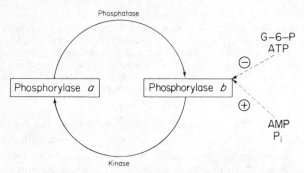

Figure 4.5. Control of phosphorylase activity. The activity of phosphorylase b is controlled by a balance of the concentrations of G-6-P, ATP, AMP and P_i. Phosphorylase can be activated by hormones via the conversion of the b form to the a form

situations phosphorylase b will be converted to the a form (by the action of adrenaline; see next section), glycogenolysis will be stimulated and the concentrations of the glycolytic intermediates will be elevated in preparation for an increased demand for energy. This is important because biological energy is not stored in its utilizable form (ATP) but has to be constantly regenerated by phosphorylation reactions (see Figure 3.8). Therefore, when an animal senses danger, the release of adrenaline will ensure a transient increase in glycolytic intermediates in the muscle cell, so that if the animal has to escape, the rate and force of contraction will not be restricted by a limitation in the ability of the muscle to regenerate ATP. The ability of an animal to travel from point A to point B in, for example, 9 seconds instead of 10 seconds (a 10% reduction in transit time) may have considerable survival value!

D. CONTROL OF PHOSPHORYLASE ACTIVITY BY ENZYMATIC INTERCONVERSIONS

Although phosphorylase b *can* be activated directly by variations in the concentrations of metabolites, the conversion of phosphorylase b to a occurs under all physiological conditions that result in increased glyco-genolysis. The theory of control which prevails at present is based on the properties of the enzymes that catalyse the interconversions (phosphorylase b kinase and phosphorylase a phosphatase) and, in particular, upon the properties of phosphorylase b kinase.

1. Phosphorylation of phosphorylase b

Phosphorylase b kinase has been shown to catalyse the following reaction

$$2 \text{ phosphorylase } b + 4\text{ATP} \rightarrow \text{phosphorylase } a + 4\text{ADP}$$

During this reaction the terminal phosphate of ATP is transferred to a specific amino acid residue on each individual monomer of phosphorylase b. The phosphate is covalently bound by esterification with the hydroxyl group of a serine residue (see Figure 4.6).

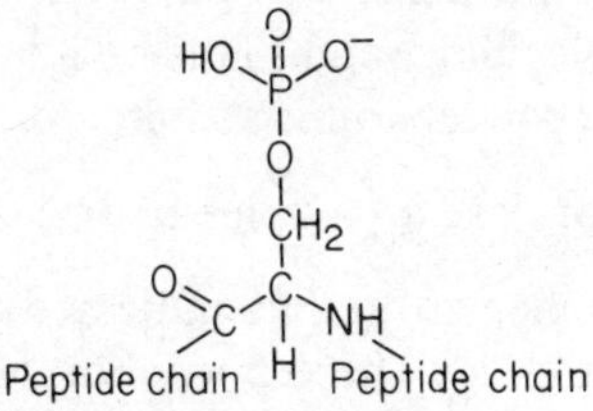

Figure 4.6. Phosphorylated serine residue

This has been demonstrated by partial proteolytic digestion of phosphorylase a (phosphorylated phosphorylase b) and the isolation from the hydrolysate of a pentapeptide containing serine phosphate. Larger fragments, containing this pentapeptide, have since been isolated from partial hydrolysates, including a tetradecapeptide which has been completely sequenced. This tetradecapeptide can be dephosphorylated by phosphorylase a phosphatase and the resulting dephospho- form can be rephosphorylated by phosphorylase b kinase.[15] The sequence of this peptide in the phosphorylase a from rabbit skeletal muscle is as follows: Ser-Asp-Gln-Glu-Lys-Arg-Lys-Gln-Ile-Ser(P)-Val-Arg-Gly-Leu. The serine residue, which is phosphorylated during the interconversion, is in a region of the peptide chain that is highly basic. It is possible to speculate that addition of a phosphate group in this peptide sequence would have a marked effect upon the local charge of the peptide and hence on the conformation of the molecule. This peptide sequence takes no direct part in the catalytic process: the residue that remains after removal of the peptide retains phosphorylase activity. This residue resembles phosphorylase *b* in that it requires AMP for activity but, of course, it cannot be converted to phosphorylase *a*. The evidence suggests that the phosphorylated site occupies a position on the surface of the protein: it is available to both phosphorylase *a* phosphatase and phosphorylase *b* kinase and it is readily attacked by several proteolytic enzymes.

In summary, it is known that the phosphorylation site is on the surface of the protein, that a specific serine residue is phosphorylated which might modify the local (primarily) positively charged area in the molecule, and that this site is spatially distinct from the catalytic site. The molecular details that would explain the increase in catalytic activity upon phosphorylation of this serine residue are as yet unknown (for a review see reference 16).

Molecular weight studies have shown that phosphorylase *b* in its active form is a dimeric molecule consisting of two protein subunits each of molecular weight 92,500. Crystalline phosphorylase *a* from several sources has a molecular weight of 370,000 and is therefore made up of four of the 92,500 subunits. When pure phosphorylase *a* is dephosphorylated by the phosphatase, 4 moles of inorganic phosphate are released per mole of phosphorylase *a* and the molecular weight falls by a factor of two. Thus, *in vitro* the stoichiometry of the conversion is as follows,

$$\text{phosphorylase } a \rightarrow 2 \text{ phosphorylase } b + 4P_i$$

Recent work by the Fischer group has indicated that this is unlikely to be the situation in living muscle, where phosphorylase *a* is probably dimeric. *In vitro* both the *a* and *b* forms of phosphorylase can exist in monomeric, dimeric and tetrameric forms. The monomers, whose formation is reversibly effected by sulphydryl reagents, are inactive, whilst the dimeric form of both *a* and *b* can be active under the appropriate conditions. The Fischer group proposes that the phosphorylation of dimer *b* into dimer *a* takes place in two separate steps, the intermediate being a partially phosphorylated hybrid which has one phosphorylated and one unphosphorylated subunit. Each of the dimers may exist in one of two conformations which are in equilibrium (see Figure 4.7). In phosphorylase *b*, this equilibrium strongly favours the inactive conformation unless activators (AMP, P_i) are added. The equilibrium of the phosphorylated form (phosphorylase *a*) strongly favours the active conformation. Phosphorylase *b* kinase acts upon the inactive conformation while phosphorylase *a* phosphatase acts upon the active conformation. The active conformations will aggregate and this accounts for the fact that active phosphorylase *a* is isolated in the tetrameric state, as is phosphorylase *b* in the presence of AMP. Although phosphorylase *a* from human, rabbit, rat and frog skeletal muscles tetramizes readily, the enzymes from all other sources so far investigated do not. This observation supports the idea that tetramization is not essential for catalysis.

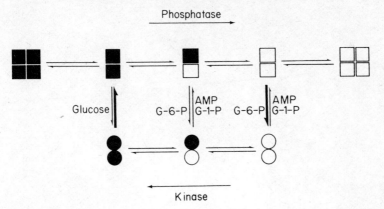

Figure 4.7. A model for the structure and conformation of phospho-dephospho-hybrids. Circles represent inactive conformations and squares represent active ones. Open and filled symbols represent non-phosphorylated and phosphorylated subunits, respectively[16]

2. Properties of phosphorylase *b* kinase

When phosphorylase *b* kinase is isolated from skeletal muscle it shows very little activity. It can be activated *in vitro* in a number of ways:

(*a*) incubation with ATP and Mg^{2+} ions,
(*b*) incubation with Ca^{2+} ions,
(*c*) treatment with a proteolytic enzyme (such as trypsin),
(*d*) increasing the pH to about 8·2.

Neither trypsin treatment nor exposure to a high pH are thought to have any physiological significance. The activation of the enzyme by partial proteolysis is an irreversible process and therefore it is difficult to see how it could be of any significance for the regulation of phosphorylase *b* kinase in the muscle cell. The enzyme, as isolated in its non-activated form, has an optimum activity above pH 8 and shows very little activity at pH 6·8. This non-activated form differs even when active at pH 8 from the enzyme which has been activated by other means (such as incubation with ATP-Mg^{2+} or with Ca^{2+}) and is in fact less active even at high pH (see Figure 4.8).* Since it is very unlikely that a large pH shift occurs intracellularly, this pH effect is probably unphysiological and the non-activated form of phosphorylase *b* kinase is always inactive in the cell.

* The differential effect of pH on the non-activated and activated forms of *b* kinase has provided a convenient experimental tool for the measurement of the degree of activation *in vivo*. Muscle is rapidly extracted and the activity of *b* kinase is measured at pH 6·8 and at pH 8·2. A low ratio of the activity at pH 6·8 to that at pH 8·2 indicates that the enzyme is in the non-activated form: as the ratio approaches unity activation approaches 100% (Figure 4.8).

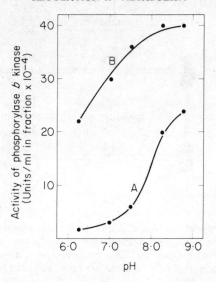

Figure 4.8. The pH profiles of inactive and active phosphorylase *b* kinase. A is the inactive form and B is the active form[17]

The activation of phosphorylase *b* kinase by ATP-Mg^{2+} and by Ca^{2+} both appear to be physiologically important. The results of much fruitful research upon these two effects may be assembled into a coherent theory of control in which the stimulation of glycogenolysis by adrenaline is mediated via the ATP-Mg^{2+}-dependent activation of phosphorylase *b* kinase, whilst the increased glycogenolysis which follows nervous stimulation of muscle is brought about by the activating effect of Ca^{2+} upon this same enzyme. These two mechanisms for activating glycogenolysis are discussed separately in Sections D.3 and D.4, despite the fact that in some conditions they may work *in concert* in the muscle cell.

3. Hormonal control of phosphorylase activity

(a) The effects of ATP-Mg^{2+} on phosphorylase b kinase

The activation of phosphorylase *b* kinase by incubation of a muscle extract with ATP and Mg^{2+} suggested that a phosphorylation reaction might be involved in the activation process. Accordingly, incubation of *b* kinase with ATP labelled with ^{32}P in the γ position resulted in the incorporation of ^{32}P into the enzyme protein as the activation proceeded (see Figure 4.9). Further evidence that phosphorylation accompanies activation was provided by an experiment with the cyclic nucleotide 3',5'-AMP, which had been implicated in the stimulation of glycogenolysis by adrenaline as early

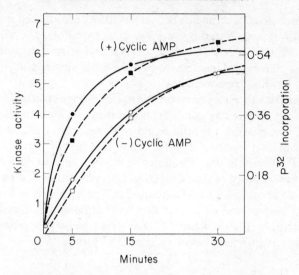

Figure 4.9. Activation of rabbit muscle phosphorylase b kinase by $AT^{32}P$ and Mg^{2+}, with and without cyclic AMP. Purified non-activated phosphorylase b kinase was incubated at pH 7·0 with 10 mM Mg^{2+} and 2 mM $AT^{32}P$, with and without 0·2 mM cyclic AMP. At intervals, aliquots were precipitated with trichloroacetic acid, washed, and counted. Other aliquots were diluted and assayed for phosphorylase b kinase activity at pH 6·8. The ordinate on the left gives kinase activity in arbitrary units. The ordinate on the right gives ^{32}P incorporation in mol/L $\times 10^5$ g protein. Broken lines represent ^{32}P incorporation; solid lines represent b kinase activity[17]

as 1958 (see Section D.3(b) for a full account of the role of cyclic AMP). The addition of cyclic AMP to the assay medium of phosphorylase b kinase caused a marked increase in activity and a parallel stimulation of ^{32}P incorporation from ATP (Figure 4.9).[17] No cyclic AMP was formed during the incubation with ATP and Mg^{2+} alone, and therefore its effect must have been separate from that of ATP-Mg^{2+}. Also, strikingly low concentrations of the cyclic nucleotide were sufficient for its stimulatory effect: 1×10^{-7} M cyclic AMP caused a 50% increase over the activation by ATP-Mg^{2+} alone. Since the cyclic AMP effects were greater with less pure preparations of phosphorylase b kinase, there was probably some other factor involved in the cyclic AMP activation which was removed during purification. It was thought that the phosphorylation of phosphorylase b kinase by ATP was enzymatic and the exciting possibility arose that cyclic AMP might exert its effect via another kinase enzyme, namely, phosphorylase b kinase kinase.[17] The existence of such an enzyme was eventually reported in 1968[18] and since that time its properties have been studied in some detail. In particular, it is activated by very low concentrations of cyclic AMP (see Section D.3(b)(v)). It has also been observed that this enzyme will phosphorylate a number of proteins other than phosphorylase *b* kinase and therefore it has been renamed, *protein kinase*.

The properties of phosphorylase *b* kinase in respect of its activation by ATP-Mg^{2+} are obviously complex, but nonetheless, on the basis of these properties, it is possible to formulate a coherent theory of control which is physiologically satisfactory. The theory is that an increase in the level of cyclic AMP in muscle tissue leads to activation of protein kinase. Active protein kinase phosphorylates inactive phosphorylase *b* kinase with the formation of active *b* kinase. Consequently, phosphorylase *b* will be converted into phosphorylase *a* and this will stimulate glycogenolysis even in resting muscle (Figure 4.10).[18,19] The experimental evidence in support of this theory is provided below (Section D.3(b)(iii)).

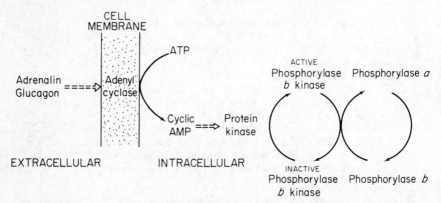

Figure 4.10. The control of phosphorylase activity by an enzyme cascade. Stimulation of adenyl cyclose increases the intracellular concentration of cyclic AMP, which stimulates protein kinase: inactive phosphorylase *b* kinase is converted to active *b* kinase, which catalyses the conversion of phosphorylase *b* into phosphorylase *a* (see also Figure 4.19)

(b) The role of cyclic 3′,5′-AMP in the regulation of phosphorylase

(i) Historical introduction. This account of the control of glycogen metabolism has so far been restricted to observations on skeletal muscle systems. A considerable amount of work was carried out during the same period on liver phosphorylase and it was this work, largely by Sutherland and his coworkers, which first gave rise to the isolation of cyclic AMP and to the elucidation of the role of this compound in the control of glycogen metabolism. In the mid-1950s Sutherland and Wosilait found that liver phosphorylase existed in an active (phosphorylated) form and in an inactive (dephosphoryl-

ated) form and that the interconversions of the two forms were catalysed by two enzymes, a kinase (requiring ATP and Mg^{2+}) and a phosphatase.

For some time it had been known that the hormones adrenaline and glucagon were potent stimulators of glycogenolysis. It was anticipated that these hormones might influence the relative proportions of active and inactive phosphorylase in liver. Accordingly, it was found that both adrenaline and glucagon caused a conversion of phosphorylase into the active form. The response to the hormones could be separated into two distinct phases: first, there occurred the formation of a heat-stable, dialysable, active factor that was produced by a particulate fraction of the cell; second, there was phosphorylation of phosphorylase b in the supernatant fraction upon which the hormones, when added directly, had no effect. Thus, the hormones stimulated the formation of the heat-stable factor which was in turn responsible for the stimulation of the phosphorylase interconversions. The identification of this factor by the Sutherland group progressed until it was known that it was an adenine nucleotide. At the same time as they were attempting to identify this unknown nucleotide, another research group was analysing a hitherto unidentified nucleotide which they had isolated from a $Ba(OH)_2$ hydrolysate of ATP. The two groups exchanged nucleotides and it turned out that they were identical[7] and that they were, indeed, cyclic 3′,5′-AMP, whose structure is shown in Figure 4.11.

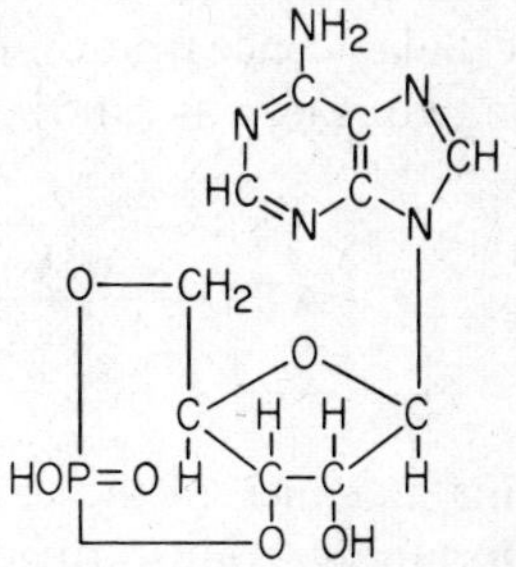

Figure 4.11. The structure of cyclic 3′,5′-AMP

Since the discovery of cyclic AMP the Sutherland group have continued their work on the enzymes that synthesize and degrade the nucleotide and on the measurement of its concentration in a variety of tissues under different conditions (for example, see references 20 and 21). These investigations have complemented those of Krebs, Fischer and colleagues on the enzymology of the phosphorylase interconversions and the result is an exciting story of the mechanism of regulation of phosphorylase activity.

(ii) *Adenyl cyclase and phosphodiesterase.* Cyclic AMP is produced from ATP in a reaction catalysed by adenyl cyclase, whose distribution and properties were first reported in 1962.[22]

$$ATP \xrightarrow[\text{cyclase}]{\text{adenyl}} 3′,5′\text{-AMP} + PP_i$$

It was observed that the activity was always associated with a particulate fraction of the cell and, initially, it was difficult to decide whether the particles in question were fragments of the cell membrane or the nuclear membrane. The advent of a special cell-fractionater made it possible, by differential centrifugation, to demonstrate clearly that adenyl cyclase is associated with the cell membrane, at least in pigeon erythrocytes and rat liver.[23] It has been tacitly assumed that the enzyme has a cell membrane location in all other tissues.

Adenyl cyclase preparations from liver are activated by adrenaline and glucagon, whereas preparations from skeletal muscle are activated only by adrenaline. The location of adenyl cyclase in the cell membrane implies that activation of this enzyme by a hormone must represent a very early molecular event in the action of the hormone on its target tissue. Unfortunately, the inability to solubilize adenyl cyclase whilst retaining its sensitivity to hormones has precluded any further advance in the knowledge of the molecular action of hormones.

Although the equilibrium constant of the adenyl cyclase reaction is unknown, it seems very likely that in the cell the reaction is non-equilibrium. Therefore cyclic AMP must be continually removed by another reaction, otherwise large quantities would accumulate in the cell. The enzyme that degrades cyclic AMP is known as cyclic AMP phosphodiesterase. The intracellular concentration of cyclic AMP is maintained in a steady state by the two reactions catalysed by adenyl cyclase and phosphodiesterase, as follows

$$ATP \xrightarrow{\text{adenyl cyclase}} cyclic\ AMP \xrightarrow[H_2O]{\text{phosphodiesterase}} AMP$$

The maintenance of the concentration of cyclic AMP by two such non-equilibrium reactions provides a very simple mechanism for the control of the concentration of this important regulator: all that is required is a change in the rate of one of the reactions. As far as is known at present, changes in concentration of cyclic AMP in muscle cells are produced physiologically only by changes in the activity of adenyl cyclase. This mechanism suffers from the disadvantage that large changes in the concentration of regulator are unlikely to occur physiologically. This is because the phosphodiesterase reaction is a first-order reaction (that is, the cyclic AMP concentration is much less than the Km of the enzyme for cyclic AMP) so that, as the cyclic AMP concentration is increased by adenyl cyclase stimulation, phosphodiesterase activity is also increased. The theoretical relationship between the change in concentration of regulator and the change in enzyme activity in this type of situation can be calculated (see Table 4.4). If such a relationship holds in vivo, the experimental modification of adenyl cyclase activity by

Table 4.4. Theoretical analysis of changes in steady-state concentrations of a compound dependent on irreversible synthesizing and degrading reactions

Activity of synthesizing system (arbitrary activity units) V_1	Concentration of B ($\times 10^3$)	
	V_2 is 10^3 (arbitrary activity units)	V_2 is 10^2 (arbitrary activity units)
1	0·1	1·0
2	0·2	2·0
5	0·5	5·0
10	1·0	11·0
20	2·0	25·0
50	5·3	100·0
100	11·1	
200	25·0	

The reaction sequence is

$$A \xrightarrow{1} B \xrightarrow{2} C$$

Both reactions are non-equilibrium and are assumed to be enzyme catalysed. The reaction A → B is zero order (that is, the substrate is present in excess) and the enzyme that catalyses the B → C reaction obeys Michaelis–Menten kinetics. The K_m for substrate B is assumed to be 0·1 arbitrary units. The equation governing this situation is

$$[B] = \frac{V_1 \times K_m}{V_2 - V_1}$$

where V_1 and V_2 are the maximal activities of enzymes catalysing reactions 1 and 2, respectively. The reaction system is considered to be similar to that controlling the intracellular concentration of cyclic AMP: reaction 1 represents the adenyl cyclase reaction, reaction 2 represents the phosphodiesterase reaction and B represents cyclic AMP (see reference 60).

physiological effectors (such as adrenaline) should result in only small changes in the intracellular concentration of cyclic AMP: that this is the case is supported by the results shown in Table 4.5. In contrast, the experimental inhibition of phosphodiesterase by non-physiological agents such as the methyl xanthines (caffeine, for example), along with the stimulation of adenyl cyclase, results in large changes in the concentration of cyclic AMP.

The limited elevation in cyclic AMP concentrations effected by hormones *in vivo* has necessitated that the sensitivity of the target enzyme to this cyclic nucleotide be increased: this is achieved by the target enzyme existing in two enzymatically interconvertible forms. At present it is known that cyclic AMP is involved in the regulation of phosphorylase, UDPG-glucosyltransferase, and adipose tissue triglyceride lipase (see reference 21), all of which exist in two enzymatically interconvertible forms. (A discussion of the theoretical aspects of the amplification provided by interconvertible forms of an enzyme is presented in Chapter 2, Section F.)

Table 4.5. The effect of hormones on the contents of cyclic AMP in various tissues[21,24]

Experimental condition	Hormone addition	Content of cyclic AMP (nmol/g fresh weight of tissue)
Liver slices (rabbit)	Control	0·4
	Adrenaline (4×10^{-5} M)	1·5
Gastrocnemius, isolated after adrenaline administered to whole animal (rat)	Control	0·3
	Adrenaline	1·6
Incubation of isolated diaphragm (rat)	Control	0·2
	Adrenaline (5×10^{-5} M)	2·2
Isolated perfused working rat heart	Control	0·4
	Adrenaline	1·4
Brain slices from 10-day-old rat	Control	0·025
	Adrenaline (10^{-5} M)	0·12
Isolated perfused rat liver	Control	0·5
	Glucagon ($1·4 \times 10^{-6}$ M)	27·0
Anti-insulin sera injected into rat, and liver freeze-clamped *in situ*	Control (normal sera)	0·6
	Experimental (anti-insulin sera)	1·6
Incubated epidydimal fat pad of rat	Control	0·18
	Adrenaline (5×10^{-6} M)	0·28
	Adrenaline ($5·5 \times 10^{-5}$ M)	0·37
Isolated fat cells of rat	Control	0·41*
	Adrenaline (5×10^{-6} M)	0·85*
	Control plus caffeine (10^{-3} M)	0·52*
	Adrenaline (5×10^{-6} M) plus caffeine (10^{-3} M)	9·80*

* nmol/g dry weight of tissue.

It may seem surprising that many processes should be regulated by the same intracellular messenger (cyclic AMP) and it might have been expected that Nature would have diversified the chemical structures of such messengers, if only for the sake of specificity in regulation. In fact, emphasis on one messenger is *not* surprising when the problems involved in controlling its concentration are considered. There are two essential requirements for the provision of a regulatory mechanism similar to the one involving cyclic AMP. First, there must be a fairly constant concentration of precursor (constant 'source') for the formation of the messenger. Second, the messenger must be converted into a compound that does not accumulate in the cell (efficient 'sink').

$$\text{'source'} \rightarrow \text{messenger} \rightarrow \text{'sink'}$$

In the case of cyclic AMP, the 'source', ATP, is always available while the 'sink', AMP, is easily removed via the adenylate kinase equilibrium. It is difficult to suggest 'sources' and 'sinks' for alternative messengers (except for other cyclic nucleotides, such as cyclic GMP).

(iii) *Evidence for the theory of control of phosphorylase by cyclic AMP.* A theory for the control of phosphorylase activity by enzymatic inter-conversions, which is based upon the properties of phosphorylase *b* kinase and protein kinase, has been presented in Section D.3(a) (see Figure 4.10). The chemical link between the hormones which accelerate glycogenolysis and the enzymes which catalyse this process would appear to be cyclic AMP. Indeed, the administration of adrenaline to intact muscle preparations has been shown to elevate the cyclic AMP content about four-fold. Since adrenaline has an activating effect upon partially purified preparations of adenyl cyclase, but has no effect upon phosphodiesterase, it is assumed that the increase in muscle cyclic AMP is brought about solely by stimulation of adenyl cyclase. A problem arises in that 50% activation of partially purified preparations of protein kinase occurs at about 1×10^{-7} M cyclic AMP[18,19] whereas the calculated intracellular concentration of cyclic AMP in most tissues almost always exceeds this value. This discrepancy may be explained in several ways: for example, non-specific binding of cyclic AMP in the cell or a decrease in the sensitivity of *in situ* protein kinase to cyclic AMP due to the presence of an inhibitor which competes with cyclic AMP.

The incubation of an intact muscle with adrenaline results in activation of phosphorylase *b* kinase (as measured by the ratio of activity at pH 6·8 to that at pH 8·2, see Section D.2) and conversion of phosphorylase to the *a* form (Table 4.6).[25] Thus, changes in the state of the enzymes involved in the control of phosphorylase and in the intracellular concentration of cyclic AMP are consistent with the proposed theory.

(iv) *Physiological significance of the sequence of activations in the control of phosphorylase.* Cyclic AMP activates protein kinase, which phosphorylates inactive *b* kinase to produce active *b* kinase, which in turn phosphorylates phosphorylase *b* to form phosphorylase *a*. This sequence of activating steps is an example of an enzyme cascade and it effects the amplification of an initial small signal into a much greater final response (Figure 4.10). The first example of cascade-amplification in biological systems was proposed by Macfarlane[26] to explain the complex activating system employed in blood-clotting (Figure 4.12). There is no doubt that the concentration of the initial blood-clotting factor (Hagemann factor or Factor XII) is several orders of magnitude smaller than that of the final target enzyme, prothrombin. Therefore, *direct* activation of prothrombin by the clotting factor would not form sufficient active prothrombin (thrombin) to produce a clot within a reasonably short space of time. Obviously, activation of a small amount of thrombin might eventually produce a satisfactory clot, but the loss of blood

Table 4.6. Effect of adrenaline and electrical stimulation on the concentration of cyclic AMP and the activities of phosphorylase b kinase and phosphorylase in rat and frog muscles

Animal	Muscle	Experimental treatment	Content of cyclic AMP (nmol/g muscle)	Phosphorylase b kinase activity ratio units pH 6·8 / units pH 8·2	Percentage phosphorylase a
Rat	Gastrocnemius	Control	0·69	0·04	10
		Administration of adrenaline to whole animal	1·82	0·25	48
	Gastrocnemius	Control	0·71	0·08	16
		Electrical stimulation of nerve supplying gastrocnemius	0·82	0·13	38
Frog	Gastrocnemius and sartorius	Control	0·59	0·29	21
		Administration of adrenaline to whole animal	1·59	0·40	39
	Gastrocnemius and sartorius	Control	0·63	0·28	15
		Electrical stimulation of nerves supplying gastrocnemius and direct stimulation of sartorius	0·55	0·45	61

Adrenaline was administered intracardiacly and a short time later (60 seconds and 12 minutes for the rat and frog, respectively) the muscles were removed and rapidly frozen. The ratio of activity at pH 6·8 to that at pH 8·2 provides an indication of the activation of b kinase (see Figure 4.8). The percentage phosphorylase a was calculated assuming that the total activity (a plus b) is measured in the presence of AMP and only the activity of phosphorylase a is measured in the absence of AMP.[25]

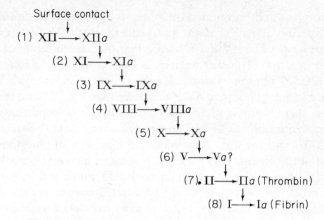

Figure 4.12. The control of blood-clotting by an enzyme
cascade

during this time would be serious if not fatal. In blood-clotting the small concentration of Factor XII initiates the activation of the cascade mechanism, in which the product of one reaction is the catalyst for the subsequent reaction. In this system amplification may occur at each catalysed reaction so that the concentrations of the activated intermediates increase at each amplification stage. If a 10-fold amplification is produced at each reaction, a system involving three such reactions could produce a 1,000-fold amplification.

The role of enzymatic interconversions in providing amplification of the response of a regulatory enzyme to a *change* in concentration of the regulator has been discussed earlier (see Chapter 2, Section F.2(a)(ii)). Enzymatic interconversions may also be important if the *actual* concentration of the regulator is lower than that of the regulatory enzyme in the metabolic pathway. In this case, direct binding of the regulator to the enzyme would not cause maximal activation since the number of regulatory molecules is smaller than the number of enzyme molecules. However, if the regulator modified the activity of the interconverting enzyme (whose concentration may be lower than that of the regulatory enzyme) this would result in almost complete activation of the regulatory enzyme, since the effect of the interconverting enzyme is catalytic. A further extension of this type of amplification, in which the actual concentration rather than the *change* in concentration of regulator is important, is found in cascade systems. In blood-clotting the absolute concentration of Factor XII is very much less than that of prothrombin and amplification is essential. The proposal that the series of activations in the control of phosphorylase activity perform an analogous function to the blood-clotting cascade system[27,28] implies that the concentration of the initial signal (cyclic AMP) is small in comparison with the concentration of phosphorylase *b* or phosphorylase *b* kinase. The concentrations of phosphorylase and phosphorylase b kinase in muscle can be calculated from the specific activities of the purified enzymes.* The concentration of phosphorylase is about 5×10^{-6} M so that the concentration of binding sites could be 10^{-5} M (assuming it is a dimeric protein). However, the concentration of phosphorylase b kinase is less than 10^{-6} M, whereas the measured content of cyclic AMP is greater than 10^{-6} M and this might suggest that there is ample cyclic AMP to activate b kinase directly. (Also, the final concentration of Ca^{2+} in the sarcoplasm is about the same as that of cyclic AMP and yet Ca^{2+} ions modify the activity of phosphorylase b kinase and not protein kinase.) If there is ample cyclic AMP available for direct activation of b kinase, protein kinase would not be required and there would be no cascade; control would be exerted by one system of inter-conversions (in a similar fashion to the glucosyltransferase system in which protein kinase catalyses directly the conversion of the I to the D form). The need for the participation of yet another enzyme becomes clear upon consideration of the mechanism for the control of the cyclic AMP concentration (see Figure 4.13).

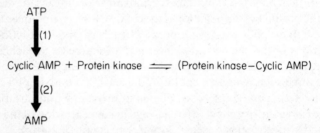

Figure 4.13. Interaction between cyclic AMP and protein kinase. (1) Adenyl cyclase, (2) Phosphodiesterase

When adenyl cyclase activity is increased there is a proportional increase in the concentration of cyclic AMP. However, if a large proportion of the total cyclic AMP were to be bound to the initial activating enzyme (protein kinase or, hypothetically, phosphorylase b kinase) the establishment of a new steady-state concentration of cyclic AMP would be a very slow process. Consequently, maximal activation of the initial activating enzyme would be slow. Furthermore the binding constant for the reaction between cyclic AMP and the initial enzyme would have to be very large in order to bind a large proportion of the cyclic AMP. Therefore the inactivation of this enzyme by destruction of cyclic AMP via the phosphodiesterase reaction would also be a very slow process (see Table 4.7). Thus, if a large proportion of

* Purified muscle phosphorylase b kinase has an activity of approximately 60×10^3 units/mg and a molecular weight of at least 10^6.[21] In crude muscle extracts, total b kinase activity is approximately 22×10^3 units/g muscle, so that 1 g of muscle contains 0·36 mg of b kinase or approximately $0·36 \times 10^{-6}$ M.

the total cyclic AMP were to be bound to the initial enzyme, there would be a serious delay between the initial stimulus (that is, modification of the activity of adenyl cyclase) and the required metabolic response (that is, a change in phosphorylase activity). In order to ensure activation of protein kinase with the minimal delay in establishing the new steady-state concentration of cyclic AMP, only a small proportion of the cyclic AMP (10–20%) must be permitted to react with the protein kinase. This can be achieved in one of two ways: either the absolute concentration of protein kinase is low (10^{-7} M compared with 10^{-6} M for cyclic AMP), or the equilibrium constant for the reaction between protein kinase and cyclic AMP is such that only 10–20% of the nucleotide is bound to the kinase (see Table 4.7). In either case, only a small amount of the initial signal (cyclic AMP) may be used to initiate the process of phosphorylase activation. Therefore, the *effective* concentration of the signal is much lower than its *actual* concentration and amplification of the cascade type is essential if the process is to be stimulated rapidly.

This discussion emphasizes the importance of the relationship between the two reactions which control the concentration of cyclic AMP in the cell—adenyl cyclase and phosphodiesterase. The mechanism provides a simple, rapid, precise and efficient system for changing the concentration of this intracellular regulator in a controlled manner. The removal of a large amount of cyclic AMP by equilibrium binding to a protein would seriously interfere with this simple control mechanism. Therefore it is suggested that protein kinase constantly samples (by equilibrium binding) only a small proportion (say, 10–20%) of the available cyclic AMP in order to detect changes in its concentration. (This is somewhat analogous to the modern radio-immunoassay of hormones in which a small amount of hormone is removed and sampled by binding to a specific antibody.) An increase in the concentration of cyclic AMP increases slightly the amount that is bound to protein kinase, increases protein kinase activity and initiates the activation of the cascade. However, a reduction in the cyclic AMP concentration decreases the amount bound to protein kinase, decreases its activity and rapidly reverses the activation process.

The need for rapid activation of phosphorylase is obviously related to its physiological function in providing energy for the fight or flight mechanism (see Section A.2). The need for rapid inactivation of the enzyme becomes clear on consideration of the properties of phosphofructokinase and the physiological role of adrenaline in the stimulation of glycogenolysis. Adrenaline is released in response to a signal of danger and it causes mobilization of glycogen to hexose phosphates and triose phosphates, which are the immediate precursors for ADP phosphorylation, prior to muscular activity. Therefore muscle is provided with an immediate energy-precursor to ensure that mobilization of energy is not limiting in the 'fight or flight' activity that may follow the danger signal. What is the metabolic response if the

Table 4.7. A theoretical analysis of a metabolic situation in which a protein molecule (P) binds reversibly a small metabolic compound (A), which is irreversibly converted to another compound (X) by a further reaction. The situation is formally analogous to the reaction between protein kinase and cyclic AMP and the conversion of the latter to 5'-AMP by phosphodiesterase[60]

Value of rate constant k_1 (s^{-1}, mol^{-1})	Equilibrium constant ([PA]/[A] × [P])	Concentration of P is 1.0×10^{-6} M		Concentration of P is 1.0×10^{-7} M	
		Initial equilibrium concentration of free A as percentage of total A	Time for conversion of 80% of total A to X (s)	Initial equilibrium concentration of free A as percentage of total A	Time for conversion of 80% of total A to X (s)
10^4	10^4	99·0	16·2	99·9	16·1
10^5	10^5	91·6	17·7	99·1	16·2
10^6	10^6	61·8	29·3	95·1	17·2
10^7	10^7	27·0	111·0	91·0	19·8
10^8	10^8	9·5	852·0	90·1	21·6
10^9	10^9	3·1	8,148·0	90·0	22·0
10^{10}	10^{10}	1·0	81,020·0	90·0	22·0

The reactions are described as follows

$$P + A \underset{k_2}{\overset{k_1}{\rightleftarrows}} PA$$
$$k_3 \downarrow$$
$$X$$

Given the initial concentrations of P and A, the system is first solved for the equilibrium attained with $k_3 = 0$. This equilibrium is then taken as the initial condition for computation of the transients which follow the switching on of the irreversible conversion of A to X. The transients are governed by the pair of differential equations.

$$\frac{d[PA]}{dt} = k_1[P][A] - k_2[PA]$$

$$\frac{d[A]}{dt} + \frac{d[PA]}{dt} = -\frac{d[X]}{dt} = -k_3[A]$$

Since interest is centred on cases for which k_3 is an order of magnitude smaller than either k_1 or k_2, an estimate of the dynamics is obtained using the pseudo-steady-state approximation for the first of the above equations. In calculating the conversion times given in the table, the second equation has been integrated numerically on a digital computer, the value of [A] at each increment of time being determined by the quasi-equilibrium distribution of the unconverted A between its bound and free states. This approximation tends to place a lower limit on the conversion times. The total concentration of P is varied between 0·1 and $1·0 \times 10^{-6}$ M as shown in the table. The total concentration of A is constant at $1·0 \times 10^{-6}$ M. The rate constant k_1 is varied as shown in the table. k_2 and k_3 are given the values 1·0 and 0·1 s^{-1}, respectively.

This system may describe the relationship between cyclic AMP, protein kinase and phosphodiesterase although it is not known if the rate constants for the various reactions are realistic for the cyclic AMP system. The analysis shows that if the concentrations of protein kinase and cyclic AMP were approximately the same, an increase in the equilibrium constant of the reaction between protein kinase and cyclic AMP would produce a very large increase in the time for destruction of cyclic AMP by the phosphodiesterase. Such an increase will lengthen the time during which protein kinase, and therefore phosphorylase, remain active after the activation of adenyl cyclase (for example, by adrenaline) has ceased. Thus, with an equilibrium constant of 10^{10}, it would take approximately 20 hours to inactivate phosphorylase but with a constant of 10^4 the inactivation time would be only 16 seconds. Note that with an equilibrium constant of 10^4 the proportion of protein kinase in the active form would be only 1%.

The equations in this table were developed and solved by Dr J. Thorson.

danger passes and the animal does not have to 'fight or fly'? Phosphorylase
is inactivated and the hexose phosphates are reconverted to glycogen. If
phosphorylase could not be rapidly inactivated, most of the glycogen would
be degraded to hexose and triose phosphates and these would accumulate
in the muscle. Under such conditions it is possible that glycolysis would be
limited by the availability of inorganic phosphate at the glyceraldehyde-3-
phosphate dehydrogenase reaction. Consequently, fructose diphosphate
would accumulate and the reaction catalysed by PFK might approach
equilibrium. (Although FDPase may be present in skeletal muscle (see
Chapter 3, Section E.4(d)) its activity will be so low in comparison to that of
PFK under these conditions as to be negligible.) Since the equilibrium
constant for the PFK reaction is approximately 10^3 (see Chapter 1, Appendix
1.1) and since a high concentration of fructose-6-phosphate will be maintained in the muscle because of continuing glycogenolysis, the result of
PFK catalysing an equilibrium (or a situation approaching equilibrium)
may be a decrease in the cytoplasmic ATP/ADP concentration ratio. (This
will depend upon the concentration ratio fructose diphosphate/fructose-6-
phosphate. For example, if this ratio is 100, the [ATP]/[ADP] ratio would
be 0·1, if the PFK reaction was at equilibrium.)

The maximal catalytic activities of phosphorylase and phosphofructokinase in skeletal muscle are very high, approximately 100 μmol/min/g
muscle (Table 4.1), so that the total glycogen reserve of the muscle (20–30 μmol)
could be degraded to hexose phosphates in less than a minute, and the PFK
reaction might approach equilibrium within several minutes. From these
simple calculations the need for a rapid reversal of the activation of phosphorylase, as well as the need for efficient resynthesis of glycogen in muscle
should be obvious.

(*v*) *Effect of cyclic 3′,5′-AMP on protein kinase.* Protein kinase is activated
by cyclic AMP. Recent work has shown that the enzyme is composed of a
regulatory subunit which binds cyclic AMP and a catalytic subunit in
which the active centre of the enzyme is located.[29] The evidence suggests
that when the regulatory and catalytic subunits are associated, the enzyme
is inactive whereas when the catalytic subunit is dissociated from the
regulatory subunit, it is active. The binding of cyclic AMP to the regulatory
subunit in the enzyme complex causes dissociation and therefore increases
the activity of the enzyme.

$$R–C + \text{cyclic AMP} \leftrightharpoons R\text{-cyclic AMP} + C$$

This equilibrium reaction provides the means by which changes in the
concentration of cyclic AMP modify the activity of protein kinase. At
present this type of mechanism is unique in metabolic regulation. However,
these are very recent findings and it is possible that in the living cell the

dissociation of the R–C complex does *not* occur upon activation of the enzyme. The conformational change that is produced by binding cyclic AMP may cause dissociation only under the conditions of the *in vitro* experiment.

(c) *Regulation of phosphorylase a phosphatase*

An entirely plausible theory for the control of muscle glycogenolysis has been constructed without reference to the regulation of phosphorylase *a* phosphatase. It has been tacitly assumed that the activity of the phosphatase is regulated solely by the concentration of its substrate, phosphorylase *a*. In this case, if the activity of the phosphatase was of the same order as that of the kinase, the conversion of a large proportion of *b* to *a* would be improbable. Obviously a concerted control mechanism, in which the phosphatase is inhibited when the kinase is activated, would be highly advantageous. Hence, phosphorylase *a* phosphatase has been the subject of several studies but these have proved far less rewarding than those on the kinase system.

(*i*) *Properties of phosphorylase a phosphatase.* Phosphorylase *a* phosphatase has so far resisted all attempts at complete purification: even after a 1,000-fold enrichment it remains heterogeneous. The enzyme sediments with a particulate fraction in which it is bound to glycogen. Hydrolysis of this glycogen releases two soluble proteins of molecular weights 66,000 and 33,000. Both of these proteins possess similar enzymic properties and they may represent different aggregates of the same protein. The only significant property of the soluble enzyme is its inhibition by AMP (or IMP). The cause of this inhibition is apparently an interaction between AMP and phosphorylase *a*. This is a rather unusual case of a regulator acting by modifying the structure of the substrate rather than the enzyme.

Preliminary work on fairly crude extracts of pigeon breast muscle implies that there are two interconvertible forms of phosphorylase *a* phosphatase: active and inactive. Activation is achieved by the addition of ATP and Mg^{2+}.[30] This activation process is inhibited by very low concentrations of cyclic AMP. These properties of the muscle enzyme are very similar to those reported for the phosphorylase *a* phosphatase from adrenal cortex, but the work on muscle is obviously in the very early stages and caution must be exerted in the interpretation of the data. Nevertheless, it is tempting to speculate that this effect of cyclic AMP on the phosphatase provides the basis for a concerted mechanism of control of both the phosphorylase interconverting enzymes.

(*ii*) *Control of phosphorylase a phosphatase in the glycogen particulate complex.* Particles may be isolated from muscle which consist of a complex of sarcoplasmic reticulum, glycogen, phosphorylase, phosphorylase *b* kinase and phosphorylase a phosphatase as well as a number of other enzymes.[16] In this complex both phosphorylase and phosphorylase b kinase are inactive. Low concentrations of Ca^{2+} ions cause activation of phosphorylase b kinase (see the following section for full discussion of Ca^{2+} and control of phosphorylase activity). The addition of 10^{-6} M Ca^{2+} and ATP-Mg^{2+} causes immediate conversion of phosphorylase b to a. When all the ATP has been utilized phosphorylase returns to the b form and addition of more ATP causes a further short-lived activation ('flash activation'). Apparently, phosphorylase a phosphatase is inhibited as much as 75% during the activation of b kinase and at the end of the activation its activity is restored and phosphorylase a is converted to phosphorylase b. It can be shown that this inhibition is not caused by AMP production (the only known regulator of the soluble enzyme).

Such a 'flash-activation' may also be triggered by the addition of 10^{-6} M cyclic AMP instead of Ca^{2+} to the system containing ATP-Mg^{2+}. Again phosphorylase a phosphatase is inhibited during the activation and this inhibition is not caused by AMP. Since purified (but not homogeneous) preparations of the phosphatase are not inhibited by cyclic AMP, ATP-Mg^{2+} or Ca^{2+}, the enzyme must either exist in two enzymatically interconvertible forms (as suggested in (i) above) or glycogen and its degradative enzymes are all involved in a highly organized complex in which the conformational changes involved in activation of b kinase automatically result in inhibition of the phosphatase. Whichever explanation is correct, it is likely that a concerted on-off mechanism for the control of glycogenolysis operates in $vivo$.

4. Nervous control of phosphorylase activity

(a) $Introduction: common control of muscle contraction and glycogenolysis$

The observation that phosphorylase b kinase could be activated by Ca^{2+} ions (see p. 162) led to the development of another theory for the control of glycogenolysis in muscle. This theory arose out of the firmly established role of Ca^{2+} as the chemical link between nervous excitation and the initiation of the contraction process in muscle (see below). The idea is that the activation of contraction and the simultaneous activation of the biochemical pathways that provide the energy for contraction (glycogenolysis and glycolysis) might both be brought about by a change in a single regulator (Ca^{2+}). The possible involvement of Ca^{2+} in the control of glycolysis has been discussed in the previous chapter (Section D.4(b)): the role of Ca^{2+} in control of muscle contraction and glycogenolysis is described below.

(b) $The regulation of muscle contraction by Ca^{2+}$

In muscle contraction, Ca^{2+} provides the link between the excitation of the muscle by the action potential and the activation of the myofibrillar

ATPase. Some knowledge of the structure of striated muscle is necessary for an appreciation of the problems involved in the control of the contraction process.

(*i*) *The morphology of striated muscle.* This description of the structure of striated muscle is extremely brief and may be supplemented with one of the many reviews on this topic (see, for example, references 31 and 32). Striated muscle is known to consist of regular arrays of two types of protein filament, A and I, which consist mainly of the proteins myosin and actin, respectively (see Figure 4.14). As the muscle contracts, the I filaments move further into

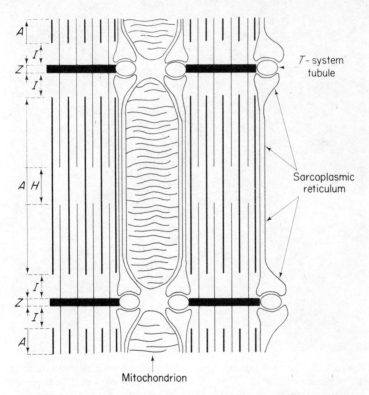

Figure 4.14. A diagrammatic representation of part of a muscle fibre

the spaces between the A filaments, so that the length of overlap is greater and there is shortening of the total length of the bundle of filaments and hence, of the muscle as a whole. A complete muscle fibre consists of many myofibrils separated from each other by longitudinal regions containing mitochondria and the vesicular sarcoplasmic reticulum. Electron micrographs of sections of striated muscle show the presence of invaginations of

REGULATION IN METABOLISM

the plasma membrane to form narrow tubules which project radially into the fibre.[31] These tubules (T-system) occur repeatedly along the length of the fibre in register with the myofibrillar striations. Closely associated with the tubules are the terminal cisternae of the sarcoplasmic reticulum. There is probably a functional link between the transverse tubules and these vesicles. The close association of the transverse tubules and a pair of cisternae produces a system of easily recognizable structural units, which are known as triads (Figure 4.15).

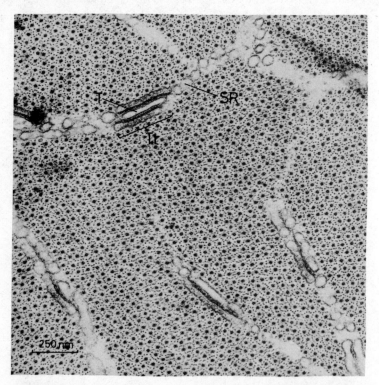

Figure 4.15. Electron micrograph of leg muscle of the water bug showing the structure of a triad. T.S. pleurotrochanteral muscle of *Lethocerus cordofanus* showing the regular array of A- and I-filaments and the T-system (T), a triad (Tr) and the sarcoplasmic reticulum (SR). The electron micrograph was kindly supplied by Dr M. Cullen of the A.R.C. Unit, Zoology Dept, Oxford

(*ii*) *The regulation of contraction and relaxation in muscle.* The discovery of the T-system provided the answer to the problem of how changes initiated by the action potential along the cell membrane could rapidly produce effects on the myofibrillar system in the interior of the fibre. A. V. Hill[33] showed that inward diffusion of an activating substance from the extracellular space could not take place sufficiently rapidly in a striated muscle cell to account for the speed of contraction following the arrival of the action potential. However, if the depolarization of the plasma membrane is conducted into the interior of the fibre along the membranes of the T-system, the rapidity of the contractile response is explained. In general, it is found that the more rapid is the response of the muscle, the more extensive is its T-system.[31]

Several lines of evidence now indicate that this depolarization of the T-system membrane somehow causes a release of Ca^{2+} from the vesicles of the sarcoplasmic reticulum which are in close contact with the tubules. As a result, the concentration of Ca^{2+} in the sarcoplasm, which surrounds the actin and myosin filaments, is increased and this causes a stimulation of the enzyme known as myofibrillar (or actomyosin) ATPase. The energy derived from ATP hydrolysis is utilized for the microscopic changes within the filaments that are responsible for the process of contraction. Relaxation of the muscle is brought about by a reduction in the sarcoplasmic Ca^{2+} concentration which decreases the activity of the myofibrillar ATPase. The fall in the sarcoplasmic concentration of Ca^{2+} occurs because there is a continual removal of these ions by the sarcoplasmic reticulum. This uptake is an energy-requiring process and Ca^{2+} ions are accumulated within the reticulum against a concentration gradient. The effect of the action potential may cause a transitory increase in the permeability of the sarcoplasmic reticulum to Ca^{2+} ions so that their passive release down the massive concentration gradient is markedly accelerated for a very short period of time. The result is that a pulse of Ca^{2+} is released into the sarcoplasm. Immediately after the action potential has passed, the *status quo* is restored: the rate of active uptake of Ca^{2+} once more exceeds the rate of release and the sarcoplasmic concentration gradually falls (see references 34, 35 and 36 for reviews). The sarcoplasmic reticulum has the ability to reduce the concentration of Ca^{2+} in the sarcoplasm to 10^{-8} M or lower. The effect of the action potential is to increase the concentration of Ca^{2+} in the sarcoplasm to 10^{-6} M or higher. This range of Ca^{2+} concentration (10^{-8} M to 10^{-6} M) is precisely the range which *in vitro* activates myofibrillar ATPase. Therefore, there is strong evidence for a physiological role of this activating effect of Ca^{2+}.

It may seem somewhat incongruous that changes in Ca^{2+} concentration in a specific compartment of the cell (the sarcoplasm) can be accurately determined when it is not possible to determine the changes in many other cellular constituents (such as ATP) in that compartment. However, the process of muscular contraction is unusual in that the control mechanism is fairly amenable to experimental investigation. In particular, three types of experiment provide information on the magnitude of the changes in Ca^{2+} concentration during contraction and relaxation.

(*a*) A number of *in vitro* preparations of the contractile system of muscle (for example, purified actomyosin, glycerol extracted fibres and myofibrils) can be made to contract and to perform work if provided with ATP and Ca^{2+}. In particular, they respond to an increase in Ca^{2+} concentration from 10^{-8} to 10^{-6} M (see reference 37 and Figure 4.16).

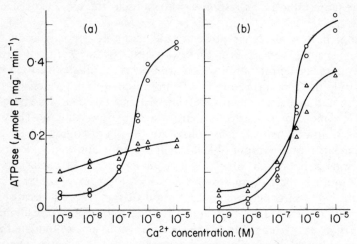

Figure 4.16. Effect of Ca^{2+} concentration on the ATPase activity of myofibrils from the honey-bee (a) and the locust (b). Protein concentrations, honey-bee leg 0·17 mg/ml, flight 0·11 mg/ml; locust leg 0·26 mg/ml, flight 0·27 mg/ml. Triangles, flight muscle; circles, leg muscle. (Reproduced from R. Tregear, *Proc. Roy. Soc.*, **B169**, 229 (1968) (Figure 2) by permission of The Royal Society, London)

(*b*) It is possible to buffer the Ca^{2+} concentration by the use of a compound with a high affinity for Ca^{2+} (for example, EGTA). Such buffers are similar in principle to H^+ buffers and are particularly useful for maintaining a reasonably precise concentration of Ca^{2+} when the absolute concentration is very low. Buffered solutions of Ca^{2+} have been injected into single muscle fibres in the crab *Maia squinado*.[38] These classic experiments demonstrated that contraction of the intact muscle fibre occurs when the injected solutions contained Ca^{2+} buffered at about 10^{-6} M. Also, the application of similar concentrations of Ca^{2+} to the surface of frog muscles, which had had the sarcolemma removed by microdissection (skinned fibres), caused contraction: this effect was reversible, indicating that the applied Ca^{2+} was rapidly removed from the myofibrillar region.[39]

(*c*) Two calcium 'indicators' have been extremely useful in providing evidence for the intracellular role of Ca^{2+}. They are known as murexide, whose absorption spectrum changes upon binding Ca^{2+}, and aequorin, a compound which fluoresces when it binds Ca^{2+}. If murexide is injected into toads it finds its way into the muscle fibres; aequorin, on the other hand, has been microinjected into large barnacle muscle fibres. Isolated preparations of muscle fibres that contain these indicators can be electrically stimulated and the spectral or fluorescence change in the specific compound followed. Such experiments have shown that the spectral or fluorescence change occurs before the increase in tension and the extent of this change is proportional to the amount of tension that is developed.[40,41]

Finally, calculations show that the concentration of Ca^{2+} inside the reticulum during relaxation must be about 10^{-3} M in order to account for the size of the Ca^{2+} pulse when the muscle is stimulated. *In vitro* experiments with the sarcoplasmic reticulum have shown that it is indeed able to accumulate Ca^{2+} to such a concentration. Also the rate of removal of Ca^{2+} by the sarcoplasmic reticulum *in vitro* (about 60 μmol Ca^{2+}/min/mg protein) is sufficient to account for the speed of relaxation observed *in vivo*.[34,35,36] Thus, there can be little doubt that Ca^{2+} is responsible for the control of contraction and relaxation in muscle.

(c) The control of phosphorylase b kinase by Ca^{2+}

Electrical stimulation of isolated muscle preparations results in accelerated glycogenolysis which is accompanied by an increase in the proportions of both phosphorylase and phosphorylase *b* kinase in the active forms. Since there is no change in the intracellular content of cyclic AMP under these conditions, this compound cannot be responsible for the activation of *b* kinase (Table 4.6).[25] The earlier work on the activation of *b* kinase by Ca^{2+} *in vitro*[6] coupled with the knowledge that changes in the intracellular Ca^{2+} concentration control the contraction process of muscle (see above), suggested that the increase in activity of *b* kinase caused by electrical stimulation was due to the increase in the concentration of Ca^{2+} in the sarcoplasm. Unfortunately there were two major problems associated with this simple extrapolation of *in vitro* properties to the control of phosphorylase *b* kinase within the muscle fibres. First, the concentration of Ca^{2+} that caused activation of phosphorylase *b* kinase *in vitro* was about 10^{-3} M, whereas an extremely low concentration of Ca^{2+} (10^{-7} to 10^{-6} M) is required for the stimulation of muscle contraction (see above). Second, the activation of phosphorylase *b* kinase by Ca^{2+} was irreversible: after incubation with Ca^{2+}, addition of chelating agents (EDTA, EGTA) did not decrease phosphorylase *b* kinase activity. At this stage of the investigations it was questionable whether this Ca^{2+} effect on *b* kinase had a physiological basis. Such doubts were reinforced when it became apparent that the protein factor that was necessary for the activation by Ca^{2+} (a so-called 'kinase activating factor' or KAF) was probably an intracellular proteolytic enzyme dependent upon Ca^{2+} for its activity. (The *in vitro* effect of 10^{-3} M Ca^{2+} was probably similar to the effect of trypsin—see p. 162.)

If the Ca^{2+} effect was unphysiological, there remained the question of the factor responsible for the increased b kinase activity when muscle was electrically stimulated. The problem was solved by Ebashi and his coworkers.[42] They found that phosphorylase b kinase *is* activated by Ca^{2+} at about 10^{-7}–10^{-6} M. In order to show this it was necessary to remove all traces of contaminating Ca^{2+} from the assay system. In all previous experiments there must have been sufficient Ca^{2+} present to cause complete activation so that any further activation was not detected until the Ca^{2+} concentration reached 10^{-3} M, when proteolytic activation occurred. The use of Ca^{2+}–EGTA buffers allowed the concentration of added Ca^{2+} to be carefully controlled in the range 10^{-8}–10^{-5} M. The effect of increasing the concentration of added Ca^{2+} is shown in Figure 4.17. This activation by

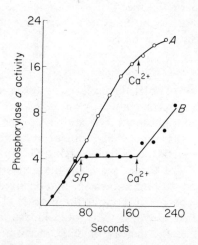

Figure 4.17. Ca^{2+}-dependent reversal of the inhibition of phosphorylase b kinase by sarcoplasmic reticulum. The initial reaction mixture contained the following components: phosphorylase b, 100,000 Cori units per ml; ATP, 1·4 mM; magnesium acetate, 4·6 mM; Tris, 20 mM; and glycerol-P, 30 mM. The mixture was warmed to 30 °C and the reaction started by the addition of 2·0 μg/ml of nonactivated phosphorylase b kinase. The reaction was run at pH 7·6 with aliquots being taken at intervals for the determination of phosphorylase a activity. At 70 s of reaction time freshly isolated sarcoplasmic reticulum (SR) was added at a final concentration of 2·7 mg of protein per ml. Curve A represents a control without added sarcoplasmic reticulum. Curve B represents the effect of sarcoplasmic reticulum upon phosphorylase b kinase before and after the addition of 5×10^{-4} M Ca^{2+}. The latter curve is corrected for a control run in the absence of added phosphorylase b kinase[43]

low concentrations of Ca^{2+} (unlike the effect at 10^{-3} M) is reversible and does not require any additional protein factor. The early results of Ebashi and coworkers were confirmed and extended by Krebs and coworkers.[43]

They have shown that both active and inactive phosphorylase b kinases are stimulated by low concentrations of Ca^{2+}. Thus, there is substantial evidence that the *in vitro* effects of 10^{-7}–10^{-6} M Ca^{2+} on phosphorylase b kinase activity are of physiological importance.

5. Summary

There are three main mechanisms by which the activity of phosphorylase is controlled in muscle: metabolite control, hormonal control and nervous control.

(a) Metabolite control

Phosphorylase b can be controlled by changes in the concentrations of ATP, AMP, P_i or glucose-6-phosphate. This is considered to be a primitive mechanism of control in which factors that increase the utilization of energy by the muscle (such as contraction) will increase phosphorylase activity in concert with the change in activity of PFK, so that glycogenolysis and glycolysis will be stimulated simultaneously. The mechanism is therefore independent of hormonal or nervous control.

(b) Hormonal control

Muscle phosphorylase activity is controlled by adrenaline, whose action mobilizes the carbohydrate stores for anticipated mechanical activity (such as flight from a predator). This is brought about by a stimulation of adenyl cyclase which results in an increase in cyclic AMP and activation of protein kinase. Active protein kinase catalyses the phosphorylation of inactive phosphorylase b kinase to form active phosphorylase b kinase, which in turn catalyses the phosphorylation of phosphorylase b to phosphorylase a. Hence, glycogenolysis is stimulated. Thus, for a short period of time, the primitive control of phosphorylase is bypassed and glycogen is degraded despite high concentrations of ATP and glucose-6-phosphate.

(c) Nervous control

The conduction of a nervous impulse to a muscle results in the generation of an action potential along the plasma membrane and this is conducted into the interior of the muscle by means of the T-system. Information is then transferred (by some mechanism as yet unknown) to the sarcoplasmic reticulum causing the release of Ca^{2+} which simultaneously activates the myofibrillar ATPase system (resulting in contraction) and phosphorylase b kinase. Thus, the cyclic AMP-protein kinase system is bypassed and both inactive phosphorylase b kinase and active phosphorylase b kinase (which may already have been formed in response to adrenaline secretion) are stimulated by Ca^{2+} ions. As a result phosphorylase b is converted to phosphorylase a and glycogenolysis is stimulated.

E. CONTROL OF GLYCOGEN SYNTHESIS IN MUSCLE

1. Historical introduction

The reactions involved in the pathway of glycogen synthesis and the evidence which indicates that glucosyltransferase is a regulatory enzyme for this pathway have been described in Section A. Only two years after glucosyltransferase was discovered it was found to be activated by glucose-6-phosphate.[44] This property provided the basis for a theory of control of the enzyme activity through changes in the intracellular concentration of glucose-6-phosphate. More recently this enzyme has been shown to exist in two enzymatically interconvertible forms, one of which requires glucose-6-phosphate for activity, whilst the other is active in its absence. The proportion of the enzyme in either form depends upon the activities of the interconverting enzymes and these can be modified by certain hormones, particularly insulin.

As early as 1926, Best and coworkers observed that insulin could increase the amount of glycogen in muscle in an eviscerated animal. In 1940, Gemmill showed that with the incubated rat diaphragm as much as 92 % of the 'extra' glucose taken up in the presence of insulin could be converted to glycogen (see reference 45 for a review of this early work). This was the first indication that insulin could have a specific effect upon glycogen synthesis. However, the demonstration that insulin could stimulate the membrane transport of glucose into the muscle cell suggested that many, if not all, of the observed effects of insulin could be explained through its action on the membrane. Consequently, the early experiments of Gemmill on glycogen synthesis were largely ignored. In 1959, Larner and colleagues confirmed the work of Gemmill and also demonstrated that increasing glucose uptake by raising the external concentration of glucose did not stimulate glycogen synthesis to the same extent as did insulin.[46] A year or so later, Villar-Palasi and Larner showed that after treatment of the rat diaphragm with insulin the activity of glucosyltransferase in extracts of the diaphragm was markedly increased. However, this stimulation was only observed when the assays were performed in the absence of glucose-6-phosphate: in the presence of this compound, the activity of the transferase was increased, but the effect of insulin was no longer apparent. The activity of the enzyme assayed in the absence of glucose-6-phosphate was concluded to be entirely due to a form of the enzyme which was independent of glucose-6-phosphate (the so-called I form), whereas the activity in the presence of the compound was due to the total enzyme activity—that is, independent plus dependent forms (I + D). The fact that insulin did not increase the total activity of the enzyme suggested that it increased the proportion of the enzyme in the independent form.[46] The two forms were eventually isolated and their characteristic properties studied (see Table 4.8). The main difference between the two forms is that, in the absence of glucose-6-phosphate, the maximum catalytic activity of the D form is very much smaller than that of the I form.[47] Since these earlier studies, research has concentrated on the isolation and properties of the interconverting enzymes. Also the properties of glucosyltransferase-D have been studied in greater detail.

Table 4.8. The effect of glucose-6-phosphate on the K_m and V_{max} values for the dependent (D) and independent (I) forms of UDPG-glucosyltransferase[47]

	Independent form		Dependent form	
		Glucose-6-phosphate		Glucose-6-phosphate
	No addition		No addition	
K_m for UDP-glucose (mM)	1·0	0·2	0·6	0·4
V_{max} (μmol/mg protein/hr)	2·3	2·3	0·27	1·80

2. Properties and theory of regulation of glucosyltransferase-D

The dependent form of glucosyltransferase is activated by low concentrations of glucose-6-phosphate ($K_a < 0.1$ mM) and, since the concentration of glucose-6-phosphate in muscle can be calculated to be between 0·2 and 0·4 mM (0·2 μmol/g fresh muscle), it would be expected that this form of the enzyme would always be active *in vivo*. However, glucosyltransferase-D is inhibited very strongly by ATP, ADP and inorganic phosphate.[48] Glucose-6-phosphate overcomes the inhibition by ATP, etc., but only when it is present at high concentrations (above 10 mM). Thus, it can be concluded that under most physiological conditions the D form of the enzyme is almost totally inactive.

In contrast, the I form of the enzyme shows only a small degree of inhibition by ATP, ADP and P_i and this inhibition appears to be independent of the concentration of glucose-6-phosphate. The maximum difference in activities between the two forms of the enzyme in the presence of 6 mM ATP occurs when the glucose-6-phosphate concentration is within the physiological range (0·2–0·4 mM).

3. Evidence for enzymatic interconversions of glucosyltransferase

The incubation of a fresh muscle extract for about 30 minutes causes a transition of glucosyltransferase-D into the I form. (The two forms are easily distinguished by their behaviour in the absence of glucose-6-phosphate, when only the I form is measured, and in the presence of glucose-6-phosphate when the activity of both forms is measured.) Addition of ATP–Mg^{2+} to incubated extracts stimulates the reverse process—that is, the I form is converted to the D form. These observations suggested that the D-to-I conversion involves a phosphatase enzyme, whilst the I-to-D conversion involves a phosphokinase enzyme. This was confirmed as follows: after centrifugation of muscle extracts at 100,000g for 1 hour, the supernatant contains the glucosyltransferase and phosphokinase activities, but the phosphatase activity (D-to-I conversion) is not present.[49] Incubation of this supernatant preparation with ATP labelled with ^{32}P in the γ (terminal) phosphate group resulted in the incorporation of ^{32}P from ATP into protein (presumably glucosyltransferase). This incorporation accompanied the I-to-D transition. The labelled protein was purified on a DEAE-cellulose column and the radioactivity was found to be in the same fractions as the glucosyltransferase activity. Finally, the incubation of this partially purified, labelled glucosyltransferase with fresh muscle extract (which contains the phosphatase activity) resulted in the transition of glucosyltransferase-D to I, and the formation of the I form paralleled the release of labelled P$_i$. Thus, the interconversions of glucosyltransferase can be summarized as follows:

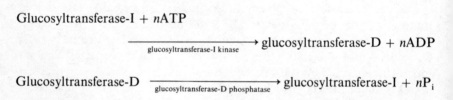

Glucosyltransferase-I + nATP

$$\xrightarrow[\text{glucosyltransferase-I kinase}]{} \text{glucosyltransferase-D} + n\text{ADP}$$

Glucosyltransferase-D $\xrightarrow[\text{glucosyltransferase-D phosphatase}]{}$ glucosyltransferase-I + nP$_i$

Two important points were established from this work. First, the activity of glucosyltransferase could be regulated by enzymatic interconversions in a similar manner to that of glycogen phosphorylase. Second, the two systems differed in one very important aspect: activation of glucosyltransferase (D-to-I conversion) occurs via a phosphatase reaction and inactivation occurs via a kinase reaction. This is the opposite situation to that in the phosphorylase system and it immediately suggests a mechanism for simultaneous activation of phosphorylase and inhibition of glucosyltransferase, and/or vice versa (see Figure 4.18).

The possibility that transferase-I kinase and phosphorylase b kinase might be the same enzyme was naturally investigated and it was established that this was not the case;[50] neither did the two phosphatases possess a common identity. Nonetheless, the exciting prospect of a common control mechanism for both phosphorylase and glucosyltransferase has now been established (see below).

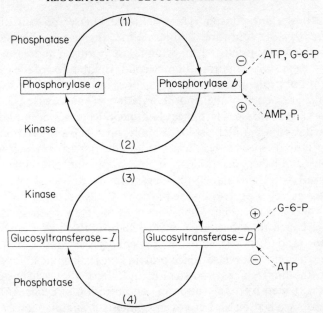

Figure 4.18. Control of phosphorylase and glucosyltransferase via enzyme interconversions and cell metabolites. (1) Phosphorylase *a* phosphatase. (2) Phosphorylase *b* kinase. (3) Glucosyltransferase-I kinase. (4) Glucosyltransferase-D phosphatase

4. Properties and theory of regulation of glucosyltransferase-D phosphatase

There has been little work done on the purification of glucosyltransferase-D phosphatase. However, one important property of the enzyme is known: its activity in crude extracts is inhibited by glycogen in a concentration-dependent manner. Such inhibition can explain the results of Danforth who demonstrated that in rat skeletal muscle there is an inverse relationship between the glycogen content of the muscle and the proportion of transferase in the I form. As the glycogen content of the muscle is increased, the activity of the phosphatase is decreased, so that more of the enzyme will exist as the inactive D form.[51] This represents a feedback regulatory mechanism for control of glycogen synthesis since, as the glycogen stores are increased, more of the glucosyltransferase is converted to the inactive form. Unfortunately, the mechanism by which glycogen is able to inhibit the phosphatase does not appear to have been studied in any detail.

5. Properties and theory of regulation of glucosyltransferase-I kinase

(a) Glucosyltransferase-I kinase and protein kinase

It has recently been discovered that protein kinase and glucosyltransferase-I kinase are the same enzyme.[52,53] The common identity of the glucosyltransferase-I kinase and phosphorylase *b* kinase kinase (protein kinase) was established by the following findings. First, the protein kinase activities towards glucosyltransferase-I, phosphorylase *b* kinase and casein increase equally at each stage of purification. Second, an inhibitor of the cyclic AMP stimulation of protein kinase activity is present in skeletal muscle and this inhibitor affects equally the phosphorylation of glucosyltransferase-I and phosphorylase *b* kinase. Third, heat treatment decreases both phosphorylation activities in a parallel fashion. Finally, both phosphorylation activities exhibit similar specificities towards cyclic nucleotide activation. It has been established also that protein kinase phosphorylates glucosyltransferase-I directly[53] (that is, no other interconverting enzyme is involved). This discovery, that protein kinase phosphorylates both glucosyltransferase and phosphorylase *b* kinase, links the control of glycogen synthesis with that of glycogen degradation: protein kinase is the enzyme which phosphorylates (and therefore activates) phosphorylase *b* kinase, and this in turn activates phosphorylase. Since protein kinase also phosphorylates (and therefore inhibits) glucosyltransferase, it follows that whenever protein kinase is activated by an elevation in concentration of cyclic AMP, glycogenolysis is switched on and glycogen synthesis is simultaneously switched off (Figure 4.19).

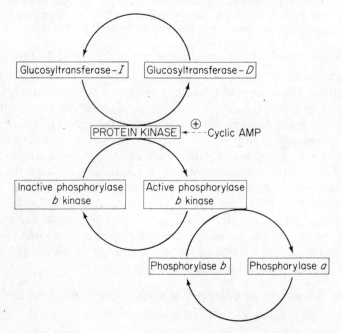

Figure 4.19. The common control of phosphorylase and glucosyl-transferase by protein kinase

This conclusion is supported by the observation that, in rat diaphragm, adrenaline causes a decrease in the amount of glucosyltransferase-I[54] and it is presumed that this is caused by the conversion of some of the I form into D form. Unfortunately, the situation is complicated by the fact that there is a decrease in *total* (I + D) glucosyltransferase in the presence of adrenaline[54] so that it cannot be claimed unequivocally that adrenaline causes the conversion of I to D. However, the fact that protein kinase, which catalyses this I-to-D conversion, is sensitive to cyclic AMP strongly supports the conclusion that adrenaline inhibits the glucosyltransferase activity by stimulation of the I-to-D conversion. The reason for the decrease in total activity (I + D) with adrenaline is unknown, although it would appear to be a physiologically important effect since it is reversed by insulin.

(b) Regulation of protein kinase by insulin

Insulin, when added to intact muscle preparations, stimulates the conversion of glucosyltransferase-D to the I form. Either a stimulation of transferase-D phosphatase or an inhibition of transferase-I kinase would explain these observations. Since little is known of the properties of the phosphatase, it has been largely ignored and attention has been focused upon the properties of transferase-I kinase (protein kinase). The significant property of this enzyme is that it is activated by cyclic AMP. However, it seems unlikely that insulin influences the activity of protein kinase through direct effects on the intracellular concentration of cyclic AMP. First, insulin does not change the cyclic AMP content of muscle,[55,56] although it has been observed to decrease the content in adipose tissue and liver. Second, insulin does not antagonize the action of adrenaline on the conversion of phosphorylase *b* to *a*.[54]

Nevertheless, insulin somehow modifies the catalytic activity of protein kinase in muscle. The first clue to the nature of this effect was provided by the work of Villar-Palasi and Wenger,[57] who obtained evidence for the existence of two forms of protein kinase (glucosyltransferase-I kinase) in muscle. They found that one form of protein kinase was active only in the presence of cyclic AMP, whereas the other form was active even in the absence of cyclic AMP. The proportion of the two forms of the enzyme in the muscle could be altered by the administration of insulin: the amount of the cyclic-AMP-dependent form is increased by insulin. Since insulin does not change the total concentration of cyclic AMP in muscle, the result is a decrease in the activity of protein kinase, a conversion of transferase-D into transferase-I and a consequent increase in glycogen synthesis.

The work of Villar-Palasi and Wenger was carried out before it was known that glucosyltransferase-I kinase was the same enzyme as protein kinase. When this common identity was discovered, it became apparent that insulin could modify the activity of protein kinase via the changes in the equilibrium which probably exists between the associated complex of the regulatory and catalytic subunits and the dissociated subunits.

$$RC + \text{cyclic AMP} \leftrightarrows R\text{–cyclic AMP} + C$$

This reaction has been described in Section D.3(b)(v): RC represents the inactive protein kinase complex and C represents active protein kinase. The two forms of glucosyltransferase-I kinase isolated by Villar-Palasi and Wenger might be equivalent to RC and C, and the effect of insulin would be to modify the equilibrium of this reaction so that the formation of RC was favoured. This mechanism of control by insulin is consistent with the action of adrenaline in overcoming the insulin effect upon glucosyltransferase: as long as the cyclic AMP concentration is elevated sufficiently, it does not matter whether the transferase-I kinase is originally in the RC form or the C form, since conversion to the C form automatically results from the elevation in cyclic AMP.

However, a number of questions remain unanswered even by these latest developments. Why does insulin counteract the effect of adrenaline on the total content of glucosyltransferase (I + D), when it does not appear to modify the effect of adrenaline upon the phosphorylase b to a conversion? Why is there no effect of insulin upon transferase-I kinase in cell-free preparations? This area of enzymology is currently being studied in a number of laboratories and there is little doubt that many problems like these will be clarified in the next few years.

Although the mechanism of the adrenaline-insulin relationship in the control of glycogen metabolism is not yet fully understood at a molecular level, the effects of the hormones fit coherently into a physiological control theory. When carbohydrate is available for the replenishment of the glycogen stores, the circulating levels of insulin are high. Thus, the greater proportion of glucosyltransferase is in the I form (active form) and glycogen is synthesized. In any stress-inducing situation, it is essential that the synthesis of glycogen should cease (at least temporarily) so that it can be mobilized to provide energy for contraction. Adrenaline is released in response to stress and it both overcomes the stimulatory effects of insulin upon glycogen synthesis and switches on glycogenolysis. If the danger passes, the adrenaline stimulus is removed and, since the insulin levels remain high, glycogen synthesis is immediately restored. When the carbohydrate intake is decreased (for example, during the diurnal fast), the circulating insulin levels fall and glycogen synthesis is depressed. The supreme importance of the 'flight or fight' response explains why insulin plays a subservient role in the control of glycogen metabolism: it neither inhibits the activation of phosphorylase by adrenaline nor does it stimulate glycogen synthesis if the adrenaline levels are high.

REFERENCES FOR CHAPTER 4

1. Potter, V. R. & Ono, T. (1961). *Cold Spring Harbor Symp. Quant. Biol.* **26,** 355.
2. Rohr, P., Saint-Saens, M. & Monod, H. (1966). *J. Physiol. Paris,* **58,** 5.
3. Xenophon. *Anabasis III,* Books I–VII, p. 47. Translated into English by Carleton L. Brownson. Trans. publd. London: Heinemann (1922).
4. Hornbrook, K. R., Burch, H. B. & Lowry, O. H. (1966). *Molecular Pharmacology,* **2,** 106.
5. Stetten, D. & Stetten, M. R. (1960). *Physiol. Rev.* **40,** 505.
6. Krebs, E. G. & Fischer, E. H. (1962). *Adv. Enzymol.* **24,** 263.
7. Sutherland, E. W. (1962). *Harvey Lectures,* **57,** 17.
8. Cori, G. T. & Cori, C. F. (1945). *J. biol. Chem.* **158,** 321; and Green, A. A. & Cori, G. T. (1943). *J. biol. Chem.* **151,** 21.
9. Fischer, E. H. & Krebs, E. G. (1955). *J. biol. Chem.* **216,** 113, 121.
10. Bergmeyer, H. U. (1963). In *Methods of Enzymatic Analysis.* Ed. H. U. Bergmeyer. London: Academic Press.
11. Lyon, J. B. & Porter, J. (1963). *J. biol. Chem.* **238,** 1.
12. Danforth, W. H. & Lyon, J. B. (1964). *J. biol. Chem.* **239,** 4047.
13. Morgan, H. E. & Parmeggiani, A. (1964). In *Control of Glycogen Metabolism,* p. 254. Ed. W. J. Whelan. London: Churchill.
14. Morgan, H. E. & Parmeggiani, A. (1964). *J. biol. Chem.* **239,** 2440.
15. Nolan, C., Novoa, W. B., Krebs, E. G. & Fischer, E. H. (1964). *Biochemistry,* **3,** 542.
16. Fischer, E. H., Pocker, A. & Saari, J. C. (1970). *Essays in Biochem.* **6,** 23. Ed. P. N. Campbell & F. Dickens. London: Academic Press.
17. Krebs, E. G., Gonzalez, C., Posner, J. B., Love, D. S., Bratvold, G. E. & Fischer, E. H. (1964). In *Control of Glycogen Metabolism,* p. 200. Ed. W. J. Whelan. London: Churchill.
18. Walsh, D. A., Perkins, J. P. & Krebs, E. G. (1968). *J. biol. Chem.* **243,** 3763.
19. Walsh, D. A., Perkins, J. P., Brostrom, C. O., Ho, E. S. & Krebs, E. G. (1971). *J. biol. Chem.* **246,** 1968; and Reimann, E. M., Walsh, D. A. & Krebs, E. G. (1971). *J. biol. Chem.* **246,** 1968.
20. Sutherland, E. W., Øye, I. & Butcher, R. W. (1965). *Rec. Progr. Horm. Res.* **21,** 623.
21. Robison, G. A., Butcher, R. W. & Sutherland, E. W. (1971). *Cyclic AMP.* New York & London: Academic Press.
22. Sutherland, E. W., Rall, T. W. & Menon, T. (1962). *J. biol. Chem.* **237,** 1220.
23. Davoren, P. R. & Sutherland, E. W. (1963). *J. biol. Chem.* **238,** 3016.
24. Drummond, G. I., Harwood, J. P. & Powell, C. A. (1969). *J. biol. Chem.* **244,** 4235.
25. Posner, J. B., Stern, R. & Krebs, E. G. (1965). *J. biol. Chem.* **240,** 982.
26. Macfarlane, R. F. (1964). *Nature, Lond.* **202,** 498.
27. Bowness, J. M. (1966). *Science, N.Y.* **152,** 1370.
28. Holzer, H. (1969). *Advances in Enzymology,* **32,** 297.
29. Brostrom, C. O., Corbin, J. D., King, C. A. & Krebs, E. G. (1971). *Proc. Nat. Acad. Sci. U.S.* **68,** 2444.
30. Chelala, C. A. & Torres, H. N. (1969). *Biochim. Biophys. Acta,* **178,** 423.
31. Smith, D. S. (1966). *Progr. Biophys. Mol. Biol.* **16,** 107.
32. Franzini-Armstrong, C. & Porter, K. R. (1964). *Nature, Lond.* **202,** 355.
33. Hill, A. V. (1949). *Proc. Roy. Soc. B,* **136,** 399.
34. Weber, A. (1966). *Current Topics in Bioenergetics,* vol. 1, p. 203. Ed. D. R. Sanadi. New York: Academic Press.
35. Ebashi, S. & Endo, M. (1968). *Progr. Biophys. Mol. Biol.* **18,** 123.
36. Hasselbach, W. (1964). *Progr. Biophys. Mol. Biol.* **14,** 167.

37. Pringle, J. W. S. (1967). *Progr. Biophys. Mol. Biol.* **17**, 1.
38. Portzehl, H., Caldwell, P. C. & Rüegg, J. C. (1964). *Biochim. Biophys. Acta*, **79**, 581.
39. Podolsky, R. J. & Costantin, L. L. (1964). *Fed. Proc.* **23**, 933.
40. Jöbsis, F. F. & O'Connor, M. J. (1966). *Biochem. Biophys. Res. Commun.* **25**, 246.
41. Ashley, C. C. (1971). *Endeavour*, **30**, 18.
42. Ozawa, E., Hosoi, E. & Ebashi, S. (1967). *J. biochem.* (*Tokyo*), **61**, 531.
43. Brostrom, C. O., Hunkeler, F. L. & Krebs, E. G. (1971). *J. biol. Chem.* **246**, 1961.
44. Leloir, L. F., Olavarria, J. M., Goldemberg, S. H. & Carminatti, H. (1959). *Arch. Biochem. Biophys.* **81**, 508.
45. Villar-Palasi, C. & Larner, J. (1968). *Vitamins & Hormones*, **26**, 65.
46. Larner, J., Rosell-Perez, M., Friedman, D. L. & Craig, J. W. (1964). In *Control of Glycogen Metabolism*, p. 273. Ed. W. J. Whelan. London: Churchill.
47. Rosell-Perez, M., Villar-Palasi, C. & Larner, J. (1962). *Biochemistry*, **1**, 763.
48. Piras, R., Rothman, L. B. & Cabib, E. (1968). *Biochemistry*, **7**, 56.
49. Friedman, D. L. & Larner, J. (1963). *Biochemistry*, **2**, 669.
50. Friedman, D. L. & Larner, J. (1965). *Biochemistry*, **4**, 2261.
51. Danforth, W. (1965). *J. biol. Chem.* **240**, 588.
52. Schlender, K. K., Wei, J. H. & Villar-Palasi, C. (1969). *Biochim. Biophys. Acta*, **191**, 272.
53. Soderling, T. R., Hickenbottom, J. P., Reimann, E. M., Hunkeler, F. L., Walsh, D. A. & Krebs, E. G. (1970). *J. biol. Chem.* **245**, 6317.
54. Craig, J. W. & Larner, J. (1964). *Nature, Lond.* **202**, 971.
55. Craig, J. W., Rall, T. W. & Larner, J. (1969). *Biochim. Biophys. Acta*, **177**, 213.
56. Goldberg, N. D., Villar-Palasi, C., Sasko, H. & Larner, J. (1967). *Biochim. Biophys. Acta*, **148**, 665.
57. Villar-Palasi, C. & Wenger, J. I. (1967). *Fed. Proc.* **26**, 563.
58. Crabtree, B. & Newsholme, E. A. (1972). *Biochem. J.* **126**, 49.
59. Start, C. & Newsholme, E. A. (1970). *FEBS Letters*, **6**, 171.
60. Crabtree, B. & Newsholme, E. A. (1972). *Biochem. J.* **130**, 697.

CHAPTER 5

ADIPOSE TISSUE AND THE REGULATION OF FAT METABOLISM

A. GENERAL INTRODUCTION

Adipose tissue is a highly specialized tissue which has developed particularly in mammals and birds for the purpose of storing fat to supply energy for the whole animal. White adipose tissue consists of aggregates of spherical cells whose most striking feature is a single large lipid droplet which in the fed state fills most of the cell (Figure 5.1). The somewhat flattened nucleus is found in the narrow band of cytoplasm around the periphery. These lipid-containing cells are found in many parts of the body but tend to be concentrated in certain regions—for example, under the skin (subcutaneous adipose

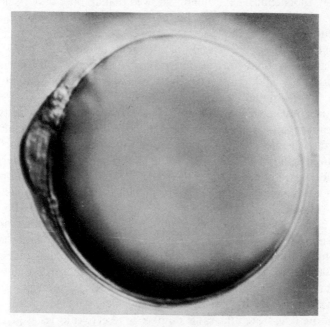

Figure 5.1. Interference contrast photograph of a white adipose tissue cell. Note the spherical lipid droplet which fills most of the cell. The photograph was kindly supplied by Professor C. N. Hales, Department of Chemical Pathology, The Welsh National School of Medicine, Cardiff

tissue) and around internal organs (heart, kidneys). The amount of sub-cutaneous adipose tissue varies considerably from species to species (and even between individuals from the same species according to the dietary intake) but it is approximately inversely proportional to the amount of body hair.

Adipose tissue was recognized as a lipid-rich tissue many years ago, but until the 1930s the general view was that it consisted of connective tissue in which droplets of fat had been deposited. It was thought that adipose tissue was metabolically inert, since it appeared to possess only a meagre supply of nerves and blood capillaries. During the following twenty years or so evidence began to accumulate which suggested that, on the contrary, the tissue was metabolically active and had a highly specialized role to play in caloric homeostasis of the animal. This evidence was collated and discussed in a classic review by Wertheimer and Shapiro[1] in 1948 and is only briefly reiterated here.

The transplant studies of Hauseberger showed that adipose tissue cells were not derived from connective tissue but from special primitive fat cells. Microscopy showed that the tissue possessed a liberal supply of nerves and capillaries. Biochemical experiments showed that adipose tissue was capable not only of taking up fat from the blood, but also of releasing fat (in the form of fatty acids) into the blood. Moreover the mobilization of fat was not dependent upon the concentration of fatty acids in the blood, but was under nervous and hormonal control. The turnover studies of Schoenheimer and Rittenberg[2] showed that although the total amount of depot fat may remain constant, it is continually being synthesized and degraded.

Thus the present view of adipose tissue is that it is a highly active tissue whose main functions are on the one hand lipid synthesis and storage, and on the other the mobilization of this stored fuel for the provision of energy. The accumulation of fat is a highly efficient means of storing energy since more calories are released upon the oxidation of one gram of fat (9·3 kcal) than one gram of carbohydrate (3·7 kcal). This is because energy is released when $C-C$ and $C-H$ bonds are oxidized to $C-O$ and $O-H$ bonds and, since fat contains proportionately more $C-C$ and $C-H$ bonds than carbo-hydrate, more energy is obtained from the oxidation of fat. Since fat is not water soluble it needs no associated water for storage and fat stores contain almost 100% lipid. These two factors contribute to the fact that fat is almost nine-fold more efficient than carbohydrate as a biological energy store.[3] This means that an average 70 kg man may store sufficient fuel for at least 40 days of starvation. If he stored the same number of reserve calories as glycogen he would weight approximately 140 kg! The stored fat can supply energy not only for periods of prolonged starvation or hibernation, but also for sustained muscular activity. In man, the latter may be for an inessential activity (such as marathon-running), but in many animals it is essential in the constant search for food and in certain species of birds, fish and insects it is vital for migration. It may also be important in dispersal and in mating. Although adipose tissue is not generally found in lower orders of animals, fat may be stored in large quantities in the liver, in muscle or in specialized organs like the insect fat body: the latter performs the combined functions of liver and adipose tissue.

Apart from its function as an energy storehouse, adipose tissue acts as a mechanical buffer for the protection of delicate internal organs like the heart and kidneys, and as a lubricant in the joints. The subcutaneous fat provides not only energy but also insulation against heat loss. The distribution and ease of mobilization of subcutaneous fat is governed not only by nervous and hormonal influences but also by hereditary and sexual factors. In addition to white adipose tissue, there occurs in certain species (for example, hibernators and rodents) a brown adipose tissue which is both histologically and metabolically different from white adipose tissue. The metabolism of brown adipose tissue is discussed in Section D.

1. Origins of stored triglyceride

(a) Dietary fat

(i) *Absorption in the gut.* The exogenous triglyceride of the diet is a major source of stored fat. Since the dietary triglyceride may amount to 150 g per day in man, the absorption of this fat through the gut, and its assimilation into the depot stores, is of obvious quantitative importance. Current theories of the mechanism of dietary fat absorption and assimilation are discussed in a recent review by Johnston.[4] In the duodenum the dietary fat is mixed with pancreatic lipase and bile salts. Monoglycerides and fatty acids are the main products of triglyceride hydrolysis and, with their production, the mixture separates into two phases: the oil phase contains unhydrolysed diglyceride and triglyceride while the clear solution contains minute (50 Å diameter) polymolecular aggregates termed micelles. These micelles consist of monoglycerides, fatty acids and bile salts. The lipase continues to act upon the remaining triglyceride in the oil phase, most of which is eventually degraded to monoglycerides and fatty acids. The micelles interact in some way with the coating on the villi of the intestinal epithelial cells and the monoglycerides and fatty acids enter the cells by passive diffusion, apparently in the free form rather than as intact micelles (although this point is still debated). Small quantities of diglyceride and triglyceride may also be absorbed into the epithelial cells, without further hydrolysis, by virtue of their slight solubility in the micellar solution.

Inside the epithelial cells triglycerides are resynthesized mainly from the monoglycerides and fatty acids. This is achieved by direct esterification involving monoglycerides and fatty acyl-CoA (Figure 5.2). Another fate is open to fatty acids upon entry into the epithelial cell: they may escape esterification and enter the portal blood unchanged. The proportion of any

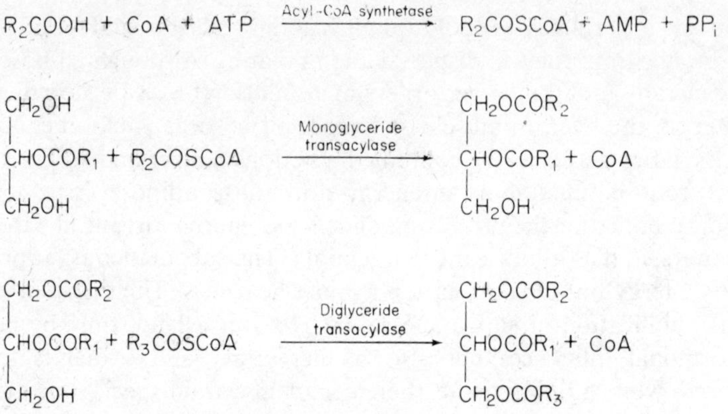

$$R_2COOH + CoA + ATP \xrightarrow{\text{Acyl-CoA synthetase}} R_2COSCoA + AMP + PP_i$$

$$\begin{array}{c} CH_2OH \\ | \\ CHOCOR_1 \\ | \\ CH_2OH \end{array} + R_2COSCoA \xrightarrow[\text{transacylase}]{\text{Monoglyceride}} \begin{array}{c} CH_2OCOR_2 \\ | \\ CHOCOR_1 \\ | \\ CH_2OH \end{array} + CoA$$

$$\begin{array}{c} CH_2OCOR_2 \\ | \\ CHOCOR_1 \\ | \\ CH_2OH \end{array} + R_3COSCoA \xrightarrow[\text{transacylase}]{\text{Diglyceride}} \begin{array}{c} CH_2OCOR_2 \\ | \\ CHOCOR_1 \\ | \\ CH_2OCOR_3 \end{array} + CoA$$

Figure 5.2. The monoglyceride shunt pathway

particular fatty acid which is esterified depends upon its affinity for the esterifying enzymes. It appears that in general the longer chain fatty acids (above C_{10}) are esterified whilst the shorter chain ones (which are found in high proportion in certain foods, such as butter) tend to be conveyed to the liver in the portal blood.

The triglycerides formed in the epithelial cells collect in the endoplasmic reticulum of these cells where they acquire a coat composed largely of protein and phospholipid. The resulting particles, which are commonly called *chylomicrons*, leave the cell by a process which is not clearly understood. They are *not* removed by the portal blood but enter the intestinal lymph vessels. Chylomicron formation and transport in the lymphatic system is quantitatively the more important pathway of fat absorption since 90% of the ingested lipid probably enters the circulation in the form of chylomicrons, the remaining 10% being absorbed in the form of fatty acids.[5]

Any fatty acids which escape esterification within the epithelial cell could theoretically either diffuse into the lymph vessels or into the blood capillaries. The available evidence suggests that only a small proportion of the fatty acids enter the lymph vessels: most of them enter the blood where they combine with albumin and are transported to the liver. In the liver these fatty acids may be either oxidized or utilized in the synthesis of triglyceride or phospholipid (see Figure 5.3). In a well-fed animal it is likely that most of these fatty acids will be esterified. However, the liver has a limited capacity for storage of triglyceride and any excess is secreted into the blood in the form of very-low-density lipoprotein (VLDL). The latter is a complex of triglyceride and a special protein that is synthesized in the liver. Thus, it is in these two forms (VLDL and chylomicrons) that the dietary lipid is made available via the blood stream to adipose tissue for storage.

(ii) *Uptake of triglyceride by tissues.* The lymphatic fluid in the thoracic duct is emptied into the left subclavian vein and here the chylomicrons enter the

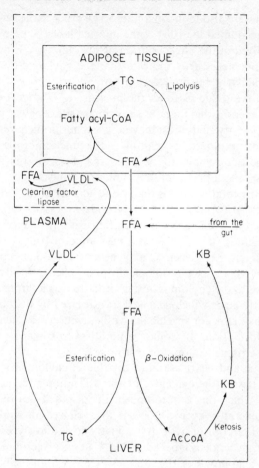

Figure 5.3. Role of the liver in the uptake and esterification of fatty acids derived from the gut or adipose tissue. TG represents triglyceride; FFA represents fatty acid; KB represents ketone bodies

plasma, giving it a milky appearance which clears as they are removed. The removal of the chylomicrons from the blood is a very efficient process, the half-life of the particles being about 10 minutes. The immediate fate of these particles has been in dispute for many years. One experimental approach to this problem is to inject labelled chylomicrons into the intact animal and study their distribution. Such experiments have indicated that the liver is an important site of chylomicron uptake, as much as 30% of the label appearing in the hepatic lipids only 20 minutes after injection of the chylomicrons.

Labelled lipids were also found in a number of other tissues, notably adipose tissue, which accounted for 10% of the injected label.[6] There are two major problems involved in the interpretation of such findings. First, the presence of label does not necessarily indicate that the chylomicron triglyceride is present intracellularly, but may result from adsorption or 'trapping' of the particle within the tissue. Second, the presence of labelled triglyceride in a tissue does not identify that tissue as the primary site of chylomicron removal, since recycling of fatty acids must inevitably occur during *in vivo* experiments.

Several important questions relating to the function of the liver in chylomicron metabolism remain to be answered. First, is the liver normally responsible for the uptake of chylomicron triglyceride? Second, what proportion of the total uptake is due to the activity of the liver; and finally, is extracellular hydrolysis of the triglyceride necessary for the uptake of triglyceride by the liver? After a comprehensive review of the literature, Robinson[6] concludes that in the rat a maximum of 10–15% of the injected dose of chylomicron triglyceride may be initially taken up by the liver. Indeed it would seem to be physiologically desirable that the liver should take up at least some of the chylomicrons, in order to extract from the dietary fat the *essential* fatty acids which *cannot* be synthesized by the body. Such fatty acids are then available for specific biosynthetic purposes (such as membrane phospholipid formation). It would be pointless to transport essential fatty acids to adipose tissue for long-term storage.

Adipose tissue and heart are both capable of chylomicron utilization *in vitro*. In these tissues the evidence for the utilization is conclusive, but the mechanism by which this is accomplished is disputed (see reference 6 for a review). The generally accepted view is that triglyceride molecules do not enter the cell without prior hydrolysis to fatty acids and glycerol. Thus, if the chylomicron triglyceride is labelled with ^{14}C in the glycerol moiety and with ^{3}H in the fatty acid moieties, the ratio of ^{14}C/^{3}H within the lipid fraction of the tissue is considerably less than in the chylomicrons. In fact, hardly any of the glycerol portion of the original triglyceride appears in the tissue lipids. This observation indicates hydrolysis of the triglyceride prior to its storage, but it does not show whether such hydrolysis takes place inside or outside the cell.

The enzyme, lipoprotein lipase (or clearing factor lipase), is considered to be responsible for the uptake of chylomicrons by adipose tissue, muscle and various other tissues (such as mammary gland). There is now considerable evidence that this enzyme resides outside the adipose tissue cells (and muscle cells),[6] probably in association with the endothelial cells of the capillary walls. The extracellular hydrolysis of the triglyceride contained in the chylomicrons and VLDL results in a local high concentration of fatty acids. These diffuse through the endothelial cell and into the adipose tissue (or muscle) cell for esterification or oxidation (see Figure 5.4).

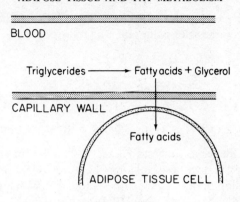

BLOOD

Triglycerides ⟶ Fatty acids + Glycerol

CAPILLARY WALL

Fatty acids

ADIPOSE TISSUE CELL

Figure 5.4

The lipoprotein lipase may be released from its location on the capillary wall and set free into the blood stream (or into the incubation medium in an *in vitro* experiment) by the presence of a variety of highly positively charged compounds (for example, heparin). This provides a useful means for measuring the activity of the enzyme: heparin is injected and the activity is measured in a sample of blood. Variations in the activity of the enzyme from some tissues correlate reasonably well with variations in the rate of triglyceride uptake (see reference 6 for discussion). During starvation the activity of lipoprotein lipase in adipose tissue is considerably decreased, while after refeeding it increases to even higher levels than in the fed state. Such observations are consistent with the proposed role of the enzyme in fat deposition.

(b) Dietary carbohydrate

Several tissues possess the complement of enzymes necessary for the synthesis of triglyceride from carbohydrate. The pathways involved are glycolysis, in which glucose is converted to acetyl-CoA; lipogenesis, in which acetyl-CoA is converted into long-chain fatty acyl-CoA; and finally esterification, in which the fatty acyl-CoA is reacted with glycerol phosphate to form triglyceride.

Glucose → → acetyl-CoA → → fatty acyl-CoA → → triglyceride

These pathways in adipose tissue have been discussed by Vaughan.[7] The process of glycolysis in adipose tissue appears to be essentially similar to that in muscle: any differences are related to the role of adipose tissue in the synthesis, storage and mobilization of triglyceride. The formation of fatty acyl-CoA from acetyl-CoA can be divided into two parts, the carboxylation of acetyl-CoA to form malonyl-CoA (catalysed by acetyl-CoA carboxylase) and the series of condensation, reduction and dehydration reactions starting with acetyl-CoA and malonyl-CoA and catalysed by a particulate enzyme complex known as fatty acyl-CoA synthetase.[8] For example, the overall reaction for the synthesis of palmitate is as follows:

(a) $CH_3CO \cdot SCoA + CO_2 + ATP$

$$\rightarrow HOOC \cdot CH_2 \cdot CO \cdot SCoA + ADP + P_i$$

(b) $7HOOC \cdot CH_2 \cdot CO \cdot SCoA + CH_3CO \cdot SCoA + 14NADPH + 14H^+$

$$\rightarrow +7CO_2CH_3(CH_2)_{14}COOH + 8CoA + 14NADP^+ + 6H_2O$$

There is some evidence to suggest that acetyl-CoA carboxylase is the regulatory enzyme for the synthesis of long-chain acyl-CoA from acetate. The theory of regulation of fatty acid synthesis together with a discussion of the origin of the reducing power (NADPH) for fatty acyl-CoA synthesis are presented below.

Long-chain fatty acyl-CoA is esterified in a series of reactions involving glycerol-1-phosphate (see Figure 5.5). The glycerol phosphate is produced

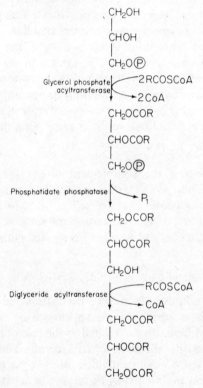

Figure 5.5. The pathway of esterification

from glucose via the glycolytic pathway. The conversion of dihydroxy-acetone phosphate to glycerol phosphate is catalysed by the enzyme glycerol-1-phosphate dehydrogenase.

$$\begin{array}{ccc}
\text{CH}_2\text{OH} & & \text{CH}_2\text{OH} \\
| & & | \\
\text{C}{=}\text{O} & + \text{NADH} + \text{H}^+ \rightleftarrows & \text{CHOH} & + \text{NAD}^+ \\
| & & | \\
\text{CH}_2\text{O}\text{\textcircled{P}} & & \text{CH}_2\text{O}\text{\textcircled{P}}
\end{array}$$

In certain tissues (in particular the liver and kidney), the enzyme glycerol kinase catalyses the formation of glycerol phosphate directly from glycerol.

$$\begin{array}{ccc}
\text{CH}_2\text{OH} & & \text{CH}_2\text{OH} \\
| & & | \\
\text{CHOH} & + \text{ATP} \rightarrow & \text{CHOH} & + \text{ADP} \\
| & & | \\
\text{CH}_2\text{OH} & & \text{CH}_2\text{O}\text{\textcircled{P}}
\end{array}$$

However, in adipose tissue this enzyme has a very low activity. Consequently, glucose provides all three precursors for triglyceride formation, namely acetyl-CoA, NADPH and glycerol phosphate.

(*i*) *Transfer of acetyl units across the mitochondrial membrane.* In the bio-synthesis of triglyceride, the conversion of glucose to pyruvate occurs in the cytoplasm of the adipose tissue cell. The conversion of pyruvate to acetyl-CoA occurs within the mitochondria, whereas the synthesis of fatty acyl-CoA occurs in the cytoplasm (probably in association with the endoplasmic reticulum). Therefore acetyl-CoA must be transported out of the mito-chondria in order to provide the substrate for the fatty-acid synthesizing enzymes. Since the mitochondrial membrane is impermeable to CoA derivatives, various transfer mechanisms have been proposed: the deacylation of acetyl-CoA to acetate, which traverses the membrane and is reacylated by acetate thiokinase in the cytoplasm; the conversion of acetyl-CoA to acetyl-carnitine (catalysed by mitochondrial carnitine-acetyl transferase), which traverses the membrane and is reconverted to acetyl-CoA in the cyto-plasm; and finally, condensation of acetyl-CoA with oxaloacetate to form citrate followed by the transfer of citrate into the cytoplasm where it is cleaved to acetyl-CoA and oxaloacetate by ATP-citrate lyase (see reference 9 for a review of these mechanisms). There is a reasonable amount of evidence to support the view that the most important transfer mechanism for acetyl-CoA is that involving citrate formation. The evidence from enzyme activity measurements and the distribution of these enzymes in the adipose tissue cell is presented in reference 10.

The enzyme, ATP-citrate lyase, which occurs outside the mitochondria, converts citrate into acetyl-CoA and oxaloacetate. The acetyl-CoA is utilized for the synthesis of fatty acyl-CoA and the oxaloacetate must re-enter the mitochondria in order to continue the transfer of acetyl-CoA. The mitochondrial membane is impermeable to oxaloacetate[11] and therefore the process of re-entry cannot be direct. It is likely that oxaloacetate enters the mitochondria by means of the pyruvate-malate cycle (see reference 10 and Figure 5.6). In the cytoplasm, oxaloacetate is converted to malate which

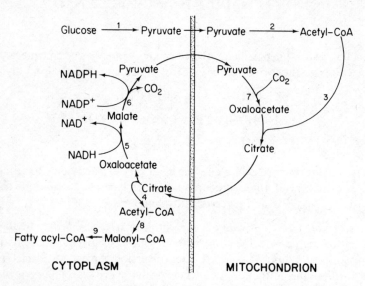

Figure 5.6. The pyruvate-malate cycle. (1) Glycolysis. (2) Pyruvate dehydrogenase. (3) Citrate synthase. (4) ATP-citrate lyase. (5) NAD^+-linked malate dehydrogenase. (6) $NADP^+$-linked malate dehydrogenase ('malic' enzyme). (7) Pyruvate carboxylase. (8) Acetyl-CoA carboxylase. (9) Fatty acyl-CoA synthetase

is oxidatively decarboxylated to pyruvate. Pyruvate enters the mitochondria where it is reconverted to oxaloacetate in a carboxylation reaction catalysed by pyruvate carboxylase, whose presence has been demonstrated in adipose tissue.[12] This cycle is obligatory for the re-entry of oxaloacetate and it results in the reduction of $NADP^+$ to NADPH which is utilized in the fatty acyl-CoA synthetase reaction. This production of NADPH in the pyruvate-malate cycle explains a paradox concerning the supply of reducing power for fatty acid synthesis (see below).

(ii) *Reducing power and the pentose phosphate pathway.* The reducing power for fatty acid synthesis is provided by NADPH, a proportion of which is formed by the oxidation of glucose in the pentose phosphate pathway. The pathways of glycolysis and the TCA cycle produce NADH (rather than NADPH) and this cannot be used for fatty acid synthesis (see Chapter 7, Appendix 7.1). In the pentose phosphate pathway, glucose-6-phosphate is oxidized to 6-phosphogluconate which is then oxidatively decarboxylated to form ribulose-5-phosphate: in both of these reactions $NADP^+$ is reduced to NADPH. The ribulose-5-phosphate can be converted back to glucose-6-phosphate in a series of transaldolase and transketolase reactions, the details of which can be found in any general biochemistry textbook. There are various ways of describing the stoichiometry of such a complex cycle of reactions; for example, the complete oxidation of one mole of glucose-6-phosphate can be described by the equation

6 glucose-6-phosphate + 12 $NADP^+$

$$\rightarrow 5 \text{ glucose-6-phosphate} + 6CO_2 + 12\,NADPH + 12H^+ + P_i$$

When glucose (in the presence of insulin) is the substrate for fatty acid synthesis, the pentose phosphate pathway appears to supply about 60% of the reducing power.[13,14] However, this pathway is not maximally stimulated under these conditions since it can be increased by the addition of an artificial electron acceptor—for example, phenazine methosulphate.[15] (The rate of this pathway may be regulated by the availability of the cofactor, $NADP^+$, which is controlled by the rate of fatty acid synthesis—see Figure 5.7. This

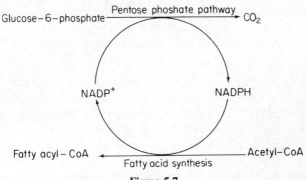

Figure 5.7

may be an example of control by cofactor availability as described in Chapter 1, Section D.1(b).) Furthermore, when adipose tissue is synthesizing fatty acids from glucose (in the presence of insulin) the addition of acetate leads to an increase in the rate of the pentose phosphate pathway and consequently increases the proportion of the NADPH provided by this pathway. Acetate is a precursor for acetyl-CoA but does not provide any reducing power so that the increase in demand for NADPH stimulates the pentose phosphate pathway.[16] If the activity of this pathway is controlled by $NADP^+$ availability and if it is not maximally stimulated during fatty acid synthesis from glucose, why should it provide only about 60% of the required reducing power? The pyruvate-malate cycle provides the answer to this question.

One turn of this cycle produces one molecule of acetyl-CoA for fatty acid synthesis and 50% of the NADPH required for the reduction of this acetate residue in the synthetic pathway. Consequently, only 50% of the NADPH need be supplied by the pentose phosphate pathway. The fact that the pathway produces about 60% is explained by the loss of some of the malate of the pyruvate-malate cycle via other processes.

(*iii*) *Control of glycolysis in adipose tissue.* The mass-action ratios for the glycolytic reactions in adipose tissue indicate that hexokinase and phosphofructokinase catalyse reactions that are removed far from equilibrium.[17,18] The properties of these two enzymes from adipose tissue are similar to those of the enzymes from other tissues, but since the content of ATP is comparatively low and that of AMP is comparatively high (the [ATP]/[AMP] ratio in adipose tissue is about 4, whereas it is about 50 in muscle), it is possible that PFK exists mainly in the de-inhibited condition. Consequently, the activity of PFK may be regulated primarily by changes in the intracellular concentration of fructose-6-phosphate.[18] Also, hexokinase may be regulated primarily by changes in the intracellular concentration of glucose. Therefore the activity of the membrane transport process for glucose may play an important role in the regulation of glycolysis in adipose tissue. In accordance with this proposal is the fact that the transport process is activated by insulin, which is known to increase the rate of glycolysis and to elevate the contents of glucose-6-phosphate and fructose-6-phosphate in the epididymal fat pad.[17,18]

(*iv*) *Control of fatty acid synthesis in adipose tissue.* The maximum catalytic activity of acetyl-CoA carboxylase is less than that of the fatty acyl-CoA synthetase complex.[19,20] This suggests that acetyl-CoA carboxylase catalyses a non-equilibrium reaction in fatty acid synthesis. However, there appears to be no evidence that it is a regulatory enzyme (according to the restricted definition given in Chapter 1, Section C.2). Nevertheless, theories on the control of fatty acid synthesis have been based upon two properties of acetyl-CoA carboxylase, namely activation by citrate[21] and inhibition by long-chain fatty acyl-CoA.[19] Thus, it has been suggested that an increase in the concentration of citrate and/or a decrease in the concentration of fatty acyl-CoA in the adipose tissue cell are responsible for increased fatty acid synthesis. However, the content of citrate in the epididymal fat pad is not changed by the presence of insulin nor is it possible to correlate changes in the contents of citrate or fatty acyl-CoA with changes in the rate of fatty acid synthesis.[22] Studies on the properties of acetyl-CoA carboxylase from liver have cast doubt on the regulatory significance of these compounds:[23] the activation by citrate was not observed in the presence of physiological concentrations of ATP; the inhibition by fatty acyl-CoA was not observed in the presence of palmitoyl-carnitine and, since these two compounds may be maintained close to equilibrium by carnitine acyl-transferase, their concentrations should always change in the same direction.

It is possible that acetyl-CoA carboxylase (and therefore fatty acid synthesis) can be regulated by substrate (that is, acetyl-CoA) availability. In this case factors that regulate glycolysis could be important in the control of fatty acid synthesis—for example, glucose transport, HK and PFK.[24] However, it has been shown recently that insulin can stimulate fatty acid synthesis from pyruvate and lactate and that this may involve control at the level of pyruvate dehydrogenase.[25] This enzyme exists in two enzymatically interconvertible forms in adipose tissue as in other tissues (see Chapter 3, Section D.7). The administration of insulin to the epididymal fat pad increases the proportion of the pyruvate dehydrogenase in the active (dephosphorylated) form. It seems likely that insulin exerts this effect by modifying the activity of one of the interconverting enzymes, possibly by an activation of the pyruvate dehydrogenase phosphatase.

(v) *Control of esterification.* The pathway of esterification has been outlined in Figure 5.5. The fact that glycerol-1-phosphate is required for esterification is of particular importance in understanding the relationship between glycolysis and fatty acid mobilization in adipose tissue. Glycerol-1-phosphate is produced from the glycolytic pathway via reduction of dihydroxyacetone phosphate in the glycerol phosphate dehydrogenase reaction. (In white adipose tissue, the enzyme glycerol kinase has a very low activity and therefore can supply little of the glycerol phosphate required in esterification.[26] Consequently esterification is dependent on glycolysis.)

Since pyruvate can function as a precursor for triglyceride synthesis in the absence of any other substrate, the glycerol phosphate that is required for esterification can be derived from pyruvate. The conversion of pyruvate to glycerol phosphate can be achieved by a partial reversal of glycolysis involving pyruvate carboxylase and phosphoenolpyruvate carboxykinase, which are both present in adipose tissue.[12,27]

$$CH_3CO \cdot COOH + CO_2 + ATP \xrightarrow{\text{pyruvate carboxylase}}$$

$$\begin{array}{l} CO \cdot COOH \\ | \\ CH_2COOH \end{array} + ADP + P_i$$

$$\begin{array}{l} CO \cdot COOH \\ | \\ CH_2COOH \end{array} + GTP \xrightarrow[\text{carboxykinase}]{\text{phosphoenolpyruvate}} \begin{array}{l} CH_2 \\ \| \\ CO\circledP \\ | \\ COOH \end{array} + GDP + CO_2$$

(vi) *Sites of lipogenesis.* The liver has long been known to synthesize fat and it used to be considered of prime importance in this respect. Only since 1950 has adipose tissue been recognized as an important site of lipogenesis. However, it has not proved possible to estimate the relative contributions of adipose tissue and liver in lipogenesis *in vivo*. The main obstacle to the interpretation of the results of *in vivo* experiments is the mobility of the lipids once they are synthesized. (For example, triglycerides synthesized in the liver are rapidly carried to adipose tissue as VLDL and therefore the measurement of the total lipid present in the tissue is meaningless.) Labelling experiments cannot provide further information since the specific activity of tissue lipids, following the injection of a labelled precursor, depends upon dilution within the tissue at all stages along the pathway as well as upon the rate of synthesis. Despite these difficulties, it has been suggested that adipose tissue is more important as a site of lipogenesis than liver.[28]

(c) Dietary protein

Amino acids derived from protein in the diet could theoretically provide precursor (acetyl-CoA) for fatty acid synthesis. *In vitro* studies show that ^{14}C from ^{14}C-labelled leucine, alanine and several other amino acids is incorporated into fatty acids in isolated fat pads.[29] Both ketogenic and glucogenic amino acids are capable of providing the acetyl-CoA required for lipogenesis. *In vivo* the main site of fatty acid synthesis from precursors derived from amino acids would be the liver, since this tissue is responsible for degradation of many of the amino acids (see Chapter 6, Section C.1). However, the extent to which amino acids may be utilized for fatty acid synthesis *in vivo* is not known. This source of precursor may be particularly important in carnivores, since such animals feed relatively infrequently and on a diet rich in protein.

2. The lipid constituents of the plasma and their function

The basic problem in transporting lipid materials in the aqueous medium of the blood is their insolubility. Living organisms have arrived at several elegant solutions to this problem, all of which depend upon the combination of the non-polar lipid molecules with certain polar compounds. Completely hydrophobic molecules like triglyceride are transported in large complex particles called micelles. These particles possess an entirely non-polar core consisting of triglycerides and esters of cholesterol. This core is surrounded by polar lipid materials (phospholipids and free cholesterol) which bind hydrophobically to the core and at the same time keep their polar groups (the phosphate groups and nitrogenous bases of phospholipids and the hydroxyl group of cholesterol) on the surface of the micelle either in contact with the polar solvent or electrostatically linked to proteins. Consequently the micelles are freely dispersed in the aqueous plasma. Indeed, Nature's solution to this problem is the envy of research workers in this field who find it impossible to mimic this situation because of lack of appropriate proteins and knowledge of the detailed architecture of such particles. Thus, triglyceride is usually dispersed ('solubilized') for experimental purposes by treatment with chemical detergents (such as polyvinyl alcohol) which are often toxic to biological systems.

(a) Triglyceride-containing particles

The chylomicrons derived from the lymph and the very low density lipoproteins secreted by the liver are only two examples of circulating lipoproteins. A brief survey of the various lipid components of the plasma and of their proposed functions may help to clarify a somewhat confusing situation. Unfortunately there are no distinct features which serve to classify a particular lipoprotein: there exists a whole spectrum of particles differing only slightly from each other in density, size and composition. An outline of the properties and composition of several groups of lipoproteins is presented in Table 5.1. Four main groups are distinguished solely on the basis of differences in density. In addition, two further classes have been identified and are given in parentheses. Bierman[30] describes 'secondary particles', differing from both chylomicrons and VLDL, which he suggests are secreted by the liver following chylomicron uptake. Very high density lipoproteins (VHDL) have also been reported but it is not clear whether these particles have a physiological role or whether they arise merely as an artefact during the preparation of high density lipoproteins (HDL).

The chylomicrons, secondary particles, VLDL and LDL are all light-scattering particles which give a turbid appearance to the plasma. They are thought to consist of a hydrophobic core of triglyceride and cholesterol esters surrounded by a coat of extended protein interacting with cholesterol-phospholipid complexes. The HDL and VHDL are much smaller and consist of pseudomolecular aggregates with a more definite quaternary structure. The only other type of plasma lipid constituent is non-esterified fatty acids (NEFA or FFA) which are solubilized by binding to albumin. The fatty acid-albumin complex is similar in density to the VHDL.

Although ideas on the functions of plasma lipids have changed radically over the years, it is now considered that the various types of triglyceride-containing particles are involved primarily in transportation. The role of phospholipids and sterols is believed to be merely that of surface-active agents and particle-stabilizers, although cholesterol may also be transported in these particles. A plausible model of lipoprotein function and metabolism has been presented by Schumaker and Adams and is summarized in a simplified and slightly modified form in Figure 5.8. The evidence on which the theory is based has been reviewed in detail and will not be discussed.[31]

Table 5.1. Properties of the various classes of plasma lipoproteins[30,31]

Class	Density g/ml	S_f*	Particle diameter (mμ)	Approximate molecular weight $\times 10^6$	Composition				
					Phospholipid (percentage)	Glyceride (percentage)	Total cholesterol (percentage)	Cholesterol ester (percentage)	Protein (percentage)
Chylomicrons	0·95	400	200–500	10^3–10^4	5–10	80	10	7	2
'Secondary particles'	1·006	400	70	—	4	—	10	—	—
VLDL	0·95–1·006	20–400	20–70	5–100	20	55	13	5	10
LDL	1·006–1·063	0–20	—	2–3	22	11	45	37	21
HDL	1·063–1·21	—	pseudo-molecular	0·25	26	6	18	15	50
Albumin-NEFA complex	>1·21	—	—	—	0	0	0	0	Up to 1 mole NEFA per mole of albumin†

* S_f is the negative sedimentation coefficient in Svedbergs in NaCl solution of density 1·063 g/ml at 26 °C.
† At physiological concentrations of NEFA.

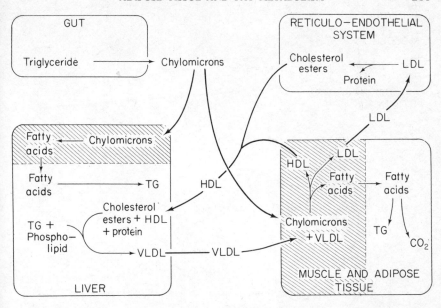

Figure 5.8. The origin and fate of plasma lipoproteins. The tissues that are principally involved in lipoprotein metabolism include gut, liver, muscle and adipose tissue. Cross-hatching represents the extracellular portion of the liver, muscle and adipose tissue

The theory of lipoprotein metabolism[31] proposes that only the liver and intestinal epithelium are involved in lipoprotein synthesis for transportation purposes. The intestines synthesize chylomicrons and the liver synthesizes VLDL, the function of both these particles being to convey triglycerides to adipose tissue (and possibly to other tissues—muscle, for example) for storage. In addition, the liver also synthesizes HDL which is probably concerned with the transport of phospholipid and cholesterol esters to the liver once these compounds have been released from the chylomicrons and VLDL. The action of lipoprotein lipase in adipose tissue and muscle removes triglyceride from the core of the chylomicrons and VLDL. The particles are therefore reduced in size and must lose some of their hydrophilic coating if they are to remain as stable particles. This is effected by the conversion of hydrophilic cholesterol into hydrophobic cholesterol ester by the action of the enzyme lecithin-cholesterol acyltransferase (LCAT). This enzyme catalyses the transfer of a fatty acid residue from lecithin to cholesterol, to form a cholesterol ester which may enter the core of the particle or may be absorbed by the adipose tissue cell (Figure 5.9).[31] The lysolecithin is lost to the particle and may be collected by the HDL (or possibly by the VHDL). The result of the loss of triglyceride and the esterification of cholesterol is the formation of LDL particles from chylomicrons and VLDL. Indirect evidence points to the

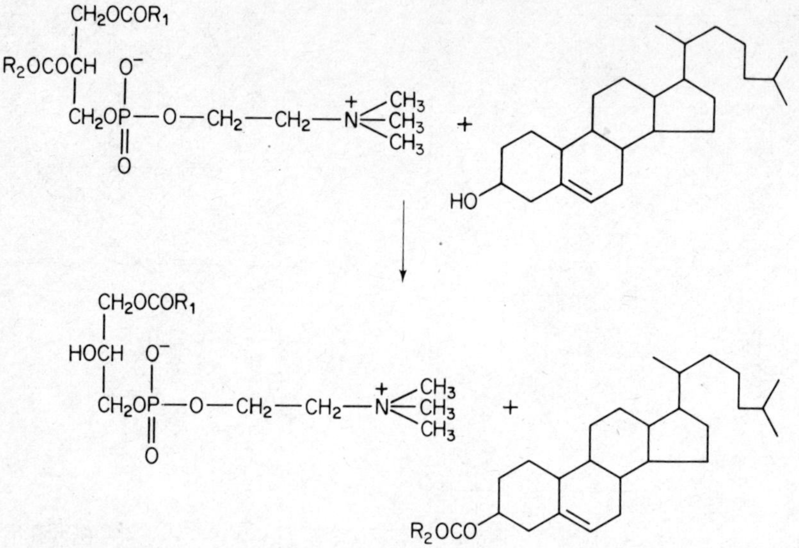

Figure 5.9. The lecithin-cholesterol acyltransferase reaction

reticulo-endothelial system* as the site of catabolism of LDL. Cholesterol esters released during the degradation of LDL are secreted by the reticulo-endothelial system into the blood where they combine with the HDL and are conveyed to the liver. In this tissue the cholesterol esters are hydrolysed releasing free cholesterol which can be used for the synthesis of VLDL.

(b) Non-esterified fatty acids: the demonstration of their significance

Non-esterified fatty acid, which is bound onto albumin, is present in the blood at a very low concentration. This complex could not be fitted readily into the scheme of fat metabolism as it was understood in the early 1950s and, since it comprised only a small proportion of the total plasma lipid (about 2%), its metabolic role was considered to be unimportant. Once it was realized that the removal of chylomicrons from the plasma entailed extracellular hydrolysis of triglyceride, attention became focused upon the non-esterified fatty acid (NEFA) fraction and methods for its assay in plasma were devised. It was anticipated that the level of plasma NEFA might rise after a fat-containing meal when the triglyceride in the chylomicrons is being hydrolysed by lipoprotein lipase. In two separate laboratories, experiments were designed to test this hypothesis.[32,33] These experiments showed, somewhat surprisingly, that the plasma NEFA level was decreased after a meal but was elevated during starvation. Furthermore, the high plasma

---

* The reticulo-endothelial system is composed of cells, lining lymph or vascular channels, which are capable of phagocytosis of bacteria, viruses or other foreign particles. They include phagocytic cells of bone marrow, spleen, liver, lymph nodes and also some mobile phagocytic cells which are found in the blood stream.

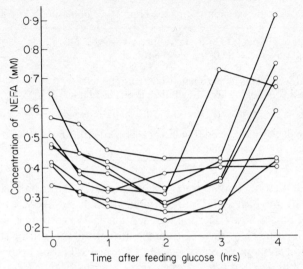

Figure 5.10. Effect of oral glucose on the plasma concentrations of fatty acids. After an overnight fast, 8 normal young men were given 100 g of glucose[33]

NEFA level observed during starvation was rapidly depressed following the administration of glucose or insulin (see Figure 5.10). Gordon and Cherkes[33] realized the full significance of such findings, namely that non-esterified fatty acids might be the form in which fat was liberated from adipose tissue and made available as an oxidizable substrate for other tissues. They also realized that the low concentration of NEFA in the plasma (0·3–1·0 mM or only 2% of the total plasma lipid) required a high turnover rate in order to supply sufficient fuel to metabolically active tissues.[34] Meanwhile Havel and Fredrickson[35] published their findings on the turnover rates of various plasma lipid components and reported a very short half-life (of the order of 2 minutes) for the plasma NEFA. From this data it can be calculated that in man 160 g fat per day at least (that is, 60% of the total caloric requirement) can be transported in the form of NEFA (see Table 5.2). Thus the physiological importance of NEFA was established.

Until this period it was not universally accepted that fatty acids could be oxidized directly by muscle tissue. Before 1930 there were two schools of thought as to how stored triglyceride was metabolized. One maintained that carbohydrate was the sole fuel for oxidation and fat must be converted into carbohydrate before oxidation. The other contended that such a conversion was improbable, since R.Q. measurements indicated the direct oxidation of fat.[36] (It is now known that fat *cannot* be converted to carbohydrate in the mammalian body.) Direct oxidation of fat could be achieved either by oxidation of NEFA or by conversion of NEFA to ketone bodies in the liver. It was

Table 5.2. A calculation demonstrating the importance of plasma NEFA in man[33,35]

Concentration of plasma NEFA in starvation is 0·6 mM
In 3 litres of plasma there are 0·6 × 3 = 1·8 mmol
                              = 0·45 g fatty acid
The fractional turnover is approximately 0·25 per minute
Therefore the flux of fatty acids through the plasma in 24 hours is

$$0·45 × 0·25 × 60 × 24 = 160 \text{ g fatty acid}$$

The oxidation of 160 g fat provides sufficient energy to satisfy 60 % of the daily energy requirements for the average man.

---

thought that ketone bodies were the important fuel for muscles during starvation, although in 1945 Stadie argued strongly in favour of the direct oxidation of fatty acids.[37] Despite the fact that in 1956 strong evidence was presented that long chain fatty acids are an important fuel during starvation, the precise physiological role of plasma fatty acids, ketone bodies and triglyceride is still debated (see Chapter 7).

B. REGULATION OF FATTY ACID MOBILIZATION FROM ADIPOSE TISSUE

1. Introduction

The fat reserves of the mammalian body are stored as droplets of triglyceride in the adipose tissue. This triglyceride must first be hydrolysed to non-esterified fatty acids (NEFA) before it can be transported from the adipose tissue to other tissues. Since the long-chain fatty acids are relatively insoluble in the aqueous plasma they are transported in combination with a plasma protein, albumin. An analogy may be drawn between the role of the albumin-fatty acid complex and the haemoglobin-oxygen complex, which is important in the transportation of a much greater quantity of oxygen than could be achieved through simple solution of oxygen in plasma.

$$\text{albumin} + \text{NEFA} \rightleftarrows \text{albumin} - \text{NEFA}$$
$$\text{haemoglobin} + O_2 \rightleftarrows \text{haemoglobin} - O_2$$

The control mechanism involved in the hydrolysis of triglyceride stores has been intensively investigated. When isolated pieces of adipose tissue (such as the extremely thin epididymal fat pads of the male rat, or very thin pieces of intra-abdominal fat) are incubated, fatty acids and glycerol are released into the medium.[38,39] There is no evidence of significant rates of triglyceride release from adipose tissue but, somewhat surprisingly, investigations do not appear to have been extensive. It is generally assumed that, even if this process occurs, it is insignificant in relation to NEFA release. The hydrolysis of the triglyceride prior to the mobilization of NEFA occurs within the adipose tissue cells and is catalysed by a lipase system. The triglyceride lipase of this system is distinct from the lipoprotein lipase, which occurs outside the adipose tissue cell.* The transport of fatty acids across the adipose tissue cell membrane seems to occur by simple diffusion and therefore the rate of their release is proportional merely to the concentration gradient. Accordingly the transport of fatty acids across the membrane of the adipose cell is not an energy-dependent process and does not appear to be influenced by metabolic or hormonal factors. (However, with *in vitro* systems it does depend upon the presence of albumin in the incubation medium.)

The hydrolysis of triglyceride to fatty acids and glycerol (lipolysis) takes place in a stepwise fashion, the intermediate products being diglyceride and monoglyceride.

$$TG \rightarrow FA + DG$$

$$DG \rightarrow FA + MG$$

$$MG \rightarrow FA + glycerol$$

The lipolysis is catalysed by at least three enzymes: triglyceride-, diglyceride- and monoglyceride-lipases. The activities of the latter two are 10–100-fold greater than the former, which suggests that triglyceride lipase is the regulatory enzyme. In accordance with this idea, the activity of the triglyceride lipase can be increased by a number of hormones (such as adrenaline, noradrenaline or glucagon) whereas the activities of the diglyceride and monoglyceride lipases are not affected.

The release of fatty acids by adipose tissue must obviously depend upon the rate of lipolysis, but this is not the only process that has to be considered. In particular, the re-esterification of fatty acids to form triglyceride can play an important role in the regulation of fatty acid mobilization. If lipolysis occurred in the absence of esterification, every molecule of glycerol released from adipose tissue would be accompanied by three molecules of fatty acid. However, experiments with isolated fat pads *in vitro* have demonstrated that in general much more glycerol is released than fatty acids (see Table 5.3). Therefore a large quantity of the fatty acids cannot be accounted for and the simplest assumption is that they are re-esterified to form triglyceride. This type of experiment, in which changes in total fatty acids and glycerol (that is, tissue + medium) are followed, has been termed the non-isotopic balance method[40] for the estimation of the rates of lipolysis and esterification. (Such estimations assume that the rates of *de novo* fatty acid synthesis and fatty acid oxidation are so low that they can be ignored.) Further experimental support for simultaneous esterification and lipolysis has been obtained from

* Lipoprotein lipase has an alkaline pH optimum, is specific for chylomicrons or VLDL and is inhibited by phosphate, protamine and a high salt concentration. Triglyceride lipase has a pH optimum of 6–7 and is not inhibited by any of these compounds.

Table 5.3. Non-isotopic balance method for measurement of lipolysis and esterification in adipose tissue from the rat[40]

	Concentration (μmol/g of adipose tissue)	
	Glycerol	Fatty acid
Initial concentration in tissue	1·8	2·0
Final concentration in tissue	0·5	0·8
Net change in tissue	− 1·3	− 1·2
Initial concentration in medium	0·0	0·2
Final concentration in medium	2·6	1·5
Net change in medium	2·6	1·3
Overall change for system	1·3	0·1

The initial concentrations in the tissue and the medium are obtained before the incubation. The final concentrations are obtained after incubation at 37 °C for one hour. The high initial concentrations of both fatty acids and glycerol in the tissue are probably explained by the effects of trauma that arise during the removal of the epididymal fat pad from the rat. The reduction in these concentrations in the tissue during the incubation is probably due to diffusion of glycerol and fatty acid into the medium. The quantity of glycerol formed during the incubation is a direct measure of the rate of lipolysis in the adipose tissue. If lipolysis were the only process under consideration, 3 molecules of fatty acid should be formed for every molecule of glycerol. However, in this experiment the formation of 1·3 μmol of glycerol is accompanied by the production of only 0·1 μmol of fatty acid. Therefore it is assumed that 3·8 μmol of fatty acid is re-esterified within the adipose tissue.

experiments in which ^{14}C from ^{14}C-glucose was incorporated into glyceride-glycerol at the same time as fatty acids and glycerol were being released into the medium. The conclusion is reached that both lipolysis and esterification occur simultaneously and therefore a triglyceride/fatty acid cycle (Figure 5.11) operates in adipose tissue.

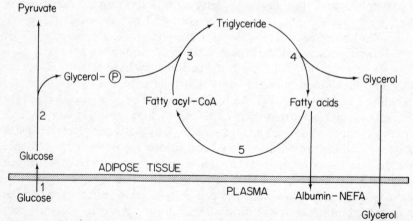

Figure 5.11. The triglyceride/fatty acid cycle in adipose tissue. (1) Glucose transport across cell membrane. (2) Glycolysis. (3) Esterification. (4) Lipolysis. (5) Activation of fatty acids (fatty acid-CoA synthetase). Normally, long chain fatty acids are found in plasma in combination with albumin and they are usually referred to as NEFA (non-esterified fatty acids)

2. The importance of the triglyceride/fatty acid cycle

At first sight simultaneous lipolysis and esterification might seem to be an unnecessarily complex system for the regulation of fatty acid storage and/or mobilization. Furthermore, the continuous activation of fatty acids to fatty acyl-CoA and the provision of glycerol phosphate to maintain the triglyceride-fatty acid cycle requires the utilization of ATP. It might be considered more economical for the tissue to possess independent means of controlling the two systems so that they would never be simultaneously active (lipolysis would be inhibited when triglyceride was being synthesized and esterification would be inhibited during the breakdown of triglyceride). Nonetheless the experimental evidence strongly indicates the existence of such a cycle in adipose tissue and therefore its possible advantages must be considered. This cycle is an example of a substrate cycle as described in Chaper 2 (Section F.2(a)(i)) and it is somewhat analogous to the fructose-6-phosphate/fructose diphosphate cycle discussed in Chapter 3. One advantage of this substrate cycle is an increase in sensitivity of the control mechanism for fatty acid mobilization (in comparison to control of the lipase alone). However, there is another advantage that is unique to this particular cycle and is best explained by consideration of a hypothetical, primitive animal which does not possess any hormonal mechanism for the control of blood glucose or fatty acid levels. As far as is known, glucose (or trehalose in some insects) is the primary fuel for respiration in almost all animals and triglyceride is the reserve fuel. If the level of blood glucose were to decrease in the hypothetical, primitive animal, the rate of entry of glucose into the adipose tissue cell would be depressed and this would decrease the rate of glycolysis and lower the content of glycerol phosphate. The rate of esterification would be decreased and, since the lipolytic rate would remain unchanged, the intracellular concentration of fatty acids would be increased, resulting in increased fatty acid mobilization. The sequence of events leading to release of fatty acids by the adipose tissue could be triggered merely by a fall in the level of blood glucose. Conversely, if the blood glucose level were to be elevated, glycolysis, the concentration of glycerol phosphate and the rate of esterification would be increased and fatty acid mobilization would be decreased. Therefore, regulation of fatty acid mobilization would be achieved without any specific regulatory mechanisms. Such a simple mechanism reduces the possibility of error to a minimum.

Although there is no evidence for such a mechanism of control in primitive animals (in fact, they do not appear to have been investigated), it does provide an explanation for the more sophisticated hormonal control that is found in higher animals. In mammals (and possibly other animals) the blood glucose concentration cannot fall by more than about 30% because of the continual demand for glucose by the brain and other tissues. Since changes in the blood glucose level are restricted, hormones must play an essential role in the regulation of fatty acid mobilization. In addition, they provide a means of regulating the mobilization of fatty acids in response to situations which are unrelated to fluctuations in blood glucose (such as stress).

3. The control of esterification

In the case of the hypothetical, primitive animal it has been shown how large changes in blood glucose concentration could automatically cause reciprocal changes in plasma fatty acid concentration. However, in the rat the blood glucose concentration does not fall by more than 30% during two days of starvation and this would appear to be insufficient to cause the marked increase in fatty acid mobilization that occurs under these conditions. During the same period the plasma insulin level is decreased by about 80%[41] (see Table 7.3) and this hormone is known to regulate esterification. Insulin stimulates the membrane transport of glucose into the adipose tissue cell and increases the rate of glycolysis and the glycerol phosphate concentration. During starvation the reduction in the plasma insulin level results in a decreased rate of glycolysis and a lowering of the glycerol phosphate concentration. This restricts esterification and consequently fatty acid mobilization is stimulated.

This theory is supported by the fact that the content of glycerol phosphate in adipose tissue is decreased during starvation and it is markedly increased when adipose tissue from a starved animal is incubated with glucose and insulin. There are a number of problems associated with the simple idea that esterification is controlled by the concentration of glycerol phosphate, which in turn is controlled by the membrane transport of glucose. First, there is no evidence that the concentration of glycerol phosphate is limiting for the process of esterification (the K_m for glycerol phosphate of the first enzyme in the pathway is not known). Second, since glycerol phosphate dehydrogenase catalyses a reaction which is close to equilibrium, the concentration of glycerol phosphate can be controlled by both the cytoplasmic $[NAD^+]$/$[NADH]$ ratio and the concentration of dihydroxyacetone phosphate.[42]

Dihydroxyacetone phosphate + NADH $\rightleftarrows$ Glycerol phosphate + NAD^+

These quantities may vary independently of the glycolytic rate.[17] Third, the addition of adrenaline, fatty acids or acetate to the incubated fat pad preparation stimulates esterification but does not increase the content of glycerol phosphate.[42] This experiment suggests that factors other than the glycerol phosphate concentration can regulate esterification. Such factors remain unidentified at present. Nonetheless, it must be emphasized that a marked decrease in the concentration of glycerol phosphate could limit the rate of esterification and therefore variations in its concentration must always remain a potential mechanism of control.

The level of circulating insulin can be decreased by about 80% during two days of starvation (in man and rat), despite the fact that the fall in blood glucose is no more than 30%. This large fall in the insulin level is explained by the fact that the release of this hormone from the pancreas is regulated by secretions from the duodenum as well as by changes in the blood glucose level. The hormones released by the duodenum include gastrin, secretin, pancreozymin and another factor, which is as yet unidentified, but which is released specifically in response to the presence of glucose in the duodenum (see reference 43 for a review). The secretion of these hormones is stimulated by the presence of protein and/or carbohydrate in the duodenum. Therefore the digestion of food indirectly causes a stimulation of the secretion of insulin from the pancreas. (This explains the somewhat surprising observation that the oral administration of glucose elicits a greater change in the insulin level than intravenously administered glucose.[44]) The absence of food in the duodenum must seriously reduce the secretion of the duodenal hormones and this will be partly responsible for the marked decrease in circulating insulin concentration during starvation.

4. The control of lipolysis

There are several hormones (or compounds that may be described as hormones) that can stimulate lipolysis both *in vivo* and *in vitro*. The physiological importance of all these compounds is uncertain and some of them will not be referred to here. This discussion centres upon hormones which might be important in the stimulation of lipolysis under certain physiological conditions, namely stress, starvation and exercise.

(a) The stimulation of lipolysis under stress

Mobilization of fatty acids is known to occur in higher animals in response to both psychological stress (such as fear or anxiety) and physiological stress (such as a sudden drop in environmental temperature). Such conditions result in an elevation of the plasma NEFA level and this implies an increased mobilization of fatty acids. The available evidence strongly suggests that this mobilization is caused by release of noradrenaline and adrenaline. Thus, injection of either of these two hormones increases the concentrations (and rates of turnover) of plasma fatty acids and glycerol. Adrenaline and noradrenaline also increase the rate of lipolysis in adipose tissue incubated *in vitro*. Electrical stimulation of the nerves supplying adipose tissue increases lipolysis and this may be due to the release of noradrenaline from the nerve endings.

Some details of the biochemical mechanism underlying the action of these two hormones on lipolysis in adipose tissue have now been established. The experimental approach follows that described in Chapter 1: the properties of the regulatory enzyme, triglyceride lipase, are studied *in vitro* and the theory based on these properties is formulated. The theory has been tested with experiments involving intact adipose tissue preparations (usually epididymal fat pads).

It was anticipated that adrenaline would stimulate adenyl cyclase and hence raise the concentration of cyclic AMP in adipose tissue, by analogy with its action on muscle and liver. Sutherland and coworkers have been successful in showing that adrenaline does indeed increase the content of cyclic AMP in isolated adipose tissue preparations.[45] Furthermore, this increase is a result of the stimulation of adenyl cyclase. (This enzyme is probably a constitutive part of the adipose cell membrane and its activity can be studied in preparations of adipose cells that have lost their contents: these are termed *fat cell ghosts* and consist primarily of intact cell membranes. If the adipose cell membranes are disrupted and presumably the adenyl cyclase is destroyed, catecholamines no longer have any effect upon lipolysis.) The adrenaline-induced increase in cyclic AMP content precedes an increase in the rate of release of fatty acids. This observation implies that cyclic AMP is responsible for the increased lipolysis. This theory is supported by the fact that other agents which increase the cyclic AMP content (for example caffeine, which inhibits cyclic AMP phosphodiesterase) also stimulate lipolysis. Incubation of epididymal fat pads with dibutyryl-cyclic AMP, a fat-soluble analogue of cyclic AMP which readily penetrates the cell membrane, also results in increased lipolysis.[46]

Recent work has indicated that triglyceride lipase may exist in more than one form.[47] In fact, it has been suggested that the lipase exists in two *enzymatically interconvertible forms*, one of which is phosphorylated and catalytically active, while the other, non-phosphorylated, form is inactive. Cyclic

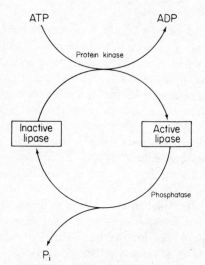

Figure 5.12. Regulation of triglyceride lipase activity via enzymatic interconversions

AMP may stimulate protein kinase in adipose tissue and hence cause phosphorylation of the lipase (see Figure 5.12). Evidence for this possibility has been obtained from a very interesting experiment: protein kinase, which was purified from skeletal muscle, increased the response of triglyceride lipase to cyclic AMP in extracts of adipose tissue.[48] In the original extract, the concentration of protein kinase would appear to be the limiting factor in the activation of triglyceride lipase by added cyclic AMP.

The advantages of a control mechanism involving interconvertible forms of an enzyme have been discussed in Chapter 2 and illustrated with reference to phosphorylase in Chapter 4. The necessity for this form of amplification may arise from the small change in concentration of cyclic AMP that is produced by adrenaline and other hormones[45] (see Chapter 4, Section D.3(b)(ii)).

(b) The stimulation of lipolysis in starvation

Starvation is another physiological situation in which an increased mobilization of fatty acids from adipose tissue can be demonstrated, both *in vivo* and *in vitro*. This effect could be explained simply by a decrease in esterification in the adipose tissue caused by the decrease in plasma insulin level (see Section B.3). However, the rise in plasma glycerol in starvation[49] and the increased glycerol release from *in vitro* preparations of adipose tissue from starved animals[50] indicate that lipolysis has been stimulated. Several hormones may be involved in this stimulation and their identification is made difficult by the fact that hormonal control of metabolism in starvation may vary from one species to another. Evidence for the involvement of growth hormone, glucagon and insulin is discussed below.

(i) Growth hormone.

The evidence that growth hormone plays a role in stimulating lipolysis during starvation stems from four lines of investigation. First, early endocrinological studies showed that the anterior pituitary was involved in the control of fat and carbohydrate metabolism. Removal of the pituitary gland ameliorates the condition of experimental diabetes (induced by alloxan administration or surgical removal of the pancreas) whereas injections of pituitary extract into such depancreatized-hypophysectomized animals restores the diabetic condition.[51] Also, when hypophysectomized animals are starved they lose less fat but more muscle glycogen and protein than control animals.[52,53] Injection of pituitary extract into such animals restores the normal response to starvation (loss of fat; maintenance of muscle glycogen and protein). If normal animals are injected with pituitary extract, their rate of fat oxidation increases and their metabolism resembles that of a starved animal.[54] By 1950 the factor in the pituitary extracts that was responsible for these changes was identified as growth hormone, and it was suggested that there would be an increased secretion of this hormone during starvation.[54] Second, the measurement of the plasma level of growth hormone, which was made possible by the development of a specific radio-immunological assay, showed that it was elevated in human subjects during starvation and immediately reduced upon refeeding.[55] (Some doubt has been cast upon the significance of this increase in growth hormone because in human subjects there is a large individual variation in response to starvation and in some species there is little change in growth hormone level.)[56,57] Third, injection of purified growth hormone into humans or rats elevates plasma levels of fatty acids and glycerol within a few hours.[58,59] Finally, it was necessary to demonstrate that growth hormone increased lipolysis in adipose tissue preparations *in vitro*. Such experiments were at first unsuccessful until it was realized that glucocorticoids were necessary for the lipolytic response to growth hormone; incubation of adipose tissue with growth hormone plus glucocorticoids for several hours results in a stimulation of lipolysis.[60]

There is always a delay of about an hour before the response to growth hormone can be detected, whereas the catecholamines cause increased lipolysis in under a minute. Therefore, it would appear that the primary effects of these two types of hormone are different. Adrenaline increases the lipase activity by raising the intracellular concentration of cyclic AMP through a stimulatory effect on the activity of adenyl cyclase. The stimulation of lipolysis by growth hormone is blocked by inhibitors of RNA synthesis[60] and this suggests that protein synthesis may be involved in the lipolytic action of growth hormone. The fact that treatment with growth hormone and glucocorticoids increases the extent of the cyclic AMP-elevation by adrenaline has led to the proposal that growth hormone stimulates the synthesis of adenyl cyclase.[61] The mechanism by which growth hormone selectively increases the concentration of this enzyme is unknown, but the effect is consistent with its slow action on lipolysis and with its physiological role in the gradual process of adaptation to starvation.

(*ii*) *Lack of insulin.* The effect of insulin in the suppression of fatty acid mobilization could be explained by stimulation of esterification and this would not involve any change in the rate of lipolysis. However, a direct antilipolytic effect of insulin has been demonstrated. The injection of insulin into starved[62] or diabetic[63] dogs decreases both the concentration and turnover of plasma glycerol and this indicates a suppression of lipolysis in adipose tissue. Also, insulin decreases glycerol output by epididymal fat pads[64] or isolated fat cells.[65] This inhibitory effect of insulin may minimize or restrain the effects of the more direct lipolytic agents so that the latter can exert pronounced effects on lipolysis when the level of insulin is depressed. Thus the large fall in plasma insulin level during starvation may permit the lipolytic hormones to exert their effects on lipolysis in the early stages of starvation before their concentrations in the plasma are actually increased. The observation that insulin inhibits lipolysis in adipose tissue from fed or 24-hour starved rats but not in adipose tissue from rats starved for two days or more[66] is consistent with this suggestion. Furthermore, the diurnal variations in plasma insulin may play an important role in the mobilization of fatty acids during an overnight fast.

The work of Butcher and colleagues[67] on the epididymal fat pad has shown that insulin decreases the intracellular level of cyclic AMP, when it has been raised by the presence of catecholamines. This explains how insulin can antagonize the action of catecholamines (and possibly growth hormone) on fatty acid mobilization. However, it is uncertain whether insulin can lower the normal level of cyclic AMP when it has not already been elevated by catecholamines. The low concentrations of cyclic AMP in normal tissue and the imprecision of the assay method preclude meaningful measurements of small changes in its concentration. It is not known how insulin lowers the concentration of cyclic AMP: it could inhibit the activity of adenyl cyclase and/or increase the activity of phosphodiesterase. Recently insulin has been shown to stimulate phosphodiesterase in adipose tissue.[68] If this is indeed the mechanism by which insulin reduces the cyclic AMP concentration, an increase in insulin should always cause a decrease in concentration of cyclic AMP (even in the absence of adrenaline), since phosphodiesterase plays an important role in maintaining the steady-state concentration of this compound (see Chapter 4, Section D.3(b)(ii)).

(iii) Glucagon. Glucagon stimulates lipolysis in the epididymal fat pad incubated in vitro. In some of the earlier experiments high concentrations of the hormone were employed, but in recent experiments physiological concentrations have also proved to be lipolytic. The effect of glucagon on the lipolytic system is similar to that of catecholamines: it increases the cyclic AMP content of adipose tissue via stimulation of adenyl cyclase activity.[69] It has proved difficult to establish whether glucagon can influence lipolysis in the intact animal, since the injection of glucagon does not result in a clear-cut rise in plasma fatty acid level. The hormone causes an activation of liver phosphorylase and the increased glycogenolysis raises the blood glucose level and this in turn minimizes the increase in plasma fatty acid level. Glucagon injections in man cause a transient decline in fatty acid level but this is followed by its prolonged elevation. In dogs the infusion of small doses of glucagon into the portal vein increases the level of fatty acids and there is no change in that of glucose.[70] Therefore it appears that under certain conditions glucagon stimulates fatty acid mobilization in vivo. Such an effect could be important in starvation. Consistent with such a role is the finding that the plasma glucagon levels are elevated in human subjects when fasting.[71] It is possible to suggest, from its effects on glycogenolysis and lipolysis, that the physiological role of glucagon during starvation may be initially to cause mobilization of liver glycogen: once these stores are depleted its action on fatty acid mobilization becomes apparent and reinforces the effects of the other lipolytic hormones (such as growth hormone).

(c) Other factors affecting lipolysis

An increase in the concentrations of growth hormone and glucagon and a decrease in that of insulin are but three factors which may play a part in the stimulation of lipolysis in adipose tissue in starvation. It is possible that the sympathetic nervous system may also be involved in this process but the available evidence is not clear on this point. One problem is that sympathetic activity could cause vasoconstriction, and the reduction in blood flow would be expected to decrease mobilization of fatty acids.

There are several other factors (such as TSH, ACTH and 'Chalmer's factor') which can elevate the plasma NEFA level but the mechanism of these effects and/or their physiological significance is uncertain at present. Since they could not be fitted simply into any physiological situation they have not been discussed, but this must not be taken to imply that they are of no physiological importance. Steinberg[40] has commented that the list of factors that influence fatty acid release from adipose tissue is embarrassingly long for the provision of an adequate and specific response to a given physiological situation. However, a speculative proposal is put forward in Chapter 7 which may account for the indiscriminating and unselective response of adipose tissue to hormones. One final word of caution in the interpretation of data in this field is that there appears to be considerable species variation in all these lipolytic effects and therefore general conclusions based upon results from particular species may not always be valid.[72]

C. PHYSIOLOGICAL SIGNIFICANCE OF VARIATIONS IN PLASMA FATTY ACID LEVEL

The biochemical mechanisms involved in the mobilization of fatty acids from adipose tissue and the various hormonal changes involved have been discussed above. In this section the metabolic actions of the mobilized fatty acids are considered. In conditions such as stress, starvation or prolonged muscular activity, the plasma fatty acid level is raised about five-fold and provides an alternative fuel to glucose, which can be conserved for use by a number of other tissues. The plasma fatty acid level is elevated because of increased mobilization from adipose tissue rather than decreased utilization by other tissues. (There is only a slight decrease in the fractional turnover rate, despite the large increase in concentration and therefore the flux through the blood must have increased—see Table 5.4.) The raised fatty acid level provides an immediate source of available fuel for other tissues and, moreover,

Table 5.4. Concentration and turnover rate of plasma NEFA in man under various conditions

Experimental conditions	Volume of plasma (litres)	Concentration of NEFA (mmol/l)	Total amount of NEFA in plasma (g)	Half-life for plasma NEFA (min)	Turnover of NEFA (g/24 hr)	Caloric equivalent of utilized NEFA
Fasting for 12–15 hours	4·2	0·42	0·5	3·1	116	1,080
Fasting for 2–3 days	3·1	2·15	1·9	3·8	360	3,350
2 hours after administration of glucose (1 g glucose/kg body weight)	2·9	0·62	0·5	2·7	133	1,240

Healthy subjects between the ages of 20 and 35 were studied. The turnover of plasma NEFA was measured by following the disappearance of ^{14}C-fatty acids after intravenous injection of a trace dose of ^{14}C-fatty acid which was bound to albumin.[115]

the increase in concentration provides the necessary signal for tissues to oxidize these fatty acids. Support for this idea is provided by experiments with *in vitro* tissue preparations (such as perfused heart and perfused liver), in which it can be shown that the rate of uptake of fatty acids is proportional to their external concentration.[73,74] Similar conclusions have been reached from experiments with the *in situ* heart.[75,76] Such experiments demonstrate merely that the rate of *uptake* depends upon concentration but it is generally accepted that an increased uptake of fatty acids automatically results in an increased rate of oxidation.[77,78]

1. The glucose/fatty acid cycle

The presence of fatty acids or ketone bodies, at concentrations that are found in the plasma during starvation, causes inhibition of glucose utilization by muscle *in vitro* (see Chapter 3, Section D.5). These *in vitro* experiments with muscle, and the *in vitro* experiments with adipose tissue described in this chapter, provide the basis for the concept of the *glucose/fatty acid cycle*.[79] This concept explains how changes in plasma levels of glucose and fatty acids are interrelated and how they influence one another in such a manner as to provide a homeostatic control mechanism. The theory of the glucose/fatty acid cycle applies to the intact animal, but it depends upon extrapolation of the properties of the perfused heart, the incubated diaphragm and the incubated epididymal fat pad to the total musculature and adipose tissue *in vivo*. (This is not unlike the extrapolation of the *in vitro* properties of PFK to provide a theory of control of this enzyme *in the living cell*. In the present case the *in vitro* properties of the muscle and adipose tissue give rise to a theory of control of plasma glucose and fatty acid concentrations *in the whole animal*.) The theory of the cycle states that if the plasma glucose concentration is decreased, fatty acids will be mobilized from the adipose tissue, the plasma fatty acid level will increase and this will cause increased fatty acid oxidation by muscle, which will depress glucose utilization. Consequently, the plasma glucose concentration will increase. This will stimulate glucose utilization by adipose tissue and restrict fatty acid mobilization, so that the plasma fatty acid level will be decreased and fatty acid oxidation in muscle will be decreased. Consequently, the inhibition of glucose utilization will be removed and the plasma glucose concentration will decrease once more (see Figure 5.13). This is a description of the mechanism for controlling the blood levels of fatty acids and glucose in the absence of any hormonal effects. Obviously the effects of hormones (which have been described in Section B of this chapter) will modify the simple controls described above; for example, an elevation in plasma glucose will increase the plasma concentration of insulin which will also decrease fatty acid mobilization (through effects on esterification and lipolysis) and increase glucose utilization in muscle (Figure 5.14). In essence the cycle provides a

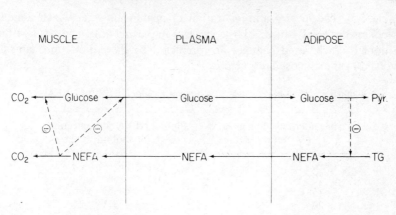

Figure 5.13. The glucose/fatty acid cycle. The inhibition of NEFA mobilization from adipose tissue by glycolysis is due to the effect of esterification (Section B.3). The inhibition of glucose utilization in muscles is described in Chapter 3

mechanism for the maintenance and conservation of the blood glucose level at the expense of variations in the plasma fatty acid level. With this cycle as a basis, it is possible to explain variations in the plasma levels of glucose and fatty acids under different dietary, physiological and pathological conditions.

Experiments which provide support for the glucose/fatty acid cycle include the following:

(*a*) The plasma fatty acid level varies over about a five-fold range in different physiological situations but the plasma glucose varies at most by 30%.

(*b*) The rise in glucose and insulin levels following a carbohydrate meal causes a 50% reduction in the plasma fatty acid level in only 30 minutes

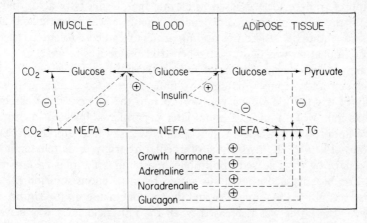

Figure 5.14. Effects of hormones on the glucose/fatty acid cycle

(Table 5.5). The *in vivo* administration of insulin antisera (which acutely lowers insulin level) causes a large increase in plasma fatty acid level within an hour.[80] Such rapid changes are predicted by the control mechanisms involved in the glucose/fatty acid cycle.

Table 5.5. Effect of refeeding glucose on the blood levels of NEFA[116]

Time after refeeding glucose (min)	Plasma NEFA concentration (μmol/ml)
0	0·79
10	0·68
15	0·52*
20	0·54*
30	0·34*
Normal fed animal	0·31*

Rats were starved for 48 hours and then force-fed glucose by stomach tube. After various time intervals blood samples were taken by cannulation of the aorta under ether anaesthesia. The concentrations are the means of five experiments and an asterisk denotes a statistically significant difference from the zero time concentration.

(c) Another prediction of the cycle is that whenever the fatty acid level is raised, glucose utilization should be depressed. There are problems involved in testing this prediction in the intact animal because techniques for artificially elevating plasma fatty acid levels are complicated by other factors. The most direct method of elevating the plasma level of fatty acids would be by intravenous injection. However, this could result in local high concentrations of fatty acids (at the site of injection) and cause haemolysis of the red cells. Injection of fatty acids bound to albumin raises the problem of injection of a foreign protein into the blood stream. Therefore in early studies, intravenous infusion of triglyceride was used to elevate the plasma fatty acids and the effect of this infusion upon oral glucose tolerance was investigated. In at least two studies[81,82] there was an impairment of glucose tolerance (that is, glucose utilization was depressed) when triglyceride was infused.

A simple and elegant means of raising the fatty acid level was devised by Schalch and Kipnis.[83] Human volunteers were fed a meal consisting mainly of triglyceride (which is absorbed into the blood stream as chylomicrons and VLDL) and 3·5 hours later heparin was injected in order to release lipoprotein lipase from the capillary walls of the adipose tissue (see Section A.1(a)(ii)). The hydrolysis of circulating triglyceride (chylomicrons and VLDL) by the released lipoprotein lipase raises the plasma fatty acid level. The blood glucose level was raised by intravenous infusion (25 g of glucose was infused in 4 minutes) and the rate of glucose disappearance was followed: the latter was decreased when the fatty acid level was elevated (see Table 5.6). In a similar study dogs, which had been starved, were infused

Table 5.6. Effect of an elevation of the plasma NEFA level on the rate of disappearance of plasma glucose in human subjects

The removal of intravenously administered glucose is an exponential process and the function for its rate of removal may be expressed as

$$K = \frac{\ln C_1 - \ln C_2}{t_2 - t_1}$$

where C_1 and C_2 are the concentrations of glucose at times t_1 and t_2 after intravenous administration.

A. The plasma NEFA was elevated by injection of heparin into eight human volunteers 3 to 4 hours after a meal containing 60 g of fat. Glucose was administered intravenously. The data are taken from reference 83.

Conditions	Plasma NEFA concentration (μmol/ml)	Disappearance of glucose K
Control	0·4–0·8	3·49 $\pm$ 0·60
Heparin	1·5–2·0	1·84 $\pm$ 0·33
Three diabetic subjects (heparin not administered)	—	1·24 $\pm$ 0·24

B. The plasma NEFA was elevated by administration of noradrenaline to six human volunteers. Also, the effect of noradrenaline on the elevation of plasma NEFA was inhibited by administration of nicotinic acid. The data are taken from reference 85.

Conditions	Plasma NEFA concentration (μmol/ml)	Disappearance of glucose K
Control	—	1·74
Noradrenaline	1·1–2·2	0·76
Noradrenaline plus nicotinic acid	0·2–0·5	1·52

with triglyceride and lipoprotein lipase was released by heparin administration. This treatment raised the plasma fatty acid level. The rate of release of glucose by the liver and the rate of peripheral glucose utilization were depressed.[84]

The infusion of noradrenaline into human subjects provides an alternative method of elevating the fatty acid level. This hormone appears to have a fairly specific effect in increasing the activity of triglyceride lipase in adipose tissue and thus increases the rate of fatty acid mobilization. The infusion of noradrenaline into human subjects also causes an impairment of the glucose tolerance[85] (Table 5.6).

In another experiment,[86] either labelled palmitate (albumin bound) or labelled glucose was infused into dogs and the rate of fatty acid or glucose oxidation and the turnover rates were measured. At a low plasma NEFA concentration the percentages of the total CO_2 derived from glucose and fatty acids were 30 and 15, respectively. At a high plasma NEFA concentration the percentages of CO_2 derived from glucose and fatty acids were 15 and 60, respectively.

(d) The theory predicts that when the fatty acid level is decreased the glucose level should fall and the glucose tolerance should improve. This prediction has been tested by the administration of nicotinic acid, which inhibits lipolysis in adipose tissue, to normal and diabetic human subjects. As predicted, the glucose concentration was lowered by nicotinic acid and the tolerance improved.[87] However, the results of this type of experiment are variable and other workers have reported hyperglycaemia and an impairment of glucose tolerance. One of the problems with nicotinic acid is that, after its antilipolytic effects have subsided, there is an elevation in plasma fatty acid level, which is known as a 'rebound' phenomenon. This could be the explanation for the conflicting results.

In another experiment, rats were made acutely diabetic with insulin antisera and were given nicotinic acid. This treatment prevented the rise in plasma level of fatty acids (and ketone bodies) and markedly reduced the hyperglycaemia which is normally associated with antisera treatment.[88]

(e) The theory predicts that inhibition of fatty acid oxidation should increase glucose utilization and lower the blood glucose concentration. Accordingly, it has been observed that certain compounds, which are known to be specific inhibitors of fatty acid oxidation, are hypoglycaemic. One such compound is 'hypoglycin' (L,α-amino, β-methylcyclopropane propionic acid) which occurs in unripe fruits of the Blighia-Sapida tree. Ingestion of such fruit causes 'Jamaican vomiting sickness', a condition which is characterized by hypoglycaemia.[89] Also, pent-4-enoic acid, which inhibits fatty acid oxidation in vitro, is hypoglycaemic whereas chemically-similar compounds, which do not inhibit fatty acid oxidation, are not hypoglycaemic.[89]

(f) Experiments have recently been performed on the human heart in situ by the use of arterial and coronary sinus catheterization techniques.[90] A negative correlation has been observed between the arterial level of NEFA and the myocardial utilization of glucose, pyruvate and lactate. This is convincing evidence that the experimental findings with the in vitro perfused heart preparation can be applied to the heart in vivo.

Despite the evidence (cited in (a) to (f) above) which supports the theory of the glucose/fatty acid cycle, there remain some doubts about the physiological significance of such a cycle. These doubts are raised by observations which appear to be inconsistent with the theory. In particular, there have been a number of experiments which demonstrate that raising the level of plasma fatty acids (or ketone bodies) decreases the plasma glucose concentration and improves glucose tolerance.[91,92,93] There is always a danger with *in vivo* experiments that the observed changes in glucose levels may be due to *indirect effects* of fatty acids (or ketone bodies) that are not predicted by the glucose/fatty acid cycle as formulated above. For example, there is some evidence that elevated levels of ketone bodies can cause stimulation of insulin secretion by the pancreas (see Chapter 7, Section E.3). The effect of insulin would be to decrease plasma fatty acid levels, increase glucose utilization and diminish glucose output by the liver. Consequently, under some conditions a rise in the plasma NEFA and ketone body levels may result in hypoglycaemia rather than hyperglycaemia. Thus, although the experimental demonstration that elevation of the plasma NEFA and ketone body levels causes hypoglycaemia is inconsistent with the original theory of the glucose/fatty acid cycle, it is consistent with the extended theory of the glucose/fatty acid cycle discussed in detail in Chapter 7 (see Section E).

2. Physiological implications of the glucose/fatty acid cycle

(a) The plasma fatty acid level as a signal for starvation

The observed increase in plasma fatty acid level in starvation should be sufficient to cause a considerable increase in the rate of their oxidation. Such an effect would decrease glucose utilization in muscle (for mechanism see Chapter 3, Section D.5) and possibly in other tissues—for example, liver and kidney cortex tissue. The oxidation of fatty acids in the liver causes the formation of ketone bodies which act as a supplementary fuel to fatty acids for muscle, kidney and possibly other tissues. Moreover, ketone bodies can function as an alternative fuel to glucose for brain and specifically reduce the glucose requirement of this tissue (see Chapters 6 and 7). The physiological result of these effects is that in starvation glucose is conserved for tissues that have some degree of dependence on this fuel (such as brain, nerves and red blood cells).

(b) Prolonged muscular activity

Prolonged muscular activity, such as occurs in migratory flights of birds and insects and in long-distance running in man, may result in a similar situation to starvation, in that reserve fuels must be utilized. It has been calculated that the energy expenditure during a marathon is of the order of 2,000 kcal, but the total reserves of carbohydrate in the average man are only about 650 kcal. Therefore the muscles must oxidize fatty acids and the energetic considerations of the marathon emphasize that glucose utilization is reduced so that the carbohydrate reserves are *not* seriously depleted.

(c) The uptake of glucose by muscle, following a carbohydrate meal

The reciprocal changes in blood glucose and fatty acid levels are predicted by the glucose/fatty acid cycle. They may be of physiological significance following a carbohydrate-containing meal. The rapid influx of glucose from the gut causes a rise in blood glucose (and insulin) level. Since the T_{max} of the kidney tubule reabsorption-system for glucose is only about twice the normal blood glucose level, it is important that the elevation in this level is restricted in order to prevent loss of carbohydrate in the urine. The liver and adipose tissue must play major roles in the removal of glucose from the circulation. However, increased glucose uptake by the large mass of skeletal muscle may also be a contributory factor. The rapid fall in the plasma level of fatty acids, which is observed after a carbohydrate meal, should ensure that glucose utilization by the musculature is increased.

(d) The absorption of fat from the gut

The absorption and assimilation of fat is a complex process consisting of a series of lipolytic and esterification reactions (see Figure 5.15). The system

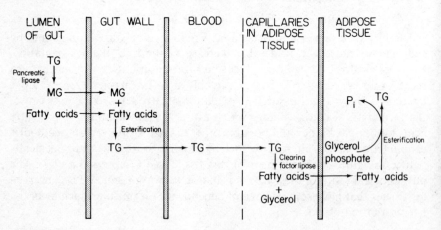

Figure 5.15. The lipolytic and esterification reactions involved in the digestion, absorption and assimilation of triglyceride

could undoubtedly be much simpler if, following the initial hydrolysis in the intestine, fatty acids were absorbed directly and transported to the adipose tissue as an albumin complex in the blood. One problem with this hypothetical mechanism for fat absorption is that the transport system in the blood (albumin/fatty acid complex) is not capable of carrying large quantities of fat in relatively short periods of time: the limit is imposed by the amount of albumin in the plasma. It has been calculated (Table 5.2) that approximately 160 g of fat can be transported in 24 hours when the concentration of the plasma fatty acid is 0·6 mM. Therefore in 6 hours (a reasonable digestive time) a maximum of 40 g of fat could be transported in this way. The fact that not even this quantity of fat is absorbed as fatty acid bound to albumin can be explained by the glucose/fatty acid cycle. If fatty acids were not esterified upon absorption, the plasma level of fatty acids would be increased. This would decrease the utilization of glucose by muscle and other tissues. Since most animals eat a mixed diet, fatty acids and glucose would be absorbed together and the utilization of the glucose would be depressed. This would result in an accumulation of glucose in the blood and its consequent loss through the kidney tubules. The process of absorption is therefore designed so that most of the ingested fatty acids enter the general circulation in an esterified form, which effectively 'conceals' them from any tissues which do not possess an active lipoprotein lipase. The only quantitatively-important tissue that contains an active lipoprotein lipase in the fed state in a normal animal is adipose tissue.

3. Pathological implications of the glucose/fatty acid cycle

It is becoming increasingly apparent that some of the symptoms (if not the basic cause) of certain pathological conditions may be related to changes in plasma fatty acid levels. High plasma levels of fatty acids (either acute or chronic) are now considered to be highly undesirable since a reasonable amount of evidence links this situation with conditions such as diabetes mellitus, obesity, thyrotoxicosis, atherosclerosis and coronary thrombosis.[94,95] Research into some of these conditions is too specialized to be discussed here, but clinical diabetes involves a disturbance of carbohydrate and fat metabolism which may be explained on the basis of the glucose/fatty acid cycle.

Diabetes mellitus

Early studies on clinical diabetes gave rise to the idea that the pathologically high blood glucose level found in this condition was caused primarily by an insufficiency of circulating insulin. The development of sensitive and specific radioimmunological assays for insulin led to the observation that in the majority of diabetic patients this was not the case. In 'growth onset' diabetes, which is usually manifest before the age of 20, the plasma insulin levels are indeed very low (less than 10% of the normal) and therefore lack of circulating insulin, presumably due to malfunction of the β-cells in the pancreatic islets, would appear to be the cause of this type of diabetes. The elevated plasma glucose level can be explained by the consequent low rate of entry of glucose into muscle and adipose tissue cells. Furthermore, the increased plasma fatty acid concentration can be explained by an increase in the rate of mobilization from adipose tissue.

The majority of diabetic patients do not develop their symptoms until 'middle age' and this type of diabetes is termed 'maturity onset'. The symptoms are similar to those of 'growth onset' diabetes: elevated plasma levels of glucose, fatty acids and ketone bodies. However, the level of plasma insulin is normal or even elevated.[96] Therefore there appear to be different primary lesions involved in these two types of diabetes. One explanation for the biochemical symptoms of maturity-onset diabetes is that a specific insulin antagonist is present in the blood of these patients so that the effect of insulin upon glucose uptake by adipose tissue and muscle is effectively reduced. This would result in increased plasma levels of glucose (and also increased fatty acid levels due to depressed esterification in adipose tissue), and this would stimulate secretion of more insulin. Consequently, the level of circulating insulin would be higher than normal. There have been several demonstrations of the presence of insulin antagonists in the blood of such patients,[97] but their importance in the aetiology of this disease is uncertain. Alternatively, it has been proposed that the primary metabolic lesion is excessive mobilization of fatty acids from adipose tissue. This would elevate the plasma level of fatty acids and stimulate their oxidation; glucose utilization would be depressed and, consequently, the plasma glucose level would be elevated. The latter would stimulate insulin secretion and increase the plasma level of the hormone. This interpretation is obviously based on the theory of the glucose/fatty acid cycle.[98] At present it is not possible at a biochemical level to distinguish between these two extreme theories. The clinical condition may be highly complex and both explanations may be partially correct. Nonetheless, in both cases treatment with exogenous insulin would be expected to restore the situation towards normal, despite the fact that an absolute deficiency of insulin is not the primary metabolic lesion.

4. Fat as a fuel for exercise

There is no longer any doubt that the oxidation of fat plays a vital role in the provision of energy for sustained muscular activity. Fat is available to the muscle either as triglyceride stored within the muscles (endogenous) or as one of the fat fuels present in the blood (long-chain fatty acids, ketone bodies and triglyceride). Fatty acids in the blood are derived from triglyceride stored in adipose tissue and ketone bodies are formed from the partial oxidation of fatty acids in the liver (see Chapter 7 for full discussion). Triglyceride is present in the blood usually in the form of VLDL and it can be oxidized for the supply of energy if the muscle possesses sufficient lipoprotein lipase activity. Unfortunately, the maximum activity of lipoprotein lipase in skeletal muscle is not known at present.

Carbohydrate is used as a fuel for supply of energy for muscular activity. However, the endogenous stores of carbohydrate in the muscle are so limited that if this were the only fuel, exhaustion would occur within minutes or even seconds from the initiation of muscular work. Indeed, it can be calculated that the rate of ATP turnover during intense muscular activity is of the order of 200 μmol per g muscle per minute (Chapter 3, Appendix 3.1). Since the glycogen stores are only of the order of 20 μmol per g muscle, the maximum amount of ATP which could be formed by the *complete oxidation* of all the muscle glycogen would be in the region of 700 μmol per g and this could support contraction for only 3·5 minutes. The *anaerobic* degradation of this glycogen could support contraction for only 20 seconds. The glucose that is available in the blood can also provide a fuel for muscles, if they possess an adequate vascular system to supply glucose at a sufficient rate. The blood glucose used during muscular activity would need to be replenished from the reservoir of liver glycogen, and this also is limited. For example, the human liver can store about 100 g of glycogen and this might provide a marathon runner with sufficient fuel for about 15 minutes running.

In contrast, the stores of fat in the body are not only large but, in certain species (notably *Homo sapiens*), their capacity appears to be virtually unlimited! The advantage of fat as a fuel rests in the fact that approximately nine times more energy can be obtained from the oxidation of one gram of stored fat than can be obtained from one gram of stored glycogen (see Section A). Thus, in order to store an equivalent amount of fuel solely in the form of glycogen, the energy reserve would have to be nine-fold heavier. This is an obvious problem for terrestrial animals but it would be insurmountable for animals such as migratory birds and insects which have to fly long distances non-stop. If such animals were to store sufficient fuel for a long migratory flight solely in the form of glycogen, they would be too heavy to lift themselves off the ground!

A number of studies have been carried out on the fat content of migratory birds and insects. Some species of migratory birds fly continuously for approximately 1,500 miles and this entails sustained muscular activity for about 60 hours (travelling at 25 miles per hour). Birds that migrate from North to Central America across the Gulf of Mexico have been studied in some detail since there is no land upon which they could rest and feed during the flight and the distances for the various routes that are taken are between 600 and 1,500 miles.[99] Some of these birds are killed by flying into a tall television transmitting tower situated on the Florida coast and, although it is unfortunate for these creatures, they do provide suitable biopsy material for the study of some aspects of their metabolism. The fat index* of non-migratory birds is usually of the order of 0·2–0·4, but for some migratory species (the ruby-throated humming bird, for example) the values reach between 3·0 and

* The 'fat index' is defined as the amount of ether-extractable fat material per gram of non-fat material (on a dry weight basis).

4·0. When these birds are captured after their migratory flight, the fat index has invariably decreased to between 0·3 and 0·6.

Many insects (butterflies, moths and locusts, for example) use fat as a source of energy during migratory flights. Detailed studies have been carried out on the use of stored fat during prolonged tethered flight by the locust in the laboratory. The insect is fixed, by some form of support to the dorsal part of the thorax, and it can be induced to fly by directing a current of air over its head. Weis-Fogh[100] has shown that there is sufficient fat stored in the locust for about 10 hours' continuous flight, that locusts can fly for approximately this length of time under laboratory conditions and that the quantity of fat consumed was sufficient to provide the energy for this flight. However, during a normal migratory flight, the use of favourable wind currents may enable the locust to remain airborne for considerably longer than 10 hours and hence to fly for several hundred miles.

There is considerable evidence that fat is utilized by man, particularly during prolonged exercise. Measurements of respiratory quotients show a shift to lower values (that is, towards increased fat oxidation) as the duration of exercise is increased and considerable attention has been focused upon the type of the lipid used for exercise in man. Sustained exercise (for example, taking part in a nine-hour ski race)[101] results in a considerable decrease in in the plasma lipoprotein concentration, in particular VLDL. However, it has been concluded that this is unlikely to be caused by an increased rate of removal by muscle, but can probably be explained by a decreased production of VLDL by the liver. Preliminary reports indicate that endogenous muscle triglyceride is decreased by prolonged exercise.[102] However, Carlson[103] has reached the conclusion that most of the energy demand during prolonged exercise in man can be satisfied by the increased mobilization of fatty acids. Calculations based upon the elevation in plasma NEFA level in man during moderate sustained exercise (walking 50 km per day on a low-calorie diet) indicate that most of the energy requirement can be derived from the oxidation of plasma fatty acids.*

The emphasis in this discussion upon lipid fuels must not be taken to imply that, under all conditions, fat is the sole, or even the most important, fuel for muscle contraction: this is certainly not the case. The proportion of the total energy which is derived from fat depends upon a variety of factors including the intensity of the work performed, the duration of the exercise period, the type of work performed (in terms of the particular muscles

* The average plasma NEFA concentration in the fasting subjects was 1·4 mM, that is 1·4 μmol/ml or a total of 4·2 mmol in the blood (taking the average blood volume as 3 litres). 4·2 mmol of long-chain fatty acid (average molecular weight approximately 250) is equivalent to 1 g fatty acids. The fractional turnover rate is 0·33 per minute, that is 0·33 g long-chain fatty acids enter and leave the blood each minute. Therefore the daily turnover is 0·33 × 60 × 24 g, equals 475 g. The average daily weight loss observed in the fasting, exercising subjects was 750 g, which is equivalent to 500 g long-chain fatty acids.

used) and lastly the species under consideration (see reference 104 for review). Apparently certain species of insects (honey-bee and blowfly, for example) rely solely upon carbohydrate (stored in the form of glycogen, trehalose or glucose) as a fuel for flight. In man a mixture of fat and carbohydrate is used at a moderate work intensity and as the muscular activity is prolonged the *RQ* decreases, suggesting that fat becomes the more important fuel. As the work *intensity* is increased so the *RQ* approaches 1·0, suggesting that the rate of glucose and/or glycogen utilization is increased. Physical exhaustion occurs more rapidly at a higher work intensity when perhaps the limiting factors are the availability of oxygen and fuel which are supplied in the blood. Presumably, if the supply of energy is limited by the oxygen availability to the muscles, anaerobic glycolysis from endogenous glycogen may provide extra energy for a short period of time. If fuel rather than oxygen is limiting, the glycogen could be completely oxidized and provide a more efficient use of this fuel for energy production. A low rate of oxidation (assuming complete oxidation) of endogenous glycogen could provide a small percentage (say 10%) of the extra energy for the mechanical work for a considerable period of time (say 15–30 minutes). However, once the endogenous glycogen has been utilized, the muscle must presumably begin to take up glucose from the blood which would result in a decrease in the blood glucose level. It is not known how far the blood glucose level could fall before the muscle would fail to obtain sufficient energy for contraction and before the onset of fatigue. However, if physical exhaustion is related to a lowering of the blood glucose concentration in the local environment of the muscle, a depletion of the muscle glycogen reserves may be the initiating factor in the development of fatigue. The experimental observation that the infusion of glucose into a previously exhausted subject allows the resumption of exercise is consistent with this idea.

In this context it is undoubtedly incorrect to consider exhaustion as being due either to a simple lack of ATP or to the accumulation of lactate in the muscle. As discussed in Chapter 3, a lack of ATP in a tissue would cause a serious disturbance in energy-transfer mechanisms and this would impair the efficiency of many metabolic reactions. In any situation in which energy levels are in danger of decreasing seriously, non-essential processes are inhibited so that activities vital to the life of the cell (ion transport, for example) can continue. For example, if the isolated perfused heart is made anaerobic, the contraction rate rapidly falls despite the fact that the ATP content is reduced by only about 10%. When the perfusion is transferred back to aerobic conditions (even after 15 minutes anaerobiosis), the heart soon regains its normal contractility.[105] In muscles which have a good blood supply (heart, for example), the lactate produced by anaerobic glycolysis from glycogen can be easily removed. Indeed, should the accumulation of lactate be the cause of fatigue, it would be anticipated to occur at an early stage of glycogen breakdown when glycolysis would be maximally stimulated, and not when the glycogen and local blood glucose pools have been depleted. It seems possible that physical exhaustion is not due to any malfunction of the biochemical process within the muscle cell itself, but perhaps is due to a failure of the nervous system supplying the muscles. Since exhaustion appears to be related to an insufficiency in the supply of glucose, and since it is known that nervous tissue has an important requirement for glucose, a temporary malfunction of the metabolism within the local nervous supply to the muscle may be an explanation of fatigue.

If fatty acids and oxygen are supplied to the muscles at a rate that is sufficient for the supply of energy from fatty acid oxidation, glycogen and glucose utilization could be reduced to a minimum and muscular activity could be continued for a long period without exhaustion. Presumably this is the situation in the migratory animals and in man when walking (an activity which can be continued for many hours without exhaustion). The role of training in increasing the amount of exercise which can be performed may be related to an improvement in blood circulation (so that more oxygen and more fuel can be supplied to the muscle) and perhaps an improved ability to mobilize and oxidize fatty acids. The effect of training on increasing the resistance to physical exhaustion is difficult to explain in biochemical terms. It may be connected with the glucose/fatty acid cycle, since an improved capacity for fatty acid oxidation will reduce the dependence on glucose and glycogen.

D. THE METABOLIC ROLE OF BROWN ADIPOSE TISSUE

1. Brown adipose tissue and thermogenesis

Brown adipose tissue is highly specialized and is found in some animals, particularly hibernating animals and the new-born of certain species. This tissue has presumably been termed 'adipose tissue' on account of its high lipid content, but it is structurally, metabolically and functionally distinct from white adipose tissue. Most of the brown adipose tissue is localized in the dorsal part of the thorax under the shoulder blades, although there are often smaller amounts around the adrenals and kidneys and in the peri-anal and inguinal regions.

The particular association of brown adipose tissue with hibernating animals, with animals whose habitat is a cold region and with neonatal infants, has given rise to the idea that this tissue might be important in heat generation.[106] Hibernating animals warm up slowly as the ambient temperature increases in spring, but many are capable of warming up rapidly despite a low ambient temperature (for example, for short periods in winter). Such animals must possess a special mechanism for the production of heat and it has been found that brown adipose tissue develops extensively prior to hibernation. In some very young animals (for example, human babies and newly born rabbits) the ability to produce heat by shivering (involuntary muscular activity which results in heat production rather than movement) is not developed, but brown adipose tissue is present. The proximity of brown adipose tissue to the vital organs (such as the heart and kidneys) is consistent with the theory that the tissue is responsible for heat generation. More direct evidence for the involvement of this tissue in heat production has been obtained from experiments on hibernating animals in which thermocouples have been placed in brown adipose tissue and in several other tissues. During the arousal period the temperature of brown adipose tissue increases before that of any other tissue and this temperature difference is maintained for some time.[107] It is now generally accepted that the function of brown adipose tissue is to generate heat. Indeed it has been calculated that at least 50% of the heat produced during arousal in hibernating animals is derived from this tissue.[108] However, the metabolic mechanism by which large quantities of heat are produced in this tissue is still disputed.

Some indication of the metabolic nature of brown adipose tissue has been obtained from investigations into its ultrastructure. The tissue is highly vascular and consists of small polygonal cells, each containing many separate lipid droplets (cf. white adipose tissue). The striking feature of these cells is the high content of mitochondria (see Figure 5.16). Thus, oxidative

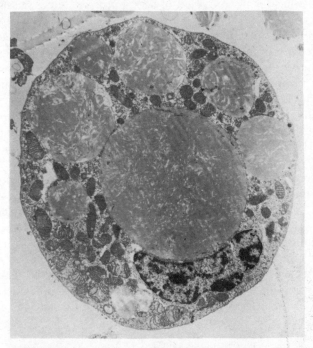

Figure 5.16. An electron micrograph of a brown adipose tissue cell. × 4,000. The electron micrograph was kindly supplied by Dr G. V. Brenchley and Professor C. N. Hales of the Department of Chemical Pathology, The Welsh National School of Medicine, Cardiff

metabolism of triglyceride is anticipated to play a vital role in heat production.

2. Mechanisms of thermogenesis

The generation of heat by shivering may be explained as follows: the increase in mechanical activity causes a stimulation of ATP hydrolysis in the muscle and this leads to an increased rate of general metabolism including mitochondrial respiration and ATP turnover. The extra heat is generated particularly by increases in the rates of *non-equilibrium* reactions of metabolism. Obviously in brown adipose tissue the stimulation of metabolism and respiration must occur by some means other than increased mechanical activity! There are at least two possible mechanisms for the increased thermogenesis in this tissue. First, mitochondrial phosphorylation might be uncoupled from respiration so that the energy of electron transport, which is normally conserved in ATP synthesis, would be lost as heat. Second, specific metabolic reactions, which involve the hydrolysis of ATP, might be stimulated so that the metabolic rate, mitochondrial respiration and ATP turnover would increase.

Both of these mechanisms for heat generation require an increased oxidation of some fuel for the provision of heat. In brown adipose tissue the fuel is, of course, triglyceride. This is hydrolysed to fatty acids which provide the substrate for mitochondrial oxidation. Therefore an increase in the catalytic activity of the triglyceride lipase in this tissue is a prerequisite for increased heat production. It has been shown that an increase in cyclic AMP content in brown adipose tissue is associated with increased lipolysis.[109] The content of cyclic AMP in brown adipose tissue is raised in response to noradrenaline[110] and there is evidence that during arousal in hibernating animals this hormone is released from sympathetic nerve endings in this tissue.[111] Therefore the sequence of events initiating heat production during arousal may be as follows: stimulation of the sympathetic nervous system raises the local concentration of noradrenaline in the brown adipose tissue, the intracellular level of cyclic AMP is raised and this activates the lipase leading to an increase in the intracellular concentration of fatty acids. The latter are oxidized by the brown adipose tissue (although some may be released into the blood).

Obviously the next question is, why should an increase in the concentration of fatty acids lead to the generation of heat? In other words, what facet of its metabolism differentiates brown adipose tissue from other tissues in its response to an increased intracellular concentration of fatty acids? There are at least two possible answers to this question.

(a) The uncoupling of phosphorylation from electron transport

Mitochondria isolated from brown adipose tissue usually convert much less inorganic phosphate to ATP per mole of oxygen consumed than those isolated from other tissues (for example, liver).[112] This strongly suggests that phosphorylation is uncoupled from electron transport in mitochondria from brown adipose tissue. Since long-chain fatty acids are known to be potent uncoupling agents,[113] this situation could result from the high concentrations of fatty acids present in the tissue homogenate during preparation of the mitochondria. The high concentration of fatty acids might be an artefact of the extraction process and bear little relation to the concentration in the cell during thermogenesis. On the other hand, activation of the lipase by noradrenaline might be sufficient to elevate the intracellular level of fatty acids to such an extent that uncoupling is a physiological response. It is difficult to distinguish between these two possibilities although, if precautions are taken to maintain a low concentration of fatty acids during the preparation of the mitochondria from brown adipose tissue, they appear to be more sensitive to the uncoupling action of externally-added fatty acids than mitochondria from other tissues (for example, liver).[112] This suggests that the uncoupling action of fatty acids might be physiologically important in initiating thermogenesis in brown adipose tissue. The effect of the uncoupling action would be to prevent conservation of the energy released from electron transport during the oxidation of fatty acids. Furthermore, uncoupling would lead to a decrease in the [ATP]/[ADP] ratio in the brown adipose tissue cell and this could increase the rate of the TCA cycle (Chapter 3, Section E.2) and the rate of electron transport (Chapter 1, Section D.2). Consequently mobilization of fatty acids within the brown adipose tissue cell could stimulate oxidative metabolism, respiration and ATP turnover as well as uncoupling oxidative phosphorylation.

(b) Substrate cycles

The significance of non-equilibrium reactions in ensuring the unidirectionality of metabolism has been discussed in Chapter 1 and it has been stressed that such reactions must liberate heat. Obviously, one mechanism for the production of heat in brown adipose tissue is to increase the flux through unidirectional reactions (provided that the non-equilibrium characteristics are maintained). However, the rate of a unidirectional process cannot be increased indefinitely unless the product of that process can be continually removed. The problem of product removal can be overcome by combining two opposing processes to form a *substrate cycle*: in this case there is no product accumulation but there *is* a net loss of energy in the form of heat. In biological systems such reactions inevitably involve ATP hydrolysis (either directly or indirectly). Therefore an increase in the activities of the enzymes catalysing a substrate cycle leads to increased ATP turnover, increased mitochondrial respiration and increased heat production. One example of such a substrate cycle, the triglyceride/fatty acid cycle, is shown in Figure 5.17. In this cycle, heat is generated by the continual operation of the lipolytic and re-esterification processes. Heat will be released in all the reactions that are non-equilibrium (for example, lipolysis, fatty acid activation, and glycerol phosphorylation).

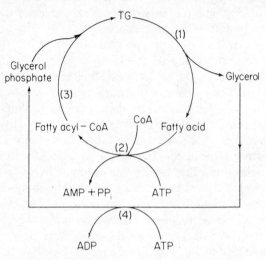

Figure 5.17. The triglyceride/fatty acid cycle in brown adipose tissue. (1) Lipolysis (lipase). (2) Fatty acid activation (fatty acyl-CoA synthetase). (3) Esterification. (4) Glycerol kinase

From experiments with isolated brown adipose tissue *in vitro*, there is evidence that this cycle is stimulated by noradrenaline. Also, experiments with whole animals have shown that the rate of this cycle is increased upon exposure to cold. An increase in the incorporation of ^{14}C from ^{14}C-labelled glucose into glyceride-glycerol has been observed in both types of experiment.[114] This implies an increase in the rate of esterification. The presence of noradrenaline or exposure to cold also leads to an increase in the activity of the triglyceride lipase, which is probably the regulatory enzyme in this cycle. In addition, brown adipose tissue contains a higher activity of glycerol kinase than white adipose tissue,[114] so that a large proportion of the glycerol released upon lipolysis can be converted to glycerol phosphate and utilized for re-esterification. Consequently, this cycle is less dependent upon a supply of glucose than the equivalent cycle in white adipose tissue.

Calculations based upon the incorporation of ^{14}C from ^{14}C-glucose into the glycerol moiety of triglyceride suggest that this cycle could account for only a small proportion of the heat produced by brown adipose tissue, even when glycerol kinase activity is taken into account.[114] Although such calculations must be very approximate, it can be concluded at the present time that the major portion of the heat released from brown adipose tissue is produced by the failure of the mitochondria to conserve the energy of electron transport.

REFERENCES FOR CHAPTER 5

1. Wertheimer, E. & Shapiro, B. (1948). *Physiol. Rev.* **28**, 451.
2. Schoenheimer, R. & Rittenberg, D. (1935). *J. biol. Chem.* **111**, 175.
3. Weis-Fogh, T. (1967). In *Insects and Physiology*, p. 143. Ed. J. W. Beament & J. E. Treherne. Edinburgh: Oliver & Boyd.
4. Johnston, J. M. (1970). In *Comprehensive Biochemistry*, **18**, 1. Ed. M. Florkin & E. H. Stotz. Amsterdam: Elsevier.
5. Kiyasu, J. Y., Bloom, B. & Chaikoff, I. L. (1952). *J. biol. Chem.* **199**, 415.
6. Robinson, D. S. (1970). In *Comprehensive Biochemistry*, **18**, 51. Ed. M. Florkin & E. H. Stotz. Amsterdam: Elsevier.
7. Vaughan, M. (1961). *J. Lipid Res.* **2**, 293.
8. Lynen, F. (1961). *Fed. Proc.* **20**, 941.
9. Srere, P. A. (1965). *Nature, Lond.* **205**, 766.
10. Martin, B. R. & Denton, R. M. (1970). *Biochem. J.* **117**, 861.
11. Lardy, H. A., Paetkau, V. & Walter, P. (1965). *Proc. nat. Acad. Sci. Wash.* **53**, 1410.
12. Ballard, F. J. & Hanson, R. W. (1967). *J. Lipid Res.* **8**, 73.
13. Flatt, J. P. & Ball, E. G. (1964). *J. biol. Chem.* **239**, 675.
14. Katz, J., Landau, B. R. & Bartsch, G. E. (1966). *J. biol. Chem.* **241**, 727.
15. McLean, P. (1960). *Biochim. biophys. Acta*, **37**, 296.
16. Flatt, J. P. & Ball, E. G. (1966). *J. biol. Chem.* **241**, 2862.
17. Halperin, M. L. & Denton, R. M. (1969). *Biochem. J.* **113**, 207.
18. Saggerson, E. D. & Greenbaum, A. L. (1970). *Biochem. J.* **119**, 193.
19. Numa, S., Bortz, W. M. & Lynen, F. (1964). *Adv. Enz. Reg.* **3**, 407.
20. Saggerson, E. D. & Greenbaum, A. L. (1970). *Biochem. J.* **119**, 221.
21. Vagelos, P. R. (1971). In *Current Topics in Cellular Regulation*, **4**, 119. Ed. B. L. Horecker & E. W. Stadtman. London & New York: Academic Press.
22. Denton, R. M. & Halperin, M. L. (1968). *Biochem. J.* **110**, 27.
23. Fang, M. & Lowenstein, J. M. (1967). *Biochem. J.* **105**, 803.
24. Del Boca, J. & Flatt, J. P. (1969). *Europ. J. Biochem.* **11**, 127.
25. Coore, H. G., Denton, R. M., Martin, B. R. & Randle, P. J. (1971). *Biochem. J.* **125**, 115.
26. Robinson, J. & Newsholme, E. A. (1967). *Biochem. J.* **104**, 2C.
27. Ballard, F. J., Hanson, R. W. & Leveille, G. A. (1967). *J. biol. Chem.* **242**, 2746.
28. Favarger, P. (1965). In *Handbook of Physiology, Section 5, Adipose Tissue*, p. 19. Ed. A. E. Renold & G. F. Cahill. Washington, D.C.: American Physiological Society.
29. Feller, D. D. (1965). In *Handbook of Physiology, Section 5, Adipose Tissue*, p. 363. Ed. A. E. Renold & G. F. Cahill. Washington, D.C.: American Physiological Society.
30. Bierman, E. L. (1965). In *Handbook of Physiology, Section 5, Adipose Tissue*, p. 509. Ed. A. E. Renold & G. F. Cahill. Washington, D.C.: American Physiological Society.
31. Schumaker, V. M. & Adams, G. H. (1969). *Ann. Rev. Biochem.* **38**, 113.

32. Dole, V. P. (1956). *J. clin. Invest.* **35,** 150.
33. Gordon, R. S. & Cherkes, A. (1956). *J. clin. Invest.* **35,** 206.
34. Gordon, R. S., Cherkes, A. & Gates, H. (1957). *J. clin. Invest.* **36,** 810.
35. Havel, R. J. & Fredrickson, D. S. (1956). *J. clin. Invest.* **35,** 1025.
36. Rapport, D. (1930). *Physiol. Rev.* **10,** 349.
37. Stadie, W. C. (1945). *Physiol. Rev.* **25,** 395.
38. Gordon, R. S. & Cherkes, A. (1958). *Proc. Soc. Exp. Biol. Med.* **97,** 150.
39. White, J. E. & Engel, F. L. (1958). *Clin. Res.* **6,** 266.
40. Steinberg, D. (1963). In *Control of Lipid Metabolism,* p. 111. Ed. J. K. Grant. London & New York: Academic Press.
41. Hales, C. N. & Randle, P. J. (1963). *Biochem. J.* **88,** 137.
42. Denton, R. M., Yorke, R. E. & Randle, P. J. (1966). *Biochem. J.* **100,** 407.
43. Unger, R. H. & Eisentraut, A. M. (1969). *Arch. int. Med.* **123,** 261.
44. Perley, M. J. & Kipnis, D. M. (1967). *J. clin. Invest.* **46,** 1954.
45. Butcher, R. W., Ho, R. J., Meng, H. C. & Sutherland, E. W. (1965). *J. biol. Chem.* **240,** 4515.
46. Sutherland, E. W, Øye, I. & Butcher, R. W. (1965). *Rec. Prog. Horm. Res.* **21,** 623.
47. Löffler, G. & Weiss, L. (1970). In *Adipose Tissue,* p. 32. Ed. B. Jeanrenaud & B. Hepp. London: Academic Press; and Jungas, R. L. & Schwartz, J. P. *ibid.* p. 37.
48. Corbin, J. D., Reimann, E. M., Walsh, D. A. & Krebs, E. G. (1970). *J. biol. Chem.* **245,** 4849.
49. Carlson, L. A. & Orö, L. (1963). *Metabolism,* **12,** 132.
50. Vaughan, M. (1962). *J. biol. Chem.* **237,** 3354.
51. Houssay, B. A. (1960). *J. Endocrinology,* **21,** 1.
52. Lee, M. & Ayres, G. B. (1936). *Endocrinology,* **20,** 489.
53. Russell, J. A. & Wilhelmi, A. E. (1950). *Endocrinology,* **47,** 26.
54. Young, F. G. (1953). *Rec. Prog. Horm. Res.* **8,** 471.
55. Roth, J., Glick, S. M., Yalow, R. S. & Berson, S. A. (1963). *Science,* **140,** 987.
56. Cahill, G. F., Herrera, M. G., Morgan, A. P., Soeldner, J. S., Steinke, J., Levy, P. L., Reichard, G. A. & Kipnis, D. M. (1966). *J. clin. Invest.* **45,** 1751.
57. Daughaday, W. H. & Kipnis, D. M. (1966). *Rec. Prog. Horm. Res.* **22,** 49.
58. Raben, M. S. & Hollenberg, C. H. (1959). *J. clin. Invest.* **38,** 484.
59. Kovacev, V. P. & Scow, R. O. (1966). *Amer. J. Physiol.* **210,** 1199.
60. Fain, J. N. (1967). *Adv. Enz. Reg.* **5,** 39.
61. Fain, J. N. & Siperstein, R. (1970). In *Adipose Tissue,* p. 20. Ed. B. Jeanrenaud & D. Hepp. New York & London: Academic Press.
62. Havel, R. J. & Carlson, L. A. (1963). *Life Sci.* **2,** 651.
63. Havel, R. J. (1965). *Ann. N.Y. Acad. Sci.* **131,** 91.
64. Jungas, R. L. & Ball, E. G. (1963). *Biochemistry,* **2,** 383.
65. Fain, J. N., Kovacev, V. P. & Scow, R. O. (1966). *Endocrinology,* **78,** 773.
66. Scow, R. O. & Chernick, S. S. (1970). In *Comprehensive Biochemistry,* **18,** 19. Ed. M. Florkin & E. H. Stotz. Amsterdam: Elsevier.
67. Butcher, R. W., Sneyd, J. G. T., Park, C. R. & Sutherland, E. W. (1966). *J. biol. Chem.* **241,** 1651.
68. Loten, E. G. & Sneyd, J. G. T. (1970). *Biochem. J.* **120,** 187.
69. Birnbaumer, L. & Rodbell, M. (1969). *J. biol. Chem.* **244,** 3477.
70. Lefèbvre, P. (1966). *Diabetologia,* **2,** 130.
71. Lawrence, A. M. (1966). *Proc. Nat. Acad. Sci.* **55,** 316.
72. Rudman, D., Di Girolamo, M., Malkin, M. F. & Garcia, L. A. (1965). In *Handbook of Physiology, Section 5, Adipose Tissue,* p. 533. Ed. A. E. Renold & G. F. Cahill. Washington, D.C.: American Physiological Society.

73. Fine, M. B. & Williams, R. H. (1960). *Amer. J. Physiol.* **199,** 403.
74. Evans, J. R., Opie, L. H. & Shipp, J. C. (1963). *Amer. J. Physiol.* **205,** 766.
75. Ballard, F. J., Danforth, W. H., Naegle, S. & Bing, R. J. (1960). *J. clin. Invest.* **39,** 717.
76. Scott, J. C., Finkelstein, L. J. & Spitzer, J. J. (1962). *Amer. J. Physiol.* **203,** 482.
77. Fritz, I. B. (1961). *Physiol. Rev.* **41,** 52.
78. Eaton, P. & Steinberg, D. (1961). *J. Lipid Res.* **2,** 376.
79. Randle, P. J., Garland, P. B., Hales, C. N. & Newsholme, E. A. (1963). *Lancet,* **1,** 785.
80. Tarrant, M. E., Mahler, R. & Ashmore, J. (1964). *J. biol. Chem.* **239,** 1714.
81. Felber, J.-P. & Vannotti, A. (1964). *Med. exp.* **10,** 153.
82. Thorell, J., Persson, B. & Sterkey, G. (1966). *Diabetologia,* **2,** 232.
83. Schalch, D. S. & Kipnis, D. M. (1964). *J. clin. Invest.* **43,** 1283.
84. Seyffert, W. A. & Madison, L. L. (1967). *Diabetes,* **16,** 765.
85. Nestel, P. J., Carroll, K. F. & Silverstein, M. S. (1964). *Lancet,* **2,** 115.
86. Paul, P., Issekutz, B. & Miller, H. I. (1966). *Amer. J. Physiol.* **211,** 1313.
87. Carlson, L. A. & Ostman, J. (1966). *Diabetologia,* **2,** 127.
88. Gross, R. C. & Carlson, L. A. (1968). *Diabetes,* **17,** 353.
89. Ruderman, N. B., Toews, C. J. & Shafrir, E. (1969). *Arch. int. Med.* **123,** 299.
90. Lassers, B. W., Wahlqvist, M. L., Kaijser, L. & Carlson, L. A. (1971). *Lancet,* **2,** 448.
91. Hawkins, R. A., Alberti, K. G. M. M., Houghton, C. R. S., Williamson, D. H. & Krebs, H. A. (1971). *Biochem. J.* **125,** 541.
92. Balasse, E. E., Couturier, E. & Franckson, J. R. M. (1967). *Diabetologia,* **3,** 488.
93. Greenough, W. B., Crespin, S. R. & Steinberg, D. (1967). *Lancet,* **2,** 1334.
94. Hales, C. N. (1968). In *The Biological Basis of Medicine,* **2,** 309. Ed. E. E. Bittar & N. Bittar. New York: Academic Press.
95. Gordon, E. S. (1970). *Adv. Metabolic Disorders,* **4,** 229.
96. Yalow, R. S. & Berson, S. A. (1960). *J. clin. Invest.* **39,** 1157.
97. Vallance-Owen, J. (1964). *Adv. Metabolic Disorders,* **1,** 191.
98. Randle, P. J., Garland, P. B., Hales, C. N. & Newsholme, E. A. (1964). *Ciba Foundation Colloquia Endocrinol.* **15,** 192.
99. Odum, E. P. (1965). In *Handbook of Physiology, Section 5, Adipose Tissue,* p. 37. Ed. A. E. Renold & G. F. Cahill. Washington, D.C.: American Physiological Society.
100. Weis-Fogh, T. (1952). *Phil. Trans. Roy. Soc. B,* **237,** 1.
101. Carlson, L. A. & Mossfeldt, F. (1964). *Acta Physiol. Scand.* **62,** 51.
102. Fröberg, S. O. (1968). In *Biochemistry of Exercise, Medicine & Sport,* **3,** 100. Ed. J. R. Poortman. White Plains, New York: Albert J. Phiebig.
103. Carlson, L. A. (1969). *Biochem. J.* **114,** 49P.
104. Asmussen, E. (1965). In *Handbook of Physiology, Section 3, Respiration,* **2,** 939. Ed. W. O. Fenn & H. Rahn. Washington, D.C.: American Physiological Society.
105. Morgan, H. E., Randle, P. J. & Regen, D. M. (1959). *Biochem. J.* **73,** 573.
106. Joel, C. D. (1965). In *Handbook of Physiology, Section 5, Adipose·Tissue,* p. 59. Ed. A. E. Renold & G. F. Cahill. Washington, D.C.: American Physiological Society.
107. Smith, R. E. & Hock, R. J. (1963). *Science,* **140,** 199.
108. Smith, R. E. & Horwitz, B. A. (1969). *Physiol. Rev.* **49,** 330.
109. Reed, N. & Fain, J. N. (1968). *J. biol. Chem.* **243,** 2843.
110. Beviz, A., Lundholm, L. & Mohme-Lundholm, E. (1968). *Brit. J. Pharmacol. Ther.* **34,** 198P.

111. Himms-Hagen, J. (1967). *Pharmacol. Rev.* **19,** 367.
112. Himms-Hagen, J. (1970). *Adv. Enz. Reg.* **8,** 131.
113. Pressman, B. C. & Lardy, H. A. (1958). *Biochem. biophys. Acta,* **21,** 458.
114. Knight, B. L. & Myant, N. B. (1970). *Biochem. J.* **119,** 103.
115. Laurell, S. (1957). *Acta Physiol. Scand.* **41,** 158.
116. Start, C. (1969). *D. Phil. Thesis*, Oxford University.

CHAPTER 6

REGULATION OF CARBOHYDRATE METABOLISM IN LIVER

A. INTRODUCTION

Liver plays a fundamental role in the metabolism of carbohydrate, fat and amino acids and in this tissue the metabolic pathways for these compounds are closely integrated and regulated. The number of metabolic reactions involved in carbohydrate metabolism within the liver is so large that it would require a whole volume to discuss them in any detail. Therefore the authors have chosen to concentrate this discussion upon areas of carbohydrate metabolism that are related to caloric homeostasis, that is, the uptake and utilization of glucose and the process of glucose formation from noncarbohydrate precursors (gluconeogenesis). The first part of the chapter describes these processes and discusses their physiological importance. The second part consists of a discussion of the regulation of the blood sugar level by the liver, and the regulation of glycolysis and gluconeogenesis in liver and kidney cortex.

Chapter 7 contains a discussion of several areas of fat metabolism in the liver and emphasizes the interrelationships between fat and carbohydrate metabolism. Amino acid metabolism is discussed only in relation to gluconeogenesis, since it would require a separate volume for a detailed description and discussion.

1. Carbohydrate utilization by the liver

The hepatic portal vein carries about 70% of the blood reaching the liver: the remainder is supplied via the hepatic artery. The hepatic portal vein drains most of the absorptive area of the gut so that, apart from triglyceride which is absorbed via the lymphatic system (see Chapter 5, Section A.1(a)), most compounds that are absorbed from the gut pass through the liver. Therefore the liver is favourably situated to function as the initial regulator of the blood levels of many compounds that enter the body through the gut (see Figure 6.1). In higher animals (ruminants being an exception) most of the ingested carbohydrate enters the blood as glucose which is produced from digestive degradation of starch, glycogen, etc., although in man, at least in many of the developed countries, much of the ingested carbohydrate enters the gut in the form of sucrose (see Section A.1(b)). Glucose plays an important role as the primary fuel of respiration for many tissues and therefore

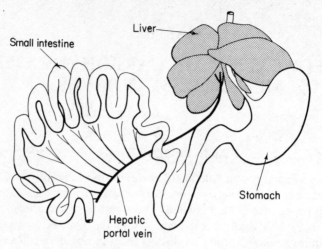

Figure 6.1. Anatomical relationship between liver, hepatic portal vein and the intestine

its concentration in the blood must be regulated. Since most animals are intermittent feeders and digestion is reasonably rapid, large quantities of glucose may enter the hepatic portal vein soon after a meal and the concentration of glucose in this vessel may increase to levels greater than 10 mM. However, if the *peripheral* blood glucose concentration exceeds about 10 mM, the threshold of the renal tubular reabsorption system is exceeded and some of the glucose is lost in the urine. The liver possesses the facility for removing large quantities of glucose from the portal vein when the concentration exceeds the normal (about 5 mM). The mechanism for this removal depends upon the presence of the enzyme glucokinase, which catalyses the phosphorylation of glucose to glucose-6-phosphate. This enzyme is similar to hexokinase but its properties are particularly related to the regulation of glucose uptake by the liver in response to changes in blood glucose concentration (see Section B.1 for a full discussion).

(a) Metabolism of glucose in the liver

Once glucose has been phosphorylated to glucose-6-phosphate, there are at least four pathways available for its utilization: glycogen synthesis, glycolysis, pentose phosphate pathway and hydrolysis to form glucose (Figure 6.2). Quantitative measurements of the relative rates of these pathways under different conditions have been attempted by the use of specifically-labelled ^{14}C-glucose, but since the pathways are complex and interrelated, the results of such experiments are difficult to interpret.[1] Nevertheless, it is possible to provide some qualitative assessment of the rates of these various pathways.

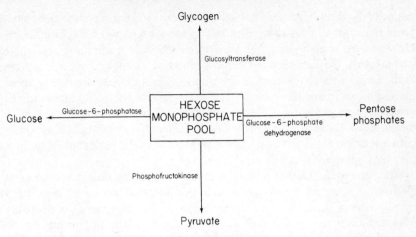

Figure 6.2. Major metabolic pathways leading from the hexose monophosphates in liver

(*i*) *Glycogen synthesis.* The pathway of glycogen synthesis and its control in liver appears to be generally similar to that in muscle (see Chapter 4). The function of liver glycogen is to provide a temporary carbohydrate reserve to maintain the blood glucose level when it is likely to be depleted (as in carbohydrate deprivation). In animals that are intermittent feeders, this reserve will be important in the periods between meals and it will be important in man during the overnight fast and in the rat during the overday fast. In the rat the glycogen stores are depleted by about 75% during the day and so the stores must be replenished, during the feeding period at night, at a rate estimated to be about $0.5\,\mu$mol of glucose residues per gram of liver per minute.[2] Comparable rates of glycogen synthesis have been observed in the isolated perfused rat liver, provided that the liver is taken from a fed animal.[3] The rate of glycogen synthesis in perfused livers from starved animals is low and this may be explained not only by glucosyltransferase existing in the inactive D form (owing to a low level of circulating insulin), but also by a decreased concentration of the enzyme. Thus, on re-feeding a 48-hour-starved rat with glucose, there is a delay in the synthesis of glycogen of about 2 hours which may be explained by the time taken for synthesis of new enzyme.[4] Nonetheless, during this two-hour period the liver is removing glucose from the portal blood and consequently this glucose must be degraded either by the pentose phosphate pathway or by glycolysis.

(*ii*) *Glycolysis.* It is generally considered that the role of glycolysis in the liver is to supply precursors for biosynthetic processes, rather than to provide pyruvate for oxidation. An important biosynthetic pathway in the liver is the formation of fatty acids (and hence triglyceride) from glucose. The pathway for the biosynthesis of triglyceride and its control appear to be similar in liver and adipose tissue (for description see Chapter 5, Section A.1(b)). However, the triglycerides that are synthesized in liver are not stored there permanently, they are secreted into the blood as VLDL and are transported to the adipose tissue for more permanent storage. In higher animals, adipose tissue and liver are the two important tissues for the biosynthesis of triglyceride from glucose, but the quantitative role of each tissue in the overall biosynthesis is still debated. Probably the distribution of fatty acid synthesis between different tissues is species dependent:[5] in the rat as much as 30 % may take place in liver.

Since glucose oxidation may provide but little of the energy requirement for liver, it is an interesting exercise to consider just what fuel is oxidized by this tissue. In starvation a large proportion of the energy is probably obtained from the β-oxidation of fatty acids, which is important for the provision of ketone bodies (Chapter 7). However, fatty acid oxidation is less important in the fed state. The oxidation of keto-acids derived from amino acid degradation may be the main process for energy formation provided that the diet contains a reasonable amount of protein.

(*iii*) *Pentose phosphate pathway.* The principal role of the pentose phosphate pathway in liver is the generation of NADPH for the reductive reactions involved in fatty acid synthesis (and also in cholesterol and steroid biosynthesis). A quantitatively less important function of the pathway is the provision of pentose phosphates for the synthesis of nucleotides required for DNA and RNA synthesis, and this function may explain why the activity of the pathway is increased in response to partial hepatectomy.[6]

It has also been suggested that the pentose phosphate pathway provides a bypass of the control of glycolysis at the phosphofructokinase reaction, since glucose-6-phosphate can be converted to triose phosphates via this pathway. It is possible that this bypass might be important in the removal of large amounts of glucose by the liver during the first two hours following re-feeding after starvation since during this time glycogen synthesis does not take place.[7]

(*b*) *Metabolism of fructose by the liver*

Fructose is metabolized by the liver according to the pathway described in Figure 6.3. Since fructose is converted via fructose-1-phosphate directly to triose phosphates by an aldolase reaction, its utilization does not require hexokinase or PFK. Since PFK is a regulatory enzyme for glycolysis in liver (see Section C.3), fructose bypasses the control of glycolysis at the PFK reaction and is able to increase the flux into the latter part of glycolysis. This latter portion of the glycolytic pathway provides acetyl-CoA for synthesis of long-chain fatty acyl-CoA and hence for synthesis of triglyceride.

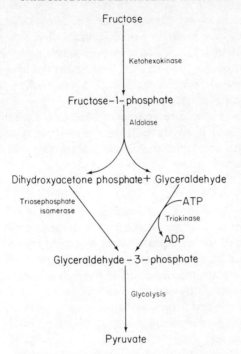

Figure 6.3. Pathway of fructose metabolism in liver

Therefore, it is possible to suggest that fructose feeding might increase the rate of hepatic lipogenesis and there is some evidence to support this idea. Feeding fructose to rats increases the activity of some of the enzymes (such as glucose-6-phosphate dehydrogenase and ATP-citrate lyase) involved in fatty acid synthesis in liver although it has no effect upon these enzymes in adipose tissue.[8] Furthermore, there is evidence linking sucrose feeding with increases in the plasma level of triglyceride in the rat and in man.[9] The precise biochemical mechanism by which fructose feeding leads to increased hepatic lipogenesis and elevated plasma triglyceride levels is unknown. Nonetheless, it is possible to link this effect of fructose with the proposal that a high consumption of sucrose is a causative factor in the occlusive arterial disease, atherosclerosis, in which there is a deposition of fatty material in the arterial walls so that their internal diameter is reduced.[10]

2. Glucose production by the liver

The normal diet for man and the natural diet for most omnivores is likely to contain sufficient carbohydrate to satisfy the needs of the whole animal. Indeed, excess carbohydrate is often ingested and this will be converted to triglyceride in the liver and adipose tissue (see above). Nevertheless, under certain conditions (starvation, low-carbohydrate diet, or sustained exercise, for example) the demand for glucose by the animal may exceed the amount that is absorbed from the gut. In these conditions the liver releases glucose into the bloodstream. This glucose release is achieved by the action of the enzyme glucose-6-phosphatase which hydrolyses glucose-6-phosphate in the liver cell. The immediate source of glucose-6-phosphate for glucose formation in the liver is glycogen. If the demand for glucose persists after the glycogen stores are depleted, glucose-6-phosphate will be produced by the process of gluconeogenesis.

(a) Glycogenolysis in the liver

In the rat, glycogen is broken down at a rate of about 0·5 μmol of glucose residues per gram of liver per minute during the diurnal fast,[2] which is similar to the rate of glucose release by the isolated perfused liver from a fed rat perfused with a glucose concentration of 6–7 mM.[3] This rate of glycogenolysis would explain the depletion of liver glycogen during the diurnal fast. However, the rate of glycogenolysis can be increased in the perfused liver by lowering the perfusate concentration of glucose or by addition of hormones (such as adrenaline and glucagon) to the perfusate.[3] These experiments demonstrate that liver phosphorylase can be controlled by hormones and possibly by factors which depend on the concentration of intracellular glucose. However, in comparison to the large amount of work that has been carried out on muscle phosphorylase, very little work has been done recently on the liver enzyme. The mass-action ratio data suggest that the enzyme catalyses a non-equilibrium reaction. Phosphorylase activity is obviously regulated by factors other than the concentration of hepatic glycogen. The early work of Sutherland established that liver phosphorylase exists in two forms, a and b, and that the effect of AMP on the activity of b is much less than on muscle phosphorylase b. This suggests that liver phosphorylase b may be an inactive form of the enzyme under all conditions in the cell. Sutherland has also demonstrated that the conversion of phosphorylase b into a is stimulated by cyclic AMP. Furthermore, adrenaline increases the content of cyclic AMP in liver slices and this increase occurs before the increase in release of glucose by the slice.[11]

Thus, it can be suggested that the increased rate of glycogenolysis in the liver in the presence of glucagon or adrenaline is due to an activation of membrane-bound adenyl cyclase, an increase in the concentration of cyclic AMP, an activation of phosphorylase b kinase and a conversion of inactive phosphorylase b to active phosphorylase a. In other words the mechanism is very similar to that described in muscle. Recently, it has been reported that protein kinase is present in rat liver and that it can be activated by cyclic AMP.[12] Apparently, it is not known whether protein kinase in liver is capable of activation of phosphorylase b directly or whether inactive phosphorylase b kinase is the substrate for this enzyme, as it is in muscle. Possibly a cascade mechanism is required for the control of phosphorylase activity in liver as in muscle (for discussion, see Chapter 4, Section D.3(b)(iv)).

It is not possible to suggest a precise biochemical mechanism which could explain the controlled increase in glycogenolysis in liver during starvation. (The effect of starvation upon liver phosphorylase has not been studied in any detail.) The hepatic content of cyclic AMP is elevated by about 60% in starvation in the rat[13] and this may be due to an increase in the glucagon level and a decrease in the insulin level in the blood (see Chapter 5, Section B.4(b)). The stimulation of glycogenolysis that occurs in the perfused liver when the perfusate concentration of glucose is reduced cannot be satisfactorily explained at the present time. A biochemical explanation may be possible when more information is available concerning the properties of phosphorylase a, phosphorylase b and the interconverting enzymes in liver.

(b) Gluconeogenesis

Certain tissues in higher animals have a continual requirement for glucose and therefore during conditions of carbohydrate deprivation it is essential that glucose is synthesized from non-carbohydrate sources by the process known as gluconeogenesis. The glucose-dependent tissues include brain, nerves, red blood cells, kidney medulla and testis. The latter three tissues derive most of their energy from the conversion of glucose to lactate since their oxidative capacities are very low. In brain and nerves the aerobic capacity (that is, TCA cycle and electron-transport chain) would appear to be adequate for the provision of biological energy and most of the glucose that is removed by the brain is completely oxidized. The interruption of the glucose supply to the brain under normal conditions results in deterioration of function within 1 minute and irreversible damage within several minutes. The reason for this dependence on glucose is not known but a speculative suggestion was put forward in Chapter 3, Section D.2(d)(i). It has recently been shown that in man the brain can adapt to prolonged starvation by reducing its requirement for glucose to only 25% of the normal: the oxidation of glucose is replaced by oxidation of ketone bodies (see below).

Gluconeogenesis is probably required in all higher animals during starvation or when the diet is deficient in carbohydrate. It may be essential in carnivorous animals on a normal diet, but unfortunately these animals have been little studied in relation to glucose requirement and carbohydrate intake. On the other hand, ruminants have been studied in detail because of the economic importance of the dairy industry and it is known that they have a constant requirement for glucose formation (see Section 2(b)(ii)).

(i) Physiological importance of gluconeogenesis in man. The information that forms the basis for the following discussion has been collated from the

Table 6.1. Tissue fuel requirements and fuel content of average diet in man[57]

Tissues	Fuel	Fuel consumption per day (g)	Oxygen uptake (moles)	CO_2 production (moles)	R.Q.	Energy released (kcal)	Average dietary intake
Brain	Glucose	120	4	4·0	1·000	423	220 g carbohydrate
Liver	Amino acids	70	3	2·4	0·801	306	
Carcass (muscle)	Glucose	100⎱	9	7·3	0·811	991	70 g protein
	Fat	60⎰					60 g fat
Total			16	13·7	0·864	1,720	

This information applies to an average man leading a sedentary life.

papers of Cahill, Owen and colleagues.[14,15,16,17] On an average diet, man eats sufficient carbohydrate to satisfy the glucose requirements of the brain and other tissues (Table 6.1). The glucose requirement for the brain has been estimated at approximately 120 g per day, and the requirement for the anaerobic tissues (kidney medulla, red cells, testis) may be about 40 g per day. Muscle also utilizes glucose, but the amount that is used depends upon the duration and extent of the mechanical activity. The total musculature of man at rest may require about 30–100 g of glucose per day, but in starvation this glucose requirement may be severely reduced owing to the oxidation of fatty acids and/or ketone bodies. Therefore, the minimal glucose requirement for an average man will be approximately 160 g per day. The carbohydrate reserves of the body (see Table 6.2) would satisfy the glucose demands

Table 6.2. The energy reserves of man

Fuel	Tissue	Fuel reserves in average man kcal	g
Triglyceride	Adipose tissue	100,000	15,000
Glycogen	Liver	200	70
	Muscle	400	120
Glucose	Body fluids	40	20
Protein	Muscle	25,000	6,000

The data are assumed to represent an 'average man' weighing 70 kg (154 pounds) and measuring 1·73 m² in body surface area. In obese subjects the triglyceride stores can weigh as much as 80,000 g.[14,57]

for about 12 hours. During this period, glycogenolysis in the liver would satisfy the requirements for glucose and it has been demonstrated (using the hepatic venous catheter technique) that glucose output from the liver is 180–350 g per day under these conditions. However, man is able to survive starvation for several months and therefore during this period glucose must be synthesized from non-carbohydrate precursors.

Quantitatively, the most important precursors for gluconeogenesis are lactate, glycerol and the amino acids. Lactate is produced from glucose degradation in such tissues as the red cells and kidney medulla and, since this is a continual process, a cycle exists between lactate production in these tissues and its conversion to glucose in the liver and kidney. Consequently, from this lactate there is no *net* production of glucose for oxidation by tissues such as the brain. During starvation the triglyceride stores in the adipose tissue are mobilized by hydrolysis to fatty acids and glycerol: the fatty acids are transported to other tissues to provide a fuel of respiration (Chapter 5). The glycerol is transported to the liver and kidneys where it acts as a very important gluconeogenic precursor. All the amino acids, except leucine, can be degraded to form compounds that can be converted to glucose (see Table 6.3). Higher animals do not possess any large reserve of either amino acids or protein and therefore during starvation the proteins of skeletal muscle are broken down to provide the amino acids that function as precursors for gluconeogenesis. Some of the amino acids are deaminated in the liver and the ammonia that is produced is excreted, mainly in the form of urea.

Table 6.3. Glucogenic and ketogenic amino acids[34,58]

Glucogenic amino acids		Ketogenic amino acid
Amino acid	Gluconeogenic precursor	
Glycine	pyruvate, succinate	Leucine
Serine	pyruvate	Isoleucine
Threonine	propionate	Phenylalanine
Valine	propionate	Tyrosine
Histidine	α-ketoglutarate	
Arginine	α-ketoglutarate	
Lysine	α-ketoglutarate	
Cysteine	pyruvate	
Proline	α-oxoglutarate	
Hydroxyproline	pyruvate	
Isoleucine	propionate	
Phenylalanine	fumarate	
Tyrosine	fumarate	

One important question is whether during prolonged starvation the amount of glucose synthesized by the liver and kidney cortex is sufficient to account for the glucose requirements of the brain and other tissues. The amount of glucose that is synthesized from glycerol and amino acids can be estimated in two ways. First, the amount of glycerol released from the adipose tissue, which depends upon the rate of lipolysis, can be estimated from the caloric expenditure of the subject while the amount of amino acids degraded can be calculated from the nitrogen excreted per day. Second, and more directly, the uptake of precursors by the liver and kidneys can be measured by catheterization techniques and the glucose equivalence can be calculated (Table 6.4).

Investigations have been carried out into the amount of glucose synthesized during prolonged therapeutic starvation of several obese subjects.[14,15,16] The amount of glucose produced from glycerol remains fairly constant throughout a 5–6 week period of starvation. However, the excretion of

Table 6.4. Calculations of glucose production from glycerol, lactate (plus pyruvate) and amino acids during starvation in man

Glucose precursor	Amount of glucose produced per day (g)	
	3 or 4 days of starvation	Several weeks of starvation
Glycerol*	19	19
Lactate + pyruvate†	39	39
Amino acids‡	41	16
	—	—
Total glucose produced from above precursors by liver and kidney cortex§	99	74
	—	—
Maximum glucose available for oxidation by the brain (i.e. glycerol and amino acid as precursors)‖	60	35
Fuel requirement of brain (Glucose equivalents)**	120	120
Suggested alternative fuel to glucose for brain††	ketone bodies	ketone bodies

* Amount of glucose produced from glycerol is estimated from the amount of triglyceride hydrolysed per day. In starvation, 190 g of triglyceride is required to satisfy the caloric needs of the subject. Since glycerol represents 10% of triglyceride it can provide 19 g of glucose per day. This amount is confirmed by measurement of glycerol uptake by liver and kidney using catheterization techniques.[15]

† Amount calculated from glucose 1-C[14] turnover studies in man which gives values between 27 and 58 g/day, and this is *not* affected by the dietary state. Also the measurement of lactate and pyruvate uptake by the liver and kidney in man by catheterization techniques estimates glucose formation as 39 g/day.[15]

‡ Amount calculated from nitrogen excreted in urine (100 g protein produces 57 g glucose; 1 g nitrogen is equivalent to 6·25 g protein).[16,34] In early stages of starvation about 12 g nitrogen is excreted per day but this is decreased in prolonged starvation to 4·7 g/day. Catheterization studies in subjects undergoing prolonged starvation indicate an uptake of amino acids by liver and kidney which could theoretically produce 26 g glucose per day.[15]

§ In prolonged starvation the hepatic-renal glucose production as measured by catheterization techniques provides an estimate of 86 g glucose per day[15] which is in good agreement with the 74 g obtained in this calculation.

‖ Catheterization techniques have been used to measure the A–V differences across the brain. In prolonged starvation, glucose oxidation by the brain (excluding glucose converted to lactate, which is converted back to glucose in the liver and kidney) is estimated as 24 g/day.[16]

** Oxygen uptake or total fuel utilization are measured by catheterization techniques.[16]

†† The rate of ketone body uptake by the brain has been estimated from A–V differences using catheterization techniques.[16] These studies strongly suggest that ketone bodies are the alternative fuel to glucose during starvation.

nitrogen progressively declines from about 12 g per day on the first day of starvation, to about 4 g per day after 4 weeks of starvation. Calculations on the amount of glucose that is synthesized from glycerol and amino acids demonstrate that, even for a short period of starvation (several days), insufficient glucose is produced to satisfy the requirement of the brain. After a prolonged period of starvation the amount of glucose synthesized accounts for only about 25% of the total fuel requirement of the brain. These studies indicate that an alternative fuel must replace glucose during prolonged starvation in humans.

This conclusion is supported by more direct studies of substrate utilization by the human brain.[17] These catheterization studies confirmed that glucose utilization by the brain is depressed by 75% during prolonged starvation. Furthermore, they showed that there is a marked A–V difference in the concentration of ketone bodies across the brain and from these data it can be calculated that the utilization of this fuel could account for about 75% of the oxygen uptake (Table 6.4). Further evidence for the ability of brain tissue to utilize ketone bodies is presented in Chapter 7.

The physiological importance of this transition of the brain towards the oxidation of ketone bodies is related to the availability of amino acids as glucose precursors. The only important source of the amino acids in starvation is skeletal muscle and, if the demand for glucose by the brain was maintained at 120 g per day during prolonged starvation, this would represent an enormous drain on the content of skeletal muscle in the body. In the natural state, skeletal muscle is of the utmost importance to an animal in capturing or foraging for food. Therefore any mechanism that conserves body protein during starvation will increase the possibility that the starvation period will be survived and therefore will be selectively advantageous.

(ii) *Physiological importance of gluconeogenesis in ruminants.* The alimentary tract of all true herbivores is adapted in one way or another so that the passage of food through the tract is delayed and bacterial fermentation of the bulky plant food (particularly cellulose) can take place. In ruminants this expanded part of the gut is represented by the rumen which is a complex fore-stomach of considerable size. In fact, the stomach of the ruminant consists of four compartments, rumen, reticulum, omasum and abomasum, and in adults the rumen accounts for about 80% of the total stomach volume: the capacity of the rumen in sheep is 4–10 litres and in cows is 100–300 litres. The rumen can be considered as a large fermentation chamber which provides a suitable environment for the continuous culture of the bacterial population. (See reference 18 for a discussion of ruminant physiology.)

The advantage of the rumen is that the animal can obtain energy from the otherwise indigestible material of the plant cell wall, which is primarily cellulose. The cellulose is degraded by a series of enzymes within the bacterial cell and the product of this hydrolytic process is thought to be glucose. (The process is not very easy to study because the enzyme responsible for the initial attack on the cellulose is very labile. Thus, no cellulase activity can be detected in the rumen fluid and the cellulase activity in extracts of rumen bacteria is rapidly lost.) The glucose produced from the hydrolysis of the cellulose is fermented by the bacteria to acetate, lactate and butyrate. The lactate is fermented further to propionate. These compounds are known collectively as the volatile fatty acids (VFAs) and they are the most important products of ruminant fermentation. They are readily absorbed from the rumen and constitute the major energy source in the ruminant.

The main disadvantage of ruminant digestion is that the starch and sugar ingested by the animal are also fermented to VFAs by the bacteria. Therefore, the amount of carbohydrate that is absorbed by the gut is very small and probably arises from digestion of bacteria and protozoa when they pass from the rumen into the small intestine. It has been calculated that the total quantity of carbohydrate from this source will not amount to more than 5 or 6 g of glucose per day. Consequently, ruminants are constantly dependent upon gluconeogenesis. The main precursors for this process are lactate and propionate absorbed from the rumen. (The pathway for the conversion of propionate to glucose is shown in Figure 6.4.)

In the very young ruminant, milk provides all the carbohydrate that is required but gradually, upon weaning, the animal ingests more plant food and relies less on the supply of milk from the mother. During the weaning period, the animal has both a partial dependence on milk and an active rumen. Milk passes directly from the oesophagus to the omasum and therefore it bypasses the rumen so that its carbohydrate is not fermented. This bypass is achieved by means of the oesophageal groove and is brought into play by a reflex action stimulated by suckling. Therefore, in the young suckling animal, sufficient carbohydrate may be absorbed from the mother's milk and gluconeogenesis is not required. However, in the fully weaned animal the glucose requirement must be satisfied by gluconeogenesis.

Measurements of the uptake of glucose by the brain and central nervous system in the sheep suggest that these tissues utilize only about 5 g of glucose per day compared with 120 g per day in man.* The low requirement for glucose could indicate that the gluconeogenic capacity in these animals is low. Somewhat surprisingly this is not the case, since it has been shown that the entry of glucose into the blood of the sheep amounts to about 86–115 g per day (not very much less than in man). Therefore the amount of glucose utilized by the brain in these animals is only about 5% of the total glucose synthesized (cf. man). What other tissues in the ruminant require large amounts of glucose? In the sheep it has been estimated that the udder requires between 60 and 80% of the total glucose produced by the animal

* It is possible that the sheep brain is able to utilize ketone bodies under fed conditions, so that normally the demand for glucose is low. However, recent measurements show that the activities of the enzymes involved in ketone body utilization (3-oxoacid-CoA transferase and acetoacetyl-CoA thiolase—see Chapter 7, Section E.2) are much lower in sheep brain (almost 10-fold) than in the brain from rat or mouse. It must remain a possibility that the brain of the sheep and other ruminants is capable of oxidation of short-chain fatty acids (VFAs) and that these fatty acids are the primary fuel of respiration for this tissue.

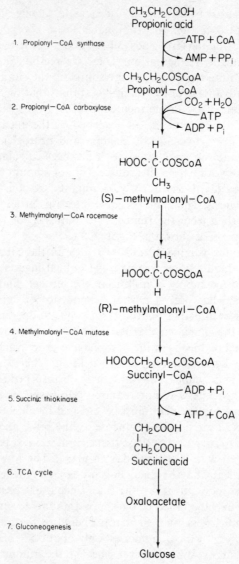

Figure 6.4. Pathway of propionate metabolism in liver

and in the cow this requirement may be as high as 90 %.[19] The udder requires glucose for milk production: glucose is necessary for the formation of lactose and it provides glycerol phosphate for triglyceride formation and glucose-6-phosphate for the pentose phosphate pathway which generates NADPH for fatty acid synthesis. In starvation (or when the quality of the food deteriorates, particularly in the winter months) the rate of gluconeogenesis will be reduced, owing to a lack of precursor, and the milk yield will suffer. Moreover, in an attempt to produce as much glucose as possible for milk formation the animals sometimes develop 'bovine ketosis', in which the ketone body levels in the plasma rise to very high values and acidosis and toxicity result.

(*iii*) *Gluconeogenesis and exhaustive exercise.* The liver glycogen provides a buffer system which can maintain the blood glucose level for periods of up to 24 hours starvation. Once these glycogen stores are depleted, gluconeogenesis must be stimulated in order to provide the glucose required by the brain and other tissues. However, liver glycogen can be acutely depleted by exhaustive exercise particularly after an overnight fast.[20] In exercise the most important precursor for glucose formation will be lactate, which is produced from glucose and glycogen metabolism in muscle. If gluconeogenesis were to be inhibited after severe exercise, hypoglycaemia with attendant malfunction of the nervous system could result. Experiments with the isolated perfused liver have demonstrated that alcohol is a potent inhibitor of gluconeogenesis.[21] Thus, the oral administration of ethanol is a simple technique for the inhibition of this process *in vivo* and one for which humans are particularly amenable experimental subjects! It has been demonstrated that the administration of alcohol to human subjects immediately after a period of exhaustive exercise prevented the subjects from maintaining the body temperature when the ambient temperature was about 14 °C and the wind speed was about 15 km per hour.[22] The average fall in the body temperature (rectal) of 7 subjects under these conditions (that is, after exercise and alcohol) was 2·22 °C. Alcohol caused a decrease in the plasma glucose level after exercise from 4·1 mM to 1·8 mM. If alcohol was not administered, the body temperature was maintained. Furthermore, the failure to maintain the body temperature after alcohol consumption could be prevented by the ingestion of glucose. These observations suggest a malfunction of some part of the nervous system which is involved in temperature regulation. Perhaps this area of the nervous system is more sensitive to lack of glucose than others. The observation that administration of alcohol to human subjects interferes in the control of body temperature may have considerable practical importance in the treatment of people who have been subjected to exposure (hill-walkers and mountaineers, for example), since this condition usually involves both starvation and exhaustion. The practice of administering alcohol to these people could be highly dangerous in that the inability to control temperature could result in hypothermia and death.[22]

B. CONTROL OF GLUCOSE UPTAKE AND RELEASE BY THE LIVER

Variations in the dietary intake of carbohydrate will result in variations in the concentration of glucose in the hepatic portal blood. The liver is ideally situated to regulate the blood glucose concentration in response to such dietary variations. The liver also has the capacity to maintain the blood glucose concentration when the dietary intake is devoid of carbohydrate, as was recognized by Claude Bernard as early as 1850 (see reference 23).

The first detailed biochemical experiments on the regulation of blood glucose by the liver were performed by Soskin and coworkers who used an *in situ* perfused dog liver preparation. They observed that, when the portal vein blood contained a high concentration of glucose, the liver removed glucose from the blood but, when the concentration was low, the liver released glucose into the blood. Moreover, the rate of uptake or release of glucose by the liver was proportional to the degree of hyper- or hypoglycaemia.[24] In other words, the higher the concentration of glucose above the normal, the more rapidly does the liver remove the glucose. Conversely, the lower the concentration below the normal, the more rapid is the release of glucose. The results of these studies have been confirmed by the use of catheterization techniques.[25] and they show that the liver must be able to respond rapidly to changes in the concentration of glucose in the portal blood.

In order to explain this physiological function of the liver at a biochemical level, one must know which reactions are responsible for the regulation of glucose uptake or release. Which reactions in the early stages of glucose metabolism can be described as regulatory? It is very unlikely that transport of glucose across the liver cell membrane is a regulatory process since it appears to be close to equilibrium. The experimental evidence in support of this is as follows. First, the liver cell membrane is generally more permeable than that of other tissues. Second, the intracellular concentration of glucose is usually very similar to the extracellular concentration (that is, the mass-action ratio approaches unity: see Chapter 3, Appendix 3.5). Third, extracellular ^{14}C-glucose rapidly equilibrates with the intracellular glucose pool and the rate of equilibration is independent of the direction of glucose flux (that is, rapid equilibration occurs on addition of ^{14}C-glucose to the perfusate despite the fact that glucose is being released by the liver).

The early reactions of glucose metabolism in the liver are obvious candidates for regulation of the blood glucose level. Glucokinase, the enzyme that phosphorylates glucose, and glucose-6-phosphatase, the enzyme that hydrolyses glucose-6-phosphate to glucose, both catalyse non-equilibrium reactions: the mass-action ratios for these reactions are much smaller than the equilibrium constants (Table 6.5), and the maximum catalytic activities of these enzymes are much lower than other glycolytic enzymes (Table 6.6). However, there is no experimental evidence to indicate that these enzymes are controlled by factors other than the substrate concentrations. Indeed, the properties of these enzymes *in vitro* are consistent with regulation by substrate concentrations *in vivo*.

Table 6.5. A comparison of the apparent equilibrium constants with mass-action ratios for reactions of glycolysis and gluconeogenesis in liver and kidney cortex

Reaction catalysed by	Apparent equilibrium constant (K')	Mass-action ratios (Γ)		Units of K' and Γ
		Liver	Kidney cortex	
Glucokinase (hexokinase)	$3.9-5.5 \times 10^3$	0.016	0.077	
Glucose-6-phosphatase	850	119.3	203.7	
Phosphoglucoisomerase	0.36–0.47	0.31	0.25	
Phosphofructokinase	$0.9-1.2 \times 10^3$	0.09	0.33	
Fructose diphosphatase	530	19.1	4.77	
Aldolase	$6.8-13.0 \times 10^{-5}$	120×10^{-8}	81.2×10^{-8}	M
Glyceraldehyde-3-phosphate dehydrogenase plus phosphoglycerate kinase	$0.2-1.5 \times 10^3$	0.3×10^3	0.2×10^3	M^{-1}
Phosphoglycerate mutase	0.1–0.2	0.12	0.10	
Enolase	2.8–4.6	2.91	4.4	
Pyruvate kinase	$2-20 \times 10^3$	0.70	1.82	
Pyruvate carboxylase plus phosphoenolpyruvate carboxykinase	7.0	1.1×10^{-3}	0.53×10^{-3}	M

The mass-action ratios are calculated from the data for liver and kidney cortex from fed rats presented in reference 32. In the calculation of the mass-action ratio for the combined pyruvate carboxylase/PEPCK reaction the combined level of GTP plus ITP in liver was obtained from reference 59. The equilibrium constants for the glycolytic reactions are taken from Chapter 3 (Table 3.2). The equilibrium constants for the glucose-6-phosphatase and fructose diphosphatase reactions were calculated from the change in standard free energies upon the hydrolysis of glucose-6-phosphate and fructose-1,6-diphosphate, respectively. The mass-action ratios for the pyruvate carboxylase plus the PEPCK reactions were calculated from the following reaction

$$\text{pyruvate} + \text{ATP} + \text{GTP} \rightarrow \text{phosphoenolpyruvate} + \text{GDP} + \text{ADP} + P_i$$

The equilibrium constant for this reaction was calculated by subtracting the standard free energy change involved in the hydrolysis of phosphoenol-pyruvate from the sum of the standard free energies of hydrolysis of ATP and GTP.
K' and Γ are dimensionless unless otherwise stated.

Table 6.6. Maximal activities of the enzymes of glycolysis and gluconeogenesis in liver and kidney

| Enzyme | Enzyme activities (μmol/min/g fresh weight at 37 °C) | | | |
| | Liver | | Kidney | |
	Rat	All species	Rat	All species
Hexokinase	0·7	0·5	7·9	5·6
Glucokinase	4·3	2·0	—	—
Glucose-6-phosphatase	17·0	12·0	13·0	—
Phosphoglucoisomerase	136·0	280·0	130·0	—
Phosphofructokinase	3·3	5·0	5·7	7·3
Fructose diphosphatase	15·0	20·0	17·0	14·0
Aldolase	10·0	6·2	10·0	8·3
Glyceraldehyde-3-phosphate dehydrogenase	170·0	150·0	200·0	200·0
3-Phosphoglycerate kinase	150·0	130·0	170·0	150·0
Enolase	17·0	53·0	53·0	53·0
Pyruvate kinase	50·0	37·0	50·0	77·0
Lactate dehydrogenase	230·0	230·0	170·0	170·0
Pyruvate carboxylase	6·7	8·3	5·8	—
Phosphoenolpyruvate carboxykinase	6·7	13·0	6·7	—

The activities are averages for the results reported in many different publications: they are presented for the rat and also for all vertebrate species for which data is available.[60]

1. Role of glucokinase in the regulation of glucose uptake by the liver

The ability of liver to remove glucose from the portal blood when the concentration increases above the normal was explained upon the discovery of the enzyme glucokinase.[26] This enzyme, like hexokinase, catalyses the phosphorylation of glucose to form glucose-6-phosphate but its activity in liver is about 10-fold higher than hexokinase.

$$\text{glucose} + \text{ATP} \rightarrow \text{glucose-6-phosphate} + \text{ADP}$$

The important differences between the two enzymes are that glucokinase, unlike hexokinase, has a high K_m for glucose (10 mM) and is not inhibited by glucose-6-phosphate (see Table 6.7). These two properties are the basis for a theory of regulation of glucose uptake which is consistent with the physiological function of the liver. After a carbohydrate-containing meal the glucose concentration in the portal blood increases from about 5 mM to 12 mM or more and, since glucose transport into the liver cell is an equilibrium process, the intracellular glucose concentration increases over a similar range. This increase in glucose concentration produces a substantial increase in the activity of glucokinase and automatically increases the uptake of glucose by

Table 6.7. Properties of glucokinase and hexokinase from rat liver[61]

Property	Glucokinase	Hexokinase
K_m for glucose	10 mM	0·01–0·1 mM
Inhibition by glucose-6-phosphate	No	Yes
Ability to phosphorylate fructose	Poor	Good
Inhibition by N-acetyl glucosamine	Strong	Weak
Approximate maximum catalytic activity in livers from fed rats (μmol/min/g fresh weight at 25 °C)	1·5	0·1

the liver. The high K_m of glucokinase for glucose is vital to the operation of this control system because hexokinase would be saturated at 1 mM glucose and a change from 5 mM to 12 mM would have no effect on its activity (see Figure 6.5). Furthermore, the absence of product inhibition of glucokinase ensures that the hepatic concentration of glucose-6-phosphate does not interfere with the process of glucose uptake. A stimulation of glucokinase activity would be expected to increase the hepatic concentration of hexose monophosphates and this in turn should stimulate PFK (Chapter 3, Section D.3(b)) and UDPG-glucosyltransferase (Chapter 4, Section E.2). Thus, the presence of glucokinase in liver can provide a control system in which an increase in the portal concentration of glucose will increase glucose uptake by the liver and stimulate glycolysis and glycogen synthesis.

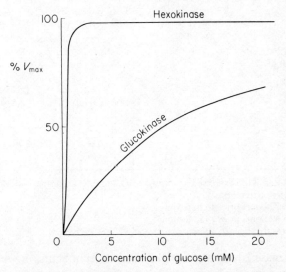

Figure 6.5. Variation of enzyme activity with substrate concentration for hexokinase and glucokinase

The function of glucokinase in liver can be seen as a bypass of the basic control mechanism of glycolysis as described for muscle (Chapter 3, Section D.3(b)). The physiological importance of this bypass is that it permits the liver to regulate glucose uptake according to the hepatic concentration of glucose and it also facilitates the conversion of the glucose residues that are removed from the blood to the storage products of glycogen (via glucosyltransferase) and triglyceride (via glycolysis and the fatty acid synthesizing system).

The indirect evidence that supports this theory for the involvement of glucokinase in the regulation of glucose uptake by the liver is summarized below.

(a) Glucokinase is found only in liver and this is the only tissue that is subjected to large variations in the extracellular glucose concentration owing to its direct link with the absorptive area of the intestine.

(b) The activity of glucokinase varies markedly with the dietary state: a diet rich in carbohydrate increases the activity whereas starvation or a low-carbohydrate diet reduces the activity (Table 6.8). These changes in activity appear to be due to changes in the concentration of the enzyme-protein and they may be controlled by insulin.[27]

Table 6.8. Activities of glucokinase in rat liver in various physiological conditions

Condition of rats	Glucokinase activities (μmol/min/g fresh weight)		
	A	B	C
Fed controls	1·46 ± 0·20 (3)	1·22 ± 0·20 (3)	—
Starved 24 hrs	1·26 ± 0·05 (6)	1·56 ± 0·06 (3)	—
Starved 48 hrs	0·86 ± 0·24 (3)	1·02 ± 0·10 (3)	1·34 ± 0·25 (4)
Starved 80 hrs	<0·05	—	—
Starved and re-fed glucose, or high glucose diet			
2 hrs	—	—	1·51 ± 0·33 (3)†
4 hrs	—	1·06 ± 0·08 (3)*	2·85 ± 0·17 (4)†
6 hrs	0·11 ± 0·04 (3)*	—	—
15 hrs	0·51 ± 0·12 (3)*	—	—
24 hrs	—	—	4·40 ± 0·32 (4)†
Alloxan diabetic	<0·05 (3)	0·21 ± 0·03 (3)	—

Activities in A and B are expressed as means ±SD and in C as means ±SEM. Numbers of animals are given in parentheses.
* Rats starved 72 hours prior to re-feeding.
† Rats starved 48 hours prior to re-feeding.
Columns A, B and C refer to references 62, 26 and 63 respectively.

(c) Glucokinase is absent from the livers of ruminants, in which only a very small amount of glucose is absorbed from the intestine (see Section 2(b)(iii)).

(*d*) Glucokinase is not present in the young rat before weaning. Thus, while the young rat is being fed by the mother the intake of carbohydrate is controlled, but once the young animal has to find food for itself, the intake of carbohydrate will vary and glucokinase will be essential for the control of the hepatic uptake of glucose.

2. Regulation of glucose uptake and release by the liver

Although the properties of glucokinase may satisfactorily explain the uptake of glucose by the liver, there is an obvious problem when the mechanism for release of glucose is considered. Liver will release glucose into the portal vein when the concentration falls below normal (about 5 mM). However, at the normal blood glucose concentration the activity of glucokinase *in vitro* is relatively high (about 25% of the maximum). At present there are no known properties of the enzyme which indicate that it would be inhibited when the portal blood glucose concentration is reduced below normal. Even the isolated perfused liver is able to respond to changes in glucose concentration and in this preparation the only factor controlling the uptake or release of glucose is the external glucose concentration. Therefore any hypothetical regulator for glucokinase (and also for glucose-6-phosphatase) would have to respond to changes in the concentration of glucose. Since a decrease from 6 mM to 4 mM glucose can produce a complete change in the *direction* of its metabolism by the liver, it is unlikely that glucose alone could directly regulate these enzymes. A metabolic intermediate related to glucose could regulate but, if it were to provide adequate activation and inhibition, an amplification mechanism would be necessary. At present there is no evidence either for the existence of such a regulator or for the operation of an amplification mechanism and any theory of control based upon possible regulators of these enzymes must be highly speculative. Two alternative hypotheses have been put forward to account for the regulation of glucose uptake and release by the liver.

(a) *A substrate cycle catalysed by glucokinase and glucose-6-phosphatase*

If glucokinase and glucose-6-phosphatase are both simultaneously active in liver, glucose will be converted to glucose-6-phosphate (with concomitant ATP hydrolysis) and glucose-6-phosphate will be converted back to glucose (and P_i). This *substrate cycle* between glucose and glucose-6-phosphate could be very sensitive to changes in the concentration of a regulator molecule. The substrate cycle can explain the physiological behaviour of the liver in the regulation of glucose uptake and release provided that the maximum activity of glucokinase exceeds that of glucose-6-phosphatase (*in vivo*) and that the activity of glucose-6-phosphatase and the concentration of its substrate (glucose-6-phosphate) remain fairly constant. The theory proposes that the activity of glucokinase varies according to the glucose concentration and that this regulates both the *direction* and the *flux* of glucose metabolism in the liver. The theory is explained quantitatively in Figure 6.6 and is described in reference 28. Qualitatively, it is explained as follows. As the glucose concentration approaches that which saturates glucokinase (approximately 50 mM) the net rate of glucose uptake by the liver is given by the V_{max} for glucokinase minus a constant rate which represents the activity of glucose-6-

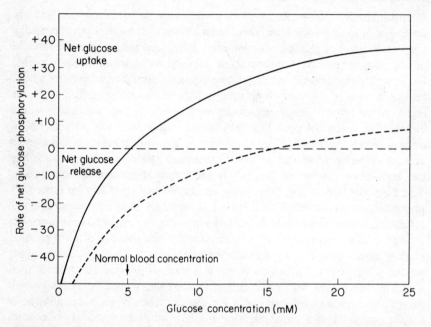

Figure 6.6. A plot of glucokinase activity against glucose concentration illustrating the role of this enzyme in the regulation of glucose uptake and the role of glucokinase and glucose-6-phosphatase in the regulation of glucose release. For simplicity it has been assumed that the K_m of glucokinase for glucose is 5 mM. In the unbroken line, glucokinase has a V_{max} of 100 units and the activity of glucose-6-phosphatase remains constant at 50. In the broken line the activity of glucokinase has been reduced to 80 while that of glucose-6-phosphatase has been increased to 60. This latter condition may represent the situation in starvation in that the sensitivity of glucose uptake to glucose has been decreased whereas that of glucose release has been increased (i.e., at concentrations below 5 mM-glucose the rate of glucose release is greater for the broken line). Net glucose phosphorylation is indicated by positive values on the ordinate whereas net glucose release is indicated by negative values. The rates of glucose phosphorylation or release are calculated from the equation

$$V = \frac{V_{max}[\text{glucose}]}{[\text{glucose}] + K_m} - V'$$

where V_{max} is the maximum activity of glucokinase, K_m is 5 mM and V' represents the constant activity of glucose-6-phosphatase (i.e. 50 or 60) phosphatase. As the glucose concentration is lowered towards the normal (5 mM), the activity of glucokinase will decrease until it approaches that of glucose-6-phosphatase. At about 5 mM glucose, the activities of both enzymes will be equal and there will be no net uptake or release of glucose by the liver. As the concentration of glucose is lowered still further (below 5 mM), the activity of glucokinase will be decreased below that of glucose-6-phosphatase and a net hydrolysis of glucose-6-phosphate will occur. Thus, the liver will release glucose into the blood stream. Therefore changes in the blood glucose level control the direction of glucose metabolism. The theory provides a biochemical explanation for the observations that the *rate* of uptake or release of glucose by the liver is proportional to the *degree* of hyperglycaemia or hypoglycaemia, respectively (see Figure 6.6). In this control system, regulation is achieved merely through changes in the blood glucose level. No specific regulator molecules are required.

At present there is no direct evidence to support or refute the theory of substrate cycling. Although the simplicity of the mechanism has been emphasized, it does, however, depend upon the activity of glucose-6-phosphatase remaining fairly constant and this in turn depends upon a constant glucose-6-phosphate concentration. Thus, the flux into the hexose monophosphate pool must be increased, when the rate of glucose release by the liver is increased, in order to maintain a constant level of glucose-6-phosphate. This could be achieved by the control of glycogenolysis *in concert* with glucose-6-phosphate hydrolysis ('control in series'; see Chapter 3, Section D.4(b)) but it is not possible to propose a satisfactory theory because of inadequate knowledge of the control of liver phosphorylase. Alternatively, the increased formation of glucose-6-phosphate could arise from a stimulation of gluconeogenesis (see later).

(b) '*Compartmentation*' *of glucokinase and glucose-6-phosphatase in the regulation of glucose uptake and release*

The 'compartmentation' theory proposes that glucokinase and glucose-6-phosphatase are never simultaneously active because they are retained in separate compartments of the cell and the substrates and products of the two enzymes are not permitted to mix. The glucose-6-phosphate produced by the action of glucokinase may function as precursor for glycolysis or for glycogen synthesis, but never as a substrate for glucose-6-phosphatase. The substrate for glucose-6-phosphatase is provided by glycogenolysis or gluconeogenesis. Also, any glucose produced by the action of the phosphatase is released into the blood and is prevented from contact with glucokinase.

There is no direct evidence to support this theory but there is some indirect evidence (for discussion of 'compartmentation' in liver see references 29 and 30). The precise intracellular location of many enzymes is a major biochemical problem at the present time and therefore it is not surprising that little information is available about the intracellular distribution of glucokinase and glucose-6-phosphatase. Glucokinase is apparently present in the soluble cytoplasm (that part of a cell homogenate that does not sediment at 100,000g), whereas glucose-6-phosphatase is associated with the endoplasmic reticulum fraction. This, however, hardly constitutes evidence for the physical separation of the two enzymes in the liver cell.

Furthermore, simple physical separation of glucokinase and glucose-6-phosphatase does not by itself provide a satisfactory theory for the control of blood glucose. For example, the membrane or membranes that separate the enzymes must be capable of distinguishing between glucose-6-phosphate produced from gluconeogenesis (or glycogenolysis) and that produced by the action of glucokinase. Alternatively, not only must these two enzymes be physically separate, but also the processes which produce glucose-6-phosphate for glucose-6-phosphatase (glycogenolysis and gluconeogenesis) must be separate from the processes that utilize glucose-6-phosphate produced by glucokinase (see Figure 6.7).

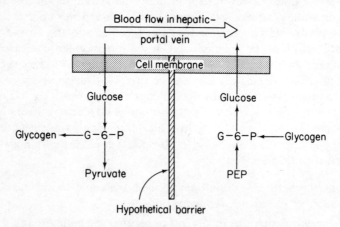

Figure 6.7. 'Compartmentation' theory for the control of glycolysis and gluconeogenesis

The 'compartmentation' theory relies upon a degree of structural organization in order to provide a satisfactory control mechanism. The substrate-cycling theory appears to be considerably more simple. This comment must not imply that structural organization ('compartmentation') does not play any role in metabolic regulation. Probably it plays a fundamental role, although not necessarily a monopolistic one. Substrate cycling is an example of chemical organization as opposed to physical organization. In the case of the control of glucose uptake and release by the liver the chemical organization appears to possess the advantage of simplicity.

C. CONTROL OF GLYCOLYSIS AND GLUCONEOGENESIS IN LIVER AND KIDNEY CORTEX

The regulation of glycolysis has not been studied as thoroughly in liver and kidney cortex as in other tissues (such as brain, muscle and red blood cells) and there are several reasons for this apparent lack of interest. The rate of glycolysis in experimental preparations of liver and kidney cortex is low and therefore difficult to measure. The process can be studied *in vitro* using either liver slices or an isolated perfused liver but both preparations present problems. The cells in the liver slices rapidly lose metabolic intermediates and cofactors to the medium and glycolysis is inhibited by lack of cofactors. A perfused liver taken from a fed animal does utilize glucose but there occurs also a degradation of endogenous glycogen to produce glucose which interferes with a precise measurement of glucose uptake. A perfused liver taken from a fasted animal readily produces glucose (even in the absence of external precursors), so that only if the external glucose concentration is considerably elevated will the liver remove glucose, but under these conditions the rate of glucose utilization cannot be measured. Nonetheless, there is no doubt that both *in vivo* and *in vitro* the liver can remove glucose from the blood and convert it into pyruvate and lactate.[31] Furthermore, under anaerobic conditions, glycogen is converted to lactate at a rate that is predicted from the maximum activity of PFK in this tissue.[32]

In contrast to glycolysis, gluconeogenesis has been studied in detail in these tissues. However, any satisfactory theory of control of gluconeogenesis must also account for the control of glycolysis.

1. Pathway of gluconeogenesis

The pathway for glucose formation in liver and kidney cortex is shown in Figure 6.8. Many of the gluconeogenic reactions are identical to those of glycolysis; such reactions are always close to equilibrium so that the rate and the direction of flow of residues can be changed by variations in the concentrations of substrates and/or products of these reactions. On the other hand, the reactions of glycolysis that are non-equilibrium (those catalysed by hexokinase, phosphofructokinase and pyruvate kinase—see Chapter 3, Section B), release a considerable amount of energy as heat and therefore cannot be easily reversed (see Chapter 1, Section B.2(d)). These specific 'energy barrier' reactions must be bypassed in the gluconeogenic pathway.[33] The reactions catalysed by hexokinase and phosphofructokinase are both bypassed by hydrolytic cleavage of the phosphate ester bond: glucose-6-phosphate is hydrolysed to glucose and inorganic phosphate, a reaction that is catalysed by glucose-6-phosphatase; fructose-1,6-diphosphate is hydrolysed to fructose-6-phosphate and inorganic phosphate, a reaction that is catalysed by fructose diphosphatase. The pyruvate kinase-bypass consists of

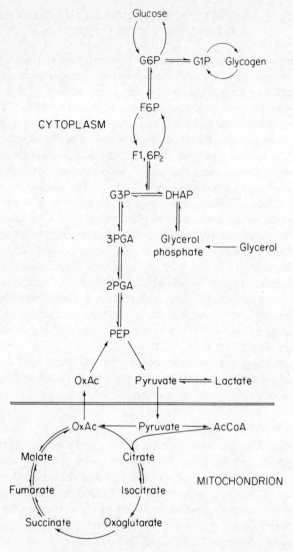

Figure 6.8. The pathways of glycolysis and gluconeogenesis in liver and kidney cortex

two separate reactions. Pyruvate is carboxylated to oxaloacetate in a reaction
involving ATP hydrolysis and catalysed by pyruvate carboxylase. Conversion
of oxaloacetate to phosphoenolpyruvate involves a decarboxylation and
phosphate transfer from either GTP or ITP, which is catalysed by phosphoenolpyruvate carboxykinase (PEPCK).

The three main precursors for gluconeogenesis are lactate, glycerol and amino acids. Lactate is converted to pyruvate by the lactate dehydrogenase reaction and enters the gluconeogenic pathway at pyruvate carboxylase. Glycerol enters the pathway by phosphorylation to glycerol phosphate and oxidation to dihydroxyacetone phosphate, catalysed by glycerol kinase and glycerol phosphate dehydrogenase, respectively. All of the amino acids except leucine can give rise to gluconeogenic precursors.[34] The points of entry into the gluconeogenic pathway of some of these amino acids are shown in Figure 6.9. The pathways by which amino acids are degraded to gluconeogenic precursors are adequately described in most general biochemistry texts (see also reference 34).

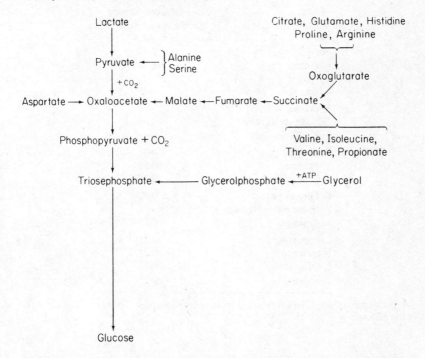

Figure 6.9. Entry of precursors into the pathway of gluconeogenesis (reproduced from H. A. Krebs, *Proc. Roy. Soc.*, **B159**, 545 (1964) (Table 6) by permission of the Royal Society, London)

Although the liver has been considered to be the main organ for the degradation and deamination of amino acids, recent work strongly suggests that extrahepatic tissues play more than a simple passive role in release of amino acids for deamination by the liver. Muscle tissue may be particularly important in the degradation of the branched-chain amino acids (such as valine and isoleucine) which form a considerable proportion of the total amino acid content of protein. These amino acids are degraded to glutamate which is either transaminated to form oxoglutarate and alanine or aminated to form glutamine. Thus, muscle tissue releases considerable amounts of alanine[35] and glutamine[36] which are transported via the blood to the liver.[35] In accordance with this role of muscle is the fact that high rates of gluconeogenesis are obtained from the perfused liver when either glutamine or alanine is the substrate (Table 6.9). The concept of a glutamine-alanine cycle has

Table 6.9. Rates of gluconeogenesis from various precursors in the perfused rat liver

Substrate added	Glucose formed (μmol/min/g fresh liver)
Nil	0·14
Lactate	1·06
Pyruvate	1·02
Glycerol	0·48
Fructose	2·68
Dihydroxyacetone	2·07
L-Serine	0·98
L-Alanine	0·66
L-Proline	0·55
L-Glutamine	0·45
L-Threonine	0·40
L-Glutamate (Na salt)	0·31
L-Arginine	0·27
L-Aspartate	0·23
L-Isoleucine	0·22
L-Ornithine	0·19
L-Valine	0·12

Female rats were used and were starved for 48 hours prior to use. Final substrate concentration in the perfusate was 10 mM.[47]

been developed to describe the roles of muscle and liver in the provision and utilization of amino acids for the process of gluconeogenesis (see Figure 6.10).

Most of the glycerol that functions as precursor for gluconeogenesis is derived from lipolysis in adipose tissue. During starvation the hydrolysis of stored triglyceride provides this important gluconeogenic precursor (glycerol) as well as the main oxidizable fuel for the body (fatty acids). It must be emphasized that in higher animals there is no net conversion of fatty acids into glucose. In some bacteria and plant seedlings, fatty acids *can* be converted to glucose via the glyoxylate cycle[37] but this pathway has never been demon-

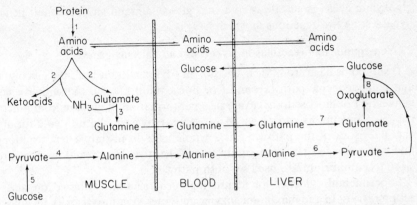

Figure 6.10. The glutamine-alanine cycle between muscle and liver. (1) Protein catabolism in muscle. (2) Degradation of amino acids in muscle. (3) Glutamine synthetase. (4) Glutamate-pyruvate transaminase in muscle. (5) Glycolysis in muscle. (6) Glutamate-pyruvate transaminase in liver. (7) Glutaminase. (8) Gluconeogenesis

strated in higher animals. The reason why fatty acids cannot give rise to glucose, in the absence of this cycle, is simply that they are degraded to 2-carbon units (acetyl-CoA) before entering the TCA cycle and in the first part of this cycle, two carbon atoms are lost as CO_2 (see Figure 6.11). In the

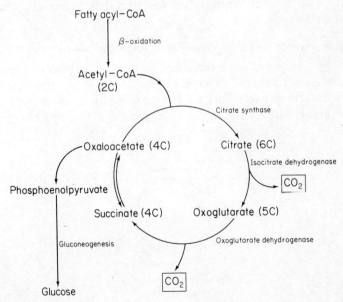

Figure 6.11. Loss of two carbon atoms during catabolism of acetate in the TCA cycle

glyoxylate cycle, isocitrate is split into glyoxylate and succinate and hence bypasses the two reactions in which CO_2 is lost.

2. Non-equilibrium reactions in glycolysis and gluconeogenesis

It should be clear from the discussion in Chapter 1 that both the glycolytic and gluconeogenic pathways must be non-equilibrium, so that either a net conversion of glucose to pyruvate or a net formation of glucose from gluconeogenic precursors can occur at any time. However, the non-equilibrium characteristics of the pathways as a whole arise from only a few reactions that are displaced far from equilibrium. The glycolytic reactions that are close to equilibrium are used by both pathways.

Experimental evidence for identifying such reactions is based on mass-action ratio data and maximum enzyme activities. A comparison of the mass-action ratios with the apparent equilibrium constants for both pathways is provided in Table 6.5. These data indicate that the reactions catalysed by glucokinase, glucose-6-phosphatase, PFK, FDPase, pyruvate kinase, PEPCK and pyruvate carboxylase are non-equilibrium. The maximal enzyme activities for the enzymes of both pathways are shown in Table 6.6. The low-activity enzymes are as follows: glucokinase, glucose-6-phosphatase, PFK, FDPase, aldolase, enolase, PEPCK and pyruvate carboxylase. Therefore the following enzymatic reactions can be classified as non-equilibrium: glucokinase, glucose-6-phosphatase, PFK, FDPase, pyruvate kinase, PEPCK and pyruvate carboxylase (cf. glycolysis in muscle, Chapter 3, Section B).

3. Regulatory enzymes in glycolysis and gluconeogenesis

A problem arises in the interpretation of data from 'crossover' experiments, in the situation where two or more enzymes catalyse a pathway reaction in opposite directions (see Figure 6.12). If the substrate of one enzyme changes in the opposite direction to the flux, the cause could be either an activation

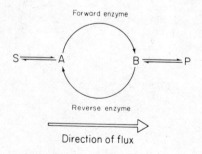

Figure 6.12

of the forward enzyme or an inhibition of the reverse enzyme. The precise interpretation has to be deferred until the properties of the two enzymes are known and a mechanism of control has been established. The simplest approach is to interpret any positive 'crossover' experiment as indicating that the *reaction system* catalysed by the two enzymes is regulatory, the actual mechanism of control depending upon the properties of the two component enzymes.

The importance of glucokinase and glucose-6-phosphatase in providing a mechanism to explain glucose uptake and release by the liver has been discussed in detail in the previous section. The experimental evidence indicating that the PFK-FDPase and pyruvate carboxylase/PEPCK/ pyruvate kinase enzyme systems are regulatory has been discussed in detail in a review article[28] and will not be repeated here. Since the publication of this review article, Williamson and coworkers have performed experiments with the perfused liver in which it has been demonstrated that perfusion with fatty acids increases the rate of gluconeogenesis from lactate, alanine and other precursors, and that the concentrations of pyruvate and fructose diphosphate (under certain conditions) are decreased.[38] These results support the conclusions that the pyruvate carboxylase/PEPCK/pyruvate kinase and PFK-FDPase enzyme systems are regulatory for glycolysis and gluconeogenesis in the liver.

Recently it has been shown that ischaemia increases the glycolytic flux in the liver and kidney *in situ*. In both tissues, ischaemia produces an increase in the contents of hexose monophosphates (presumably because phosphorylase is stimulated to a greater extent than PFK), but the content of phosphoenolpyruvate is decreased. This indicates that pyruvate kinase in these tissues is controlled by factors other than the concentration of phosphoenolpyruvate.[32]

4. Regulatory properties of glycolytic and gluconeogenic enzymes

The properties of the possible regulatory enzymes of these processes have been discussed in a review article[28] and therefore will only be briefly summarized. PFK is inhibited by ATP and citrate and this inhibition is reduced by AMP, P_i, fructose-6-phosphate and fructose diphosphate. FDPase is inhibited by AMP. Pyruvate kinase is inhibited by ATP and activated by fructose diphosphate. There are known to be two isoenzymes of pyruvate kinase in liver that are electrophoretically and immunologically distinct and whose kinetic properties are different.[39] The K_m for phosphoenolpyruvate is 0.75×10^{-4} M and 0.84×10^{-3} M for the M and L isoenzymes, respectively. The K_i for ATP is 3.5×10^{-3} M and 0.1×10^{-3} M for the M and L isoenzymes, respectively. Only the L isoenzyme is activated by fructose diphosphate. Pyruvate carboxylase is activated by acetyl-CoA and inhibited by ADP. Although there have been a number of studies on the properties of phosphoenolpyruvate carboxykinase, it appears to date to have few, if any, properties that could suggest control by feedback regulation of its activity. A number of theories for the regulation of glycolysis and gluconeogenesis, based upon some of these properties of the regulatory enzymes, have been suggested and some of these theories are discussed below.

5. Regulation of glycolysis and gluconeogenesis under anaerobic conditions

The anaerobic condition provides a very useful experimental tool with which to perturb the energy balance of a normally-aerobic cell. The resultant changes in the contents of metabolic intermediates may permit regulatory theories to be tested.

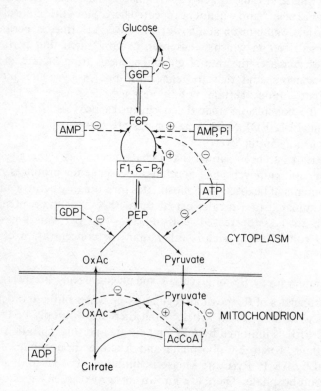

Figure 6.13. Regulation of glycolysis and gluconeogenesis by 'energy status' of the cell

Anoxia and respiratory poisons increase the rate of glycolysis in kidney cortex slices. Acute ischaemia of the liver and kidney *in situ* also increases glycolysis. The total content of ATP is decreased severely under these conditions and the content of AMP is increased. These changes would be expected to stimulate PFK and inhibit FDPase and hence stimulate glycolysis and inhibit gluconeogenesis (Figure 6.13). Experiments with the ischaemic liver provide some indirect evidence in support of this theory. The rate of lactate formation during the first few minutes of ischaemia is similar to the maximum activity of PFK as measured *in vitro*.[32] Since the maximum activity of FDPase *in vitro* is several times larger than that of PFK, this result demonstrates that ischaemia must cause severe inhibition of FDPase as well as stimulation of PFK.

In a very simple experiment it has been shown that perfusion of the isolated rat liver with 2 mM AMP causes increased glycogenolysis and glycolysis and decreased formation of glucose from lactate.[40] If it is assumed that some of the AMP enters the liver cell, the changes in glycolysis and gluconeogenesis are precisely those predicted by the theory proposed above.

A satisfactory theory for the regulation of the enzymes controlling the interconversions of pyruvate and phosphoenolpyruvate under these conditions is more difficult to find. Anoxic or ischaemic conditions may be expected to stimulate pyruvate kinase by an increase in the concentration of fructose diphosphate and a decrease in the concentration of ATP. It is also possible that an increase in the intramitochondrial concentration of ADP would inhibit pyruvate carboxylase (Figure 6.13).

Although the effects of anoxia and ischaemia on the rate of glycolysis in liver have been studied in some detail, the effects of these conditions on gluconeogenesis have not apparently been reported. In kidney cortex slices gluconeogenesis from glycerol or dihydroxyacetone is very rapidly inhibited by addition of cyanide.[41]

6. Regulation of glycolysis and gluconeogenesis by fatty acid oxidation

The stimulation of gluconeogenesis by a compound which is not itself a precursor for glucose formation was first demonstrated in 1965[42] when it was found that acetoacetate increased glucose formation from lactate and other precursors in kidney cortex slices. It has since been demonstrated that fatty acids or ketone bodies *decrease* the rate of glucose uptake by kidney cortex slices (see Table 6.10). Similarly, in the perfused liver, long-chain fatty acids have been shown to increase the rate of gluconeogenesis from lactate and other precursors (see Table 6.11), an effect which is abolished by a specific inhibitor of fatty acid oxidation.[38] These effects of fatty acids on gluconeogenesis in the perfused liver have been criticized on the grounds that concentrations of fatty acids much greater than those arising *in vivo* have been used. When the experiments have been performed at physiological levels of fatty acids there has been no stimulatory effect.[43] Such criticism may be valid, but there is no doubt that high concentrations of long-chain fatty acids stimulate gluconeogenesis in the perfused liver and this provides

Table 6.10. Effects of butyrate and acetoacetate on rates of glucose uptake and glucose formation, and on the contents of metabolic intermediates, in kidney cortex slices

Substrate	Addition to incubation	Rate of substrate removal (μmol/g wet wt/hr)	Rate of glucose formation (μmol/g wet wt/hr)	Contents in kidney cortex slice (nmol/g dry weight)						
				Glucose-6-phosphate	Fructose diphosphate	ATP	ADP	AMP	Citrate and isocitrate	Acetyl-CoA
1. Glucose	Control	8.8	—	104	60	4,092	1,327	417	576	—
	Acetoacetate (5 mM)	1.8	—							
	Butyrate (2.5 mM)	4.0	—	259	40	3,527	1,001	345	1,195	—
2. Glycerol	Control	46	7.1	129	37	3,512	1,668	365	254	—
	Acetoacetate (5 mM)	50	13.7	239	38	3,502	1,352	483	800	—
	Butyrate (2.5 mM)	46	11.4	215	59	3,607	933	182	917	—
3. Lactate	Control	—	8.6						—	24
	Acetoacetate (5 mM)	—	16.7						—	53
4. Glucose	Control	8.3	—						—	
	*48-hr starvation	5.4	—						—	
5. Glycerol	Control	—	12.5	129	37	3,512	1,668	365	254	—
	*48-hr starvation	—	19.5	250	48	4,080	1,340	271	909	—

Kidney cortex slices were incubated usually for one hour either with glucose (2 mM) in order to measure glucose uptake, or with a gluconeogenic precursor (glycerol or lactate, 5 mM) in order to measure glucose formation. The results reported below represent the mean of 4 experimental values and the differences between the control and experimental results for glucose uptake, glucose formation and the contents of glucose-6-phosphate, citrate and isocitrate and acetyl-CoA are all statistically significant.[41,42,45]

* The donor animal was starved for 48 hours; control animals had access to food.

Table 6.11. The effects of oleic acid on gluconeogenesis and the contents of metabolic intermediates in the perfused liver in the presence and absence of (+) decanoylcarnitine

| | Rates of glucose formation (μmol glucose/100 g rat) | | |
Perfusion time (min)	Control	Oleate	Oleate plus decanoylcarnitine
0	0	0	0
15	20	60	10
30	40	120	30
45	60	170	50

| | Contents in liver (μmol/g dry wt. liver) | | | |
	ATP	AMP	Citrate	Acetyl-CoA
Control	9·54	0·47	3·32	0·12
Oleate	6·73	1·13	8·04	0·21
Oleate plus decanoylcarnitine	8·52	0·74	3·05	0·13

Gluconeogenesis was measured by glucose formation from lactate, which was maintained at 8–12 mM by constant infusion. (+) Decanoylcarnitine is an inhibitor of fatty acid oxidation and it had no effect on the rate of glucose formation (or the contents of metabolic intermediates) when added to the control.[38]

a useful experimental tool for the investigation of the regulation of this process.

Fatty acid oxidation in the liver and fatty acid or ketone body oxidation in kidney cortex slices increase the contents of acetyl-CoA and citrate. Therefore the stimulation of gluconeogenesis in these two tissues can be explained by an extension of the theory of the control of glycolysis in muscle (Chapter 3, Section D.5). The same theory will of course explain the inhibition of glycolysis by fatty acid oxidation in kidney cortex slices (Table 6.10). The increased intracellular concentration of acetyl-CoA decreases pyruvate oxidation (pyruvate dehydrogenase is inhibited) and increases pyruvate carboxylation to oxaloacetate (pyruvate carboxylase is stimulated).[44] The increased intracellular concentration of citrate inhibits PFK and reduces the glycolytic flux. If it is assumed that a substrate cycle exists between fructose-6-phosphate and fructose diphosphate (catalysed by the simultaneous activities of FDPase and PFK), inhibition of PFK activity could lead to an increased rate of fructose diphosphate hydrolysis and a stimulation of gluconeogenesis (see Figure 6.14).[41,45] (A full discussion of the possible operation of such a substrate cycle is provided below.)

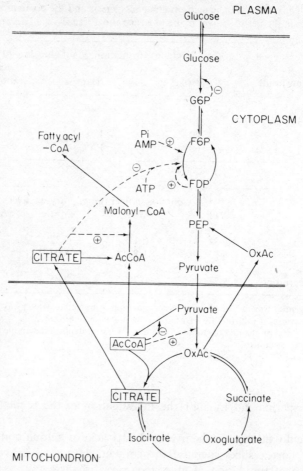

Figure 6.14. Regulation of glycolysis, glyconeogenesis and fatty acid synthesis in the liver and kidney cortex by citrate and acetyl-CoA

7. Regulation by the PFK-FDPase substrate cycle

The amplification that can be provided by a substrate cycle has been discussed in Chapter 2, Section F.2(a)(i) and possible examples of substrate cycles have been discussed in relation to the control of glycolysis in certain skeletal muscles (Chapter 3, Section D.4(e)) and in relation to the control of glucose uptake by the liver (Section B.2(a)). In liver and kidney cortex both PFK and FDPase must be present for the operation of the pathways of glycolysis and gluconeogenesis. Therefore, when there is net glycolysis, FDPase could be inactive and conversely, when there is net gluconeogenesis,

PFK could be inactive. An alternative possibility is that, under most physiological conditions, both these enzymes are simultaneously active and catalyse a substrate cycle. Although there is no direct evidence to support or refute the hypothesis of a substrate cycle at this enzymatic level in kidney cortex and liver, there is indirect evidence to support this theory.

(a) Energy consumed by the PFK-FDPase substrate cycle in liver

One of the main objections to substrate cycles in the control of metabolism is that they are energetically wasteful. In the PFK-FDPase cycle, one molecule of fructose-6-phosphate is converted to fructose diphosphate and back again at the expense of one ATP molecule. The maximum rate of cycling is determined by the activity of the enzyme that possesses the lower maximal activity as measured in vitro. For the above cycle the maximum activity of PFK in liver is about 5 μmol/min/g at 37 °C, whereas FDPase activity is three times greater than this. Thus, the highest rate of ATP utilization by the cycle would be 5 μmol/min/g at 37 °C. The rate of ATP formation in the liver may be as high as 50 μmol/min/g (calculated from the oxygen uptake of the perfused liver),[46] so that the PFK-FDPase cycle could account for no more than 10% of the total ATP production by the liver. Indeed, the properties of the two enzymes suggest that they would never be simultaneously maximally active, and therefore 10% is an overestimate.

However, in the case of this substrate cycle in liver, not all the energetic considerations are on the debit side. The substrate cycle ensures that the complex regulatory properties of PFK are available for control of both pathways (glycolysis and gluconeogenesis). If the two enzymes were to be controlled quite separately and independently (to avoid a substrate cycle) it might be expected that the properties of FDPase would be the mirror image of those of PFK—that is, FDPase would possess six regulatory properties instead of one. Since our stereospecific binding-site probably requires a peptide structure of molecular weight 10,000 or more, the energy expended in the synthesis of even one such peptide would be considerable.

(b) The extra-oxygen uptake of gluconeogenesis

In the perfused liver (or kidney) added lactate is converted almost exclusively into glucose and the amount of glucose that is synthesized can be easily measured. Since the metabolic pathway of gluconeogenesis is well established, it is possible to calculate the amount of ATP required for the synthesis of glucose and therefore the amount of oxygen required by the liver can also be calculated. However, when the oxygen uptake is actually measured, it is found to be considerably greater than that predicted from the calculation.[46] This extra-oxygen utilization can be explained by the occurrence of substrate cycles. The addition of lactate to the perfused liver (in comparison to controls to which no lactate is given) raises the concentration of glycolytic intermediates, including those that are substrates for the 'cycling' enzymes.[47] The increase in the concentration of the glycolytic intermediates initiates both glucose formation and substrate cycling so that the extra oxygen is consumed to provide the energy expended in such cycles (see Figure 6.15).

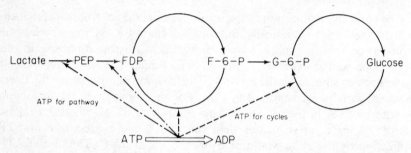

Figure 6.15. Energy expenditure in gluconeogenesis. — · — · — · →, ATP utilized in the net flux of 3-carbon residues to glucose. ————→, ATP utilized for the operation of substrate cycles

(c) Effects of fatty acids and ketone bodies on glucose utilization and glucose formation in kidney cortex slices

Kidney cortex slices take up glucose from an incubation medium at approximately $10\,\mu$mol per gram fresh weight per hour. This uptake is reduced by at least 50% when fatty acids or ketone bodies are added to the incubation medium. The rate of glucose uptake is also decreased by starvation of the donor animal. However, if glycerol (or dihydroxyacetone) replaces glucose in the incubation medium, the kidney slices form glucose at a rate of approximately $10\,\mu$mol/g/hr. This rate of glucose formation is doubled in the presence of fatty acids or ketone bodies. Starvation of the donor animal also increases the rate of glucose formation from glycerol. In both cases there is no change in the rate of glycerol uptake by the tissue. In the control condition, about 50% of the glycerol is converted to glucose, and this increases to almost 100% in the presence of fatty acids or ketone bodies, or after starvation of the animal (Table 6.10).

The effect of fatty acids, ketone bodies or starvation on kidney slices is to increase the contents of glucose-6-phosphate (fructose-6-phosphate was not measured but was assumed to be in equilibrium with glucose-6-phosphate) and citrate leaving the fructose diphosphate content unchanged (whether the substrate is glucose or glycerol). Thus, the theory that explains the inhibition of glycolysis by fatty acid oxidation in the perfused heart (Chapter 3, Section D.5) can also explain the inhibition of glycolysis in kidney cortex slices. The increase in citrate concentration inhibits PFK and this increases the glucose-6-phosphate concentration which inhibits hexokinase and restricts glucose phosphorylation and utilization.[41,45] The stimulation of gluconeogenesis (from glycerol) by fatty acids or ketone bodies can also be explained on the basis of the above theory for control of glycolysis, provided that a substrate cycle exists between fructose-6-phosphate and fructose diphosphate in kidney cortex.[41,45]

8. Regulation of hepatic phosphofructokinase during starvation

The concentrations of ketone bodies that stimulate gluconeogenesis in kidney cortex slices are within the physiological range and therefore their effect is probably physiologically important during starvation. However, the concentrations of fatty acids that stimulate gluconeogenesis in the perfused liver are much higher than occur *in vivo*. Therefore it is unlikely that this effect is physiologically important[43] and the increased fatty acid oxidation which occurs in the liver during starvation is probably *not* responsible for the stimulation of gluconeogenesis. In accordance with this idea, the hepatic content of citrate is not elevated in starvation : indeed it is markedly reduced.[48] (This situation is in contrast to that in heart muscle and kidney cortex.) Nonetheless, the rate of gluconeogenesis and hence the rate of fructose diphosphate hydrolysis is increased in the liver, but this cannot be explained by inhibition of PFK through changes in the concentration of citrate. Moreover, since the maximal activities of PFK and FDPase do not change during starvation, variations in the total catalytic capacities of these enzymes cannot be responsible.

One plausible theory of control of hepatic PFK during starvation emphasizes the critical balance between glycogenolysis and gluconeogenesis in liver.[49] The liver glycogen in the rat is depleted by about 70% after the diurnal fast and is almost completely depleted after 24 hours of starvation (Table 6.12). The rate of glycogenolysis during the first 24 hours of starvation

Table 6.12. Glycogen content of rat liver during starvation

Time of starvation (hours)	Glycogen content (μmol glucose equivalent/g fresh weight of liver)
0	218
6	231
12	56
27	9
35	2
48	4

The values given are the means of four determinations. Zero time represents the end of the overnight feeding period.[48]

may provide sufficient glucose for the demands of the whole animal. Therefore, during this period it is probably important that gluconeogenesis in the liver should be restricted in order to avoid over-production of glucose arising from the simultaneous stimulation of both glycogenolysis and gluconeogenesis. The restriction of gluconeogenesis may occur at the substrate cycle between fructose-6-phosphate and fructose diphosphate, since the maintenance of PFK activity will prevent a net hydrolysis of fructose diphosphate. However, the glycogen reserves of the liver are eventually depleted (after about 24 hours of starvation in the well-fed rat) and at this time it will be necessary to remove the restriction on the hydrolysis of fructose diphosphate. How can this be achieved? A consideration of the hexose monophosphate levels provides an answer. Although it is well known that the hexose monophosphate contents of the liver are *decreased* by starvation, it has been observed that during the early stages the hexose monophosphates are maintained at the fed levels. It is only when the glycogen reserves are near depletion that they are decreased.[48] Since fructose-6-phosphate is a substrate for PFK, a decrease in its concentration will decrease the activity of this enzyme (in effect, the ATP inhibition of PFK is increased). If a substrate cycle occurs between fructose-6-phosphate and fructose diphosphate, a decrease in PFK activity will result in an increased hydrolysis of fructose diphosphate. Thus, the maintenance of the hexose monophosphate concentration is considered to restrict gluconeogenesis at the level of FDPase *until* the glycogen store is depleted. A precise explanation for the delayed response to starvation of the hexose monophosphate concentration is not immediately apparent, but one possibility is that the gradual, long-term changes in the activities of glucokinase and glucose-6-phosphatase (together with the decreased rate of glycogenolysis) are responsible.

9. Control of gluconeogenesis by substrate availability

The main precursors for glucose formation in the liver are glycerol, amino acids and lactate. Experiments with the perfused rat liver suggest that an increase in the plasma concentration of any of these precursors could result in a stimulation of gluconeogenesis.[13] For example, the half-maximal rate of gluconeogenesis from glycerol is obtained at a concentration of 0·5 mM : the plasma level of glycerol in the fed animal is 0·1 mM and this is doubled during starvation. There is no clear-cut evidence that the plasma level of amino acids is increased during starvation. However, increased substrate availability for gluconeogenesis could also arise from a stimulation of amino acid transport into the liver cell.

There is some evidence that this transport process is modified by hormones : for example, glucagon stimulates the transport of alanine into the liver cell. It is not known if this hormone stimulates the transport of all the amino acids but the inward transport of lysine and of the non-metabolizable amino acids, α-aminoisobutyrate and cycloleucine, are also increased.

Amino acids which function as precursors for gluconeogenesis during starvation are obtained from the breakdown of protein in muscle. This catabolism is increased during starvation and changes in the circulating levels of glucocorticoids and insulin may be responsible. The lack of insulin will result in a depression of protein synthesis, whereas the glucocorticoids stimulate protein degradation. The biochemical mechanisms by which proteins are degraded are largely unexplored at present and therefore it is not possible to propose a plausible theory for the action of glucocorticoids. The subject of control of protein concentration by effects on synthesis and degradation has been reviewed by Schimke.[51]

The plasma lactate concentration is known to increase to very high values (20 mM) during vigorous exercise. This would undoubtedly stimulate gluconeogenesis. (Indeed, the liver and kidney cortex play an extremely important role in reducing the plasma level of lactate during severe exercise.) However, it seems unlikely that an increase in the concentration of lactate *alone* can lead to increased activities of all the gluconeogenic enzymes. Therefore the possibility that lactate could produce changes within the liver that could stimulate gluconeogenesis has been investigated. Administration of lactate to an intact animal raises the content of pyruvate in the liver and this should stimulate pyruvate carboxylase. The administration of lactate also increases the hepatic content of citrate and this would be expected to inhibit PFK and hence lead to stimulation of fructose diphosphate hydrolysis.[64]

10. Regulation of gluconeogenesis by hormones

In recent years a great deal of experimental work has been carried out upon the effects of hormones on gluconeogenesis both in the intact animal and in the isolated perfused liver. Unfortunately it is still not possible to formulate a satisfactory theory of control of the gluconeogenic enzymes by hormones. The effects of hormones on gluconeogenesis have been discussed in a review in 1967[28] and since then the major developments in this field stem from the work of Exton and Park who have used the isolated perfused liver to study the stimulation of gluconeogenesis by glucagon, adrenaline and glucocorticoids and its inhibition by insulin.[13,50]

(a) Effect of glucagon on gluconeogenesis

In a review article[28] it was suggested that the effects of glucagon on gluconeogenesis might be explained by a stimulation of hepatic lipolysis and that the resultant increase in fatty acid oxidation would lead to elevated concentrations of acetyl-CoA and citrate. Gluconeogenesis would be stimulated as described above. However, in careful, precise experiments with the perfused liver, Exton and Park have shown that the effect of glucagon on gluconeogenesis occurs at physiological concentrations of the hormone, whereas the effects on lipolysis and ketosis occur at concentrations that are probably not physiological. Furthermore, these workers have shown that only very high concentrations of fatty acids are effective in the stimulation of gluconeogenesis. Even at a concentration of 1·8 mM, fatty acids (bound to a physiological concentration of albumin) did not cause a stimulation of gluconeogenesis[43] although the rate of ketone body formation was increased and presumably the content of acetyl-CoA was also increased (although it was not measured). Exton and Park conclude that the acetyl-CoA effect on pyruvate carboxylase is unimportant in the control of gluconeogenesis and that glucagon must stimulate gluconeogenesis by other means.

(b) Cyclic AMP and gluconeogenesis

Both glucagon and adrenaline stimulate adenyl cyclase in liver and increase the content of cyclic AMP. Therefore the stimulatory effect of these hormones upon gluconeogenesis may be exerted through an increase in the concentration of cyclic AMP. The evidence in support of this idea is as follows. The effect of glucagon upon gluconeogenesis is very rapid: a stimulation of ^{14}C incorporation from ^{14}C-lactate into glucose is detectable within 40 seconds after the administration of glucagon to the perfused liver. The concentration of glucagon that stimulates gluconeogenesis half-maximally is the same as that which stimulates glycogenolysis and adenyl cyclase (i.e. 2×10^{-10} M).[50] The addition of cyclic AMP to the perfusate of an isolated rat liver stimulates gluconeogenesis (as measured by ^{14}C incorporation from ^{14}C-lactate into glucose).[13]

In general, the effects of glucagon, cyclic AMP and adrenaline on the contents of gluconeogenic intermediates in the perfused liver are very similar. In particular, a 'cross-over' is observed between pyruvate and phosphoenolpyruvate ([pyruvate] is decreased and [phosphoenolpyruvate] is increased). Thus the hormones (and therefore cyclic AMP) increase the conversion of pyruvate to phosphoenolpyruvate. Exton and Park rule out the possibility that this is due to an inhibition of pyruvate kinase (and an increase in phosphoenolpyruvate formation due to a substrate cycle) by demonstrating that glucagon has no effect on the conversion of fructose or dihydroxyacetone to lactate. Therefore they conclude that cyclic AMP increases the activity of either pyruvate carboxylase or PEPCK (or both).[13] Further experiments involving the incorporation of ^{14}C from ^{14}C-pyruvate into malate and phosphoenolpyruvate have suggested that PEPCK is the enzyme whose activity is modified by glucagon.[50] Unfortunately, there is no evidence that cyclic AMP has any effect upon the activity or the properties of the enzyme in vitro.

(c) Effect of insulin on gluconeogenesis

Addition of insulin to the perfused liver results in inhibition of gluco-neogenesis (and glycogenolysis). The treatment of rats with insulin antisera one hour before sacrifice for liver perfusion increases gluconeogenesis and glycogenolysis. The administration of insulin antisera to rats increases the content of cyclic AMP in the perfused liver and this is counteracted by the addition of insulin to the perfusate. Addition of insulin to the perfusate in the absence of antisera treatment leads to a small decrease in the content of cyclic AMP. Furthermore, insulin can inhibit the stimulatory effect of glucagon on gluconeogenesis (and glycogenolysis) in the liver and it prevents the rise in cyclic AMP content that is observed in the presence of glucagon alone.[13] Hence the physiological effects of insulin on the liver, like those of adrenaline and glucagon, may involve changes in the concentration of cyclic AMP.

(d) Effect of glucocorticoids on gluconeogenesis

Glucocorticoids increase the rate of gluconeogenesis by a mechanism which is at present unclear. In the rat, adrenalectomy markedly decreases the rate of ^{14}C incorporation into glucose from ^{14}C-lactate in perfused livers from fasted or diabetic animals. However, there is no effect upon the perfused livers taken from fed animals. Administration of cortisol to diabetic animals before sacrifice improves the incorporation of ^{14}C into glucose in the perfused liver. Analysis of the intermediates of gluconeogenesis shows that adrenalectomy decreases the rate of pyruvate conversion to phospho-enolpyruvate.[13] The mechanism is unknown but an interesting suggestion is that glucocorticoids may play a 'permissive role', which somehow increases the response of the gluconeogenic pathway to cyclic AMP. Glucagon is ineffective in activating gluconeogenesis in liver from fasted, adrenalectomized rats, but the response to glucagon is restored if dexamethasone (synthetic glucocorticoid) is added *in vitro* or *in vivo*. Since adrenalectomy does *not* interfere with the ability of glucagon to increase the content of cyclic AMP in the liver, corticosteroids may influence the reaction between cyclic AMP and the gluconeogenic enzyme whose activity is modified by glucagon.[13] The precise identification of this enzyme and some knowledge of how it is modified by cyclic AMP will doubtless aid the understanding of the action of both glucagon and glucocorticoids on gluconeogenesis.

11. Summary of the regulation of gluconeogenesis

(a) Non-hormonal regulation

In severe conditions of ischaemia of the liver, gluconeogenesis is prob-ably inhibited by changes in the levels of the adenine nucleotides (ATP is decreased and AMP is increased). These changes will also stimulate glycogen degradation and provide energy from anaerobic glycolysis. This situation may arise *in vivo* during severe, short-term exercise when the blood supply is diverted from the viscera to the muscles.[52]

If the liver is suddenly presented with a high concentration of a short-chain fatty acid (for example, by ingestion of a large quantity of butter which has a high content of butyrate), the hepatic concentrations of citrate and acetyl-CoA would be expected to increase and this would stimulate gluconeogenesis and inhibit glycolysis. This has been observed in the perfused liver with unphysiologically high levels of long-chain fatty acids (Section C.6). Similarly, a high level of lactate in the blood (after exercise, for example) increases the hepatic contents of citrate and pyruvate (but not acetyl-CoA) and this should stimulate pyruvate carboxylase and the hydrolysis of fructose diphosphate (Section C.9).

(b) Hormonal regulation

The effects of hormones on gluconeogenesis are summarized with reference to two physiological conditions: starvation and exercise.

(i) *Starvation.* The availability of the gluconeogenic precursors, glycerol and amino acids, is increased as a result of the effects of the lipolytic hormones and glucocorticoids. The lipolytic hormones increase glycerol release from adipose tissue. Glucocorticoids increase the catabolism of body proteins in general. The decrease in insulin level will have similar effects upon both of these processes. In starvation, the plasma level of glucagon is elevated (see Chapter 5, Section B.4(b)(iii)). These changes in insulin and glucagon may account for the 60% rise in cyclic AMP content in livers of starved animals. This elevation in cyclic AMP is probably important in the stimulation of gluconeogenesis at the level of pyruvate conversion to phosphoenolpyruvate (Section C.10). Finally, there is some evidence to indicate that the *concentrations* of the gluconeogenic enzymes are elevated during prolonged starvation and that this might be mediated by the action of glucocorticoids.[53]

(ii) *Exercise.* The hormonal changes which are known to occur during exercise are as follows: the plasma level of insulin is decreased[54] whereas that of adrenaline (also noradrenaline) is increased.[55] These changes would be expected to increase the hepatic content of cyclic AMP and consequently stimulate gluconeogenesis. Also, the increase in growth hormone[56] (and glucocorticoids) level is probably responsible for increased lipolysis in adipose tissue (Chapter 5, Section B.4(b)(i)) which increases the plasma level of glycerol.

The control of gluconeogenesis in exercise may well depend upon the severity of the exercise. In very severe exercise the blood supply to the liver may be greatly reduced and the acute ischaemia would be expected to inhibit gluconeogenesis. However, during less vigorous and more prolonged exercise, the hormonal and substrate control mechanisms are probably responsible for increased gluconeogenesis.

REFERENCES FOR CHAPTER 6

1. Landau, B. R. & Katz, J. (1965). In *Handbook of Physiology, Section 5, Adipose Tissue*, p. 253. Ed. A. E. Renold & G. F. Cahill. Washington, D.C.: American Physiological Society.
2. Potter, V. R. & Ono, T. (1961). *Cold Spring Harbor Symp. Quant. Biol.* **26**, 355.
3. Ross, B. D., Hems, R., Freedland, R. A. & Krebs, H. A. (1967). *Biochem. J.* **105**, 869.
4. Steiner, D. F. & King, J. (1964). *J. biol. Chem.* **239**, 1292.
5. Rudman, D. & Di Girolamo, M. (1967). *Adv. Lipid Res.* **5**, 35.
6. Novello, F., Gumaa, K. A. & McLean, P. (1969). *Biochem. J.* **111**, 713.
7. Newsholme, E. A. & Start, C. (1972). In *Handbook of Physiology: Endocrine Pancreas*, p. 369. Ed. D. F. Steiner & N. Freinkel. Washington, D.C.: American Physiological Society.
8. Kornacker, M. S. & Lowenstein, J. M. (1965). *Biochem. J.* **95**, 832.
9. Naismith, D. J. (1971). *Proc. Nutrition Soc.* **30**, 259; and Macdonald, I. (1971). *ibid.* **30**, 277.
10. Yudkin, J. (1968). In *Carbohydrate Metabolism and its Disorders*, **2**, 169. Ed. F. Dickens, P. J. Randle & W. J. Whelan. London: Academic Press.
11. Sutherland, E. W., Øye, I. & Butcher, R. W. (1965). *Rec. Prog. Horm. Res.* **21**, 623.
12. Chen, L.-J. & Walsh, D. A. (1971). *Biochemistry*, **10**, 3614.
13. Exton, J. H., Mallette, L. E., Jefferson, L. S., Wong, E. H. A., Friedmann, N., Miller, T. B. & Park, C. R. (1970). *Rec. Prog. Horm. Res.* **26**, 411.
14. Felig, P., Marliss, E., Owen, O. E. & Cahill, G. F. (1969). *Arch. int. Med.* **123**, 293.
15. Cahill, G. F., Herrera, M. G., Morgan, A. P., Soeldner, J. S., Steinke, J., Levy, P. L., Reichard, G. A. & Kipnis, D. M. (1966). *J. clin. Invest.* **45**, 1751.
16. Owen, O. E., Felig, P., Morgan, P. A., Wahren, J. & Cahill, G. F. (1969). *J. clin. Invest.* **48**, 574.
17. Owen, O. E., Morgan, A. P., Kemp, H. G., Sullivan, J. N., Herrera, M. G. & Cahill, G. F. (1967). *J. clin. Invest.* **46**, 1589.
18. Annison, E. F. & Lewis, D. (1959). *Metabolism in the Rumen*. London: Methuen.
19. Lindsay, D. B. (1971). *Proc. Nutrition Soc.* **30**, 272.
20. Rohr, P., Saint-Saens, M. & Monod, H. (1966). *J. Physiol. Paris*, **58**, 5.
21. Krebs, H. A. (1968). *Adv. Enz. Reg.* **6**, 467.
22. Haight, J. S. J. & Keatinge, W. R. (1973). *J. Physiol. Lond.* (In press).
23. Cahill, G. F., Ashmore, J., Renold, A. E. & Hastings, A. B. (1959). *Amer. J. Med.* **26**, 264.
24. Soskin, S., Essex, H. E., Herrick, J. F. & Mann, F. C. (1938). *Amer. J. Physiol.* **124**, 558.
25. Bondy, P. K., James, D. F. & Farrar, B. W. (1949). *J. clin. Invest.* **28**, 238.
26. Sharma, C., Manjeshwar, R. & Weinhouse, S. (1963). *J. biol. Chem.* **238**, 3840.
27. Walker, D. G. (1966). *Essays in Biochemistry*, **2**, 33. Ed. P. N. Campbell & G. D. Greville. London: Academic Press.
28. Newsholme, E. A. & Gevers, W. (1967). *Vitamins & Hormones*, **25**, 1.
29. Heath, D. F. (1968). *Biochem. J.* **110**, 313; and Heath, D. F. & Threlfall, C. J. (1968). *Biochem. J.* **110**, 337.

30. Gumaa, K. A., McLean, P. & Greenbaum, A. L. (1971). *Essays in Biochemistry*, **7**, 39. Ed. P. N. Campbell & F. Dickens. London: Academic Press.
31. Steele, R. (1966). *Ergebnisse der Physiol.* **57**, 91.
32. Hems, D. A. & Brosnan, J. T. (1970). *Biochem. J.* **120**, 105.
33. Krebs, H. A. (1964). *Proc. Roy. Soc. B*, **159**, 545.
34. Krebs, H. A. (1964). *Mammalian Protein Metabolism*, **1**, 125. Ed. H. N. Munro & J. B. Allison. New York: Academic Press.
35. Felig, P., Pozefsky, T., Marliss, E. B. & Cahill, G. F. (1970). *Science*, **167**, 1003.
36. Marliss, E. B., Aoki, T. T., Pozefsky, T., Most, A. S. & Cahill, G. F. (1971). *J. clin. Invest.* **50**, 814.
37. Kornberg, H. L. & Madsen, N. B. (1958). *Biochem. J.* **68**, 549.
38. Williamson, J. R., Browning, E. T., Scholz, R. A., Kreisberg, R. A. & Fritz, I. B. (1968). *Diabetes*, **17**, 194.
39. Tanaka, T., Harano, Y., Sue, F. & Morimura, H. (1967). *J. Biochem. Japan*, **62**, 71.
40. Hunter, A. R. & Jefferson, L. S. (1969). *Biochem. J.* **111**, 537.
41. Newsholme, E. A. & Underwood, A. H. (1966). *Biochem. J.* **99**, 24C.
42. Krebs, H. A., Speake, R. N. & Hems, R. (1965). *Biochem. J.* **94**, 712.
43. Exton, J. H. & Park, C. R. (1967). *J. biol. Chem.* **242**, 2622.
44. Utter, M. F. & Fung, C. H. (1971). In *Regulation of Gluconeogenesis*, p. 1. Ed. H.-D. Söling & B. Willms. New York: Academic Press.
45. Underwood, A. H. & Newsholme, E. A. (1967). *Biochem. J.* **104**, 300.
46. Hems, R., Ross, B. D., Berry, M. N. & Krebs, H. A. (1966). *Biochem. J.* **101**, 284.
47. Ross, B. D., Hems, R. & Krebs, H. A. (1967). *Biochem. J.* **102**, 942.
48. Start, C. & Newsholme, E. A. (1968). *Biochem. J.* **107**, 411.
49. Start, C. & Newsholme, E. A. (1970). *FEBS Letters*, **6**, 171.
50. Exton, J. H., Ui, M., Lewis, S. B. & Park, C. R. (1971). In *Regulation of Gluconeogenesis*, p. 160. Ed. H.-D. Söling & B. Willms. New York: Academic Press.
51. Schimke, R. T. (1969). In *Current Topics in Cellular Regulation*, **1**, 277. Ed. B. L. Horecker & E. W. Stadtman. New York: Academic Press.
52. Wade, O. L. & Bishop, J. M. (1962). *Cardiac Output and Regional Blood Flow*, pp. 87 & 107. Oxford: Blackwell Scientific Publications.
53. Ashmore, J. & Weber, G. (1968). In *Carbohydrate Metabolism and its Disorders*, **1**, 336. Ed. F. Dickens, P. J. Randle & W. J. Whelan. London: Academic Press.
54. Wright, R. H. & Malaisse, W. J. (1968). *Amer. J. Physiol.* **214**, 1031.
55. Vendsalu, A. (1960). *Acta Physiol. Scand.* **49**, Suppl. 173.
56. Fonseka, C. C., Hunter, W. M. & Passmore, R. (1965). *J. Physiol. Lond.* **177**, 10P.
57. Cahill, G. F. & Owen, O. E. (1968). In *Carbohydrate Metabolism and its Disorders*, **1**, 497. Ed. F. Dickens, P. J. Randle & W. J. Whelan. London: Academic Press.
58. Bartley, W., Birt, L. M. & Banks, P. (1968). *The Biochemistry of the Tissues*, p. 139. London: John Wiley.
59. Williamson, D. H. (1973). In *Methods of Enzymatic Analysis*, 2nd edition (in press). Ed. H.-U. Bergmeyer. New York: Academic Press.
60. Scrutton, M. C. & Utter, M. F. (1968). *Ann. Rev. Biochem.* **37**, 249.
61. Sols, A. (1968). In *Carbohydrate Metabolism and its Disorders*, **1**, 53. Ed. F. Dickens, P. J. Randle & W. J. Whelan. London: Academic Press.
62. Salas, M., Viñuela, E. & Sols, A. (1963). *J. biol. Chem.* **238**, 3535.
63. Blumenthal, M. D., Abraham, S. & Chaikoff, I. L. (1964). *Arch. Biochem. Biophys.* **104**, 215.
64. Start, C. (1969). D. Phil. Thesis, Oxford University.

CHAPTER 7

REGULATION OF FAT METABOLISM
IN LIVER

A. INTRODUCTION

The liver is able to carry out most of the known reactions involved in fatty acid metabolism. Such reactions constitute the pathways of fatty acid synthesis from acetyl-CoA, esterification of fatty acids and storage of triglyceride, secretion of triglyceride into the blood in the form of VLDL, synthesis of phospholipids and cholesterol esters, lipolysis of triglyceride, oxidation of fatty acids and the formation of ketone bodies. Liver also possesses the capacity to increase the chain length and/or to desaturate certain fatty acids. Detailed analysis of all these pathways will not be attempted here. This discussion will focus upon esterification of fatty acids and their oxidation to form ketone bodies. In particular, the physiological significance of ketone bodies and the mechanism for the regulation of ketosis will be discussed in detail.

The role of adipose tissue in the control of the plasma fatty acid level and the relationship between muscle and adipose tissue in the control of the plasma glucose level have been emphasized (Chapters 3 and 5). On the basis of the metabolic relationship between muscle and adipose tissue the concept of the glucose/fatty acid cycle was developed. However, it is becoming increasingly apparent that the liver plays a fundamental role in the control of the oxidation of fat by peripheral tissues and therefore it is necessary to extend the glucose/fatty acid cycle to include the metabolism of the liver.

In general, liver and adipose tissue are the two tissues primarily responsible for the storage of triglyceride and there is usually a reciprocal relationship between the amount of triglyceride stored in these two tissues in any given species (that is, if there is only a small amount of adipose tissue, the liver has a large capacity for triglyceride storage and vice versa).[1] Mammals usually have large amounts of adipose tissue and therefore the mammalian liver contains only a small amount of triglyceride. If the triglyceride in the mammalian liver is to be made available for other tissues, it is released into the blood either as triglyceride (VLDL) or as ketone bodies. Long-chain fatty acids are released into the blood only by adipose tissue and the metabolic consequence of this release has already been discussed in Chapter 5. In animals that store most of their triglyceride in the liver (fish, for example), it is not known in what form the fat is released into the blood for utilization by other tissues (ketone bodies, fatty acids and triglyceride are all possibilities) and this would appear to be an extremely important problem in comparative biochemistry and physiology. The contents of this chapter are related only to metabolism in the mammalian liver.

B. PHYSIOLOGICAL IMPORTANCE OF FATTY ACID ESTERIFICATION IN LIVER

The enzymatic reactions of the esterification process appear to be similar in liver to those in adipose tissue (see Chapter 5, Section A. 1(b)). Long-chain fatty acyl-CoA is combined with glycerol phosphate to form phosphatidic acid, which is hydrolized to diglyceride. The latter is combined with another molecule of long-chain fatty acyl-CoA to form triglyceride. (The regulation of this process at an enzymatic level is considered in Section C.1.) Once triglyceride has been produced in the liver it can either be stored within this tissue or secreted into the bloodstream as VLDL. There appears to be a delay in the secretion of the newly-synthesized triglyceride into the blood (30–40 minutes in rat and 1–3 hours in man), despite the fact that esterification can occur very rapidly. This delay in secretion presumably represents the time necessary for formation of the lipoprotein.

1. Esterification and the uptake of plasma fatty acid by the liver

In the fasting state the plasma fatty acids are derived exclusively from the hydrolysis of triglyceride within the adipose tissue and the rate of mobilization of fatty acids from this tissue controls their concentration in the blood (see Chapter 5). It has been established that up to 50 % of these fatty acids can be taken up by the liver and, therefore, this tissue could influence considerably the concentration of fatty acids in peripheral blood.[2] The rate of oxidation of fatty acids by peripheral tissues is controlled by their concentration in the blood and consequently the liver, with its capacity to take up and esterify fatty acids, could modify the rate of their peripheral oxidation. However, the liver can only store a limited amount of triglyceride and any excess is secreted into the blood as VLDL. The secretion of VLDL must be regulated in relation to the rate of its removal from the blood and therefore the liver cannot continue to secrete VLDL into the plasma at a rate greatly in excess of the rate of removal by extrahepatic tissues. Consequently the ability of the liver to influence the plasma fatty acid level will depend upon the rate of mobilization of the fatty acids from adipose tissue and the rate of utilization of plasma VLDL. If the rate of mobilization is high, the liver may be able to influence the plasma fatty acid level for only short periods of time. Nevertheless, the liver has the capacity to override the control of the plasma fatty acid concentration exerted by the lipolytic hormones at the level of the adipose tissue cell and this may be of considerable physiological importance (see later).

2. The importance of plasma triglyceride derived from liver

Triglyceride, long-chain fatty acids and ketone bodies provide three separate 'fat fuels' in the blood for use by the various tissues. The problem of why Nature has provided three fuels when only one might be sufficient is discussed later in this chapter. The importance of long-chain fatty acids and ketone bodies is discussed in Section E.4 and triglyceride is discussed below.

Triglyceride is present in the blood under almost all physiological conditions but it can be utilized only by tissues that possess an active lipoprotein lipase. In a normal well-fed animal, dietary fat is absorbed as triglyceride (chylomicrons and VLDL) which is taken up and assimilated into the adipose tissue stores by virtue of the active lipoprotein lipase in the capillaries of this tissue. Indeed, in the fed state, the activity of this enzyme ensures that triglyceride utilization is directed towards adipose tissue. In the pregnant rat the plasma triglyceride levels are elevated about sixfold, approximately 5 days before parturition. This increase is due to a lowering of the activity of lipoprotein lipase in the adipose tissue. The triglyceride level returns to normal by parturition; but this is due to an increase in the activity of lipoprotein lipase in the *mammary gland*. Thus, in this condition, the uptake of the triglyceride fatty acids has been directed towards mammary glands and away from adipose tissue by changes in the activity of lipoprotein lipase.[2] Since the change in plasma triglyceride levels in pregnancy occurs on a low-fat diet as well as on a normal diet, the plasma triglyceride must originate in the liver. Thus, in pregnant rats some of the triglyceride content of the milk is derived from triglyceride originally synthesized in the liver and made available *specifically* to the mammary gland in the form of plasma VLDL.

The rate of release of triglyceride from the liver has been measured in the rat and is approximately 100 mg per hour per kg body weight in the starved animal. If this is completely oxidized it could account for 10–20% of the caloric requirement of the rat.[2] In starvation this triglyceride will probably be oxidized by muscle, since the activity of lipoprotein lipase in adipose tissue is markedly reduced in this condition. Little work has been done on the lipoprotein lipase activity of skeletal muscle and therefore the quantitative importance of this substrate in relation to glucose or plasma fatty acids is not known. However, it is unlikely that plasma triglyceride fatty acids play a *major* role in the provision of energy and the 10–20% of the caloric requirement may represent a maximum value.

The output of triglyceride from the liver is higher by about 50% in rats fed a high-carbohydrate diet. Such diets lead to synthesis of fatty acids from glucose within the liver, which is the primary source of plasma triglyceride on fat-free diets. In man, a high-carbohydrate diet can lead to a marked elevation in the plasma triglyceride level and it has been suggested that lipogenesis in the liver is the primary factor contributing to this hypertriglyceridaemia.[2] The possible biochemical links between atherosclerosis and hypertriglyceridaemia have already been mentioned and the possible effects of fructose (and sucrose) feeding on hepatic lipogenesis and plasma triglyceride levels have been described (Chapter 6, Section A.1(b)).

C. REGULATION OF FATTY ACID ESTERIFICATION AND OXIDATION IN LIVER

The liver has the capacity to remove a large proportion of plasma fatty acids from the circulation and these fatty acids can be either esterified to form triglyceride or oxidized to form ketone bodies (Figure 7.1). Somewhat

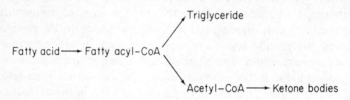

Figure 7.1

surprisingly, the problem of whether the liver cell can regulate the fate of the fatty acids has been neglected until recently. In view of the metabolic importance of ketone bodies (see below) and the possible pathological importance of hypertriglyceridaemia, it is the authors' view that this problem is of considerable importance.

It has been generally accepted that at low plasma levels of fatty acids the rate of uptake by the liver is low and the pathway of esterification competes effectively with that of oxidation. At high plasma levels of fatty acids the rate of uptake by the liver is high and the esterification pathway becomes saturated, so that oxidation increases and ketosis results. A recent investigation provides some quantitative data which support this general idea.[3] Fatty acids labelled with ^{14}C were infused into the media of perfused livers and it was found that in livers from fed animals, at a low perfusate fatty acid concentration (0·3 mM), almost all the fatty acid taken up by the liver was esterified: as the concentration of fatty acid was increased, ketone body formation occurred. This suggests that at high concentrations of external fatty acids their uptake rate exceeds the esterification capacity and that the surplus fatty acids are oxidized. In the same study it was shown that the liver can exert some specific control over the fate of the fatty acids. The proportion of fatty acids esterified was greater and the proportion oxidized was less in livers from fed rats than in livers from starved rats (Table 7.1). This suggests that starvation can increase the rate of oxidation in comparison to that of esterification.

Table 7.1. Fate of fatty acid in the perfused rat liver

Condition of animal	Concentration of fatty acid (mM)	Percentage of ^{14}C-fatty acid utilized in:		
		Esterification	CO_2	Ketone bodies
Fed	0·3	76·0	0·6	0·2
	0·9	79·4	5·2	0·9
	1·9	57·7	8·6	5·8
Starved 24 hours	0·4	24·3	27·0	5·4
	0·9	27·2	11·3	38·0
	1·75	31·0	7·2	23·5

The fatty acid (1-^{14}C-oleate) concentration was maintained constant in the perfusate by infusion. The measurements were performed over a period 90–120 minutes from the start of infusion when the pathways of fatty acid utilization were in a steady state.[3]

1. Regulation of esterification

The pathway of esterification of fatty acyl-CoA (see Figure 7.2) has not been investigated in any systematic manner in order to determine whether any of the reactions are non-equilibrium. It has generally been assumed that the glycerol phosphate concentration may regulate the rate of this process via substrate availability (cf. adipose tissue). In accordance with this view, there is some evidence that the content of glycerol phosphate in liver is decreased in starvation, although there is considerable variation in the reported values.[4] In liver, the glycerol phosphate concentration depends upon the concentration of triose phosphate, the cytoplasmic [NAD$^+$]/ [NADH] ratio and also the rate of phosphorylation of glycerol by glycerol kinase. However, in starvation or carbohydrate deprivation, it is important that the plasma glycerol, which is taken up and phosphorylated by the liver, is converted quantitatively to glucose (see Chapter 6, Section C.1). Hence, glycerol phosphate is a precursor for at least *two* biosynthetic pathways (esterification and gluconeogenesis) and therefore both pathways would be expected to be regulated independently of the concentration of this common precursor (that is, specific regulation of one of the esterification enzymes).

It has been suggested that a substrate cycle between triglyceride and fatty acids (catalysed by simultaneous activities of triglyceride lipase and the esterification enzymes) may operate in liver.[5] If this were so, the rate of lipolysis could control the apparent rate of esterification. However, studies with ^{14}C-fatty acids in the perfused liver[3] suggest that the process of esterification has a greater capacity than that of lipolysis, so that changes in the latter process would have little effect on the rate of esterification.

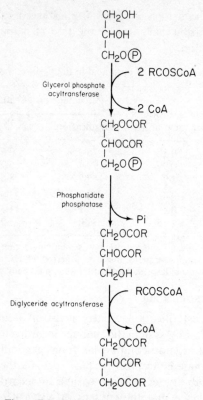

Figure 7.2. Pathway of esterification
of fatty acids

2. Regulation of fatty acid oxidation

The reactions involved in fatty acid oxidation are shown in Figure 7.3. Fatty acids are activated to fatty acyl-CoA by acyl-CoA synthetase. Since the mitochondrial membrane (probably the inner membrane) is impermeable to acyl-CoA derivatives, fatty acyl-CoA has to be converted (by carnitine acyltransferase) to fatty acyl-carnitine which can freely cross the inner mitochondrial membrane. On the inner side of the mitochondrial membrane, fatty acyl-carnitine is reconverted to fatty acyl-CoA which is oxidized by the enzymes of the β-oxidation process.[6] Any one of the enzyme-catalysed reactions shown in Figure 7.3 could be regulatory for fatty acid oxidation. However, there has been no systematic study to determine whether any of these reactions is non-equilibrium. Nonetheless, several studies have been carried out, each of which indicates a different site for regulation. These are as follows:

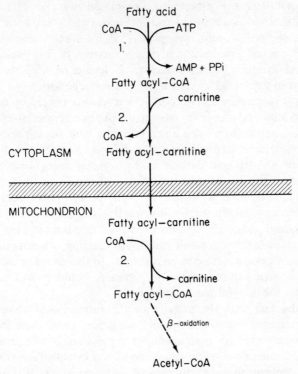

Figure 7.3. The early reactions involved in fatty acid oxidation in liver. (1) Fatty acyl-CoA synthetase. (2) Carnitine acyltransferase

(a) In 1964, Bode and Klingenberg[7] showed that isolated mitochondria oxidized palmitoyl-carnitine faster than palmitate, in the presence of ATP and CoA. Therefore they concluded that formation of acyl-CoA may limit fatty acid oxidation in the liver. A major objection to this theory is that the site of regulation arises *before* the metabolic branch point between esterification and oxidation. Consequently this would not provide independent control of either process.

(b) In 1965, Bunyan and Greenbaum[8] assayed the enzymes of the β-oxidation pathway and showed that the activity of the first enzyme (acyl-CoA dehydrogenase) was at least 10-fold less than those of the subsequent enzymes in the pathway. They concluded that this reaction was rate-limiting for fatty acid oxidation.

(c) In 1966, Garland and colleagues[9] measured the activities of acyl-CoA synthetase and palmitoyl-carnitine transferase in mitochondria isolated from rat liver. The activity of the palmitoyl-carnitine transferase was about half that of the synthetase. Furthermore, in isolated mitochondria the rate of oxygen uptake with palmitoyl-carnitine was twice that with palmitoyl-CoA plus carnitine (or palmitate, plus ATP, CoA and carnitine). In these experiments oxygen uptake was a direct measure of fatty acid oxidation and the final product was acetoacetate. It was concluded that the rate-limiting step in fatty acid oxidation by the mitochondria was the activity of carnitine acyltransferase. This conclusion was supported by the inability to detect any intermediates of the fatty acid oxidation system: the β-oxidation process would appear to possess a much greater catalytic capacity than that of the intramitochondrial carnitine acyltransferase. Since this study measured the oxidation of fatty acid derivatives by isolated mitochondria, it seems likely that the *intramitochondrial* carnitine acyltransferase limited fatty acid oxidation. (This enzyme is present in both the cytoplasm and the mitochondria in order to facilitate the mitochondrial transport of fatty acyl-CoA.) If mitochondrial carnitine acyltransferase is rate-limiting for fatty acid oxidation, it will catalyse a non-equilibrium reaction, whereas the reaction in the cytoplasm may be close to equilibrium. In this case any measurement of the *total* contents of reactants and products would be of little value in determining a meaningful mass-action ratio.

Despite the fact that the activity of the intramitochondrial carnitine acyltransferase may regulate fatty acid oxidation, there is no information available concerning the mechanism of regulation of this enzyme. Undoubtedly the rate of oxidation can be regulated by substrate availability—that is, the concentration of intracellular fatty acids, which is assumed to vary in the same direction as the concentration of plasma fatty acids. If the plasma concentration of fatty acid is lowered, the rate of oxidation is reduced, and vice versa (see Chapter 5 and reference 3).

D. INTRODUCTION TO KETONE BODIES

Ketone bodies consist of acetoacetate (CH_3COCH_2COOH), D-3-hydroxybutyrate ($CH_3CHOH \cdot CH_2COOH$) and acetone (CH_3COCH_3). The latter is of no physiological importance since it is usually present only in very small quantities and probably arises from spontaneous decarboxylation of acetoacetate. Ketone bodies were originally discovered in the urine of diabetic patients,[10,11] and this early association with a pathological condition led to the belief that they were merely useless products of metabolism that only accumulated in the blood under abnormal conditions. However, in the 1930s it was established that ketone bodies could be oxidized by certain extrahepatic tissues and it was suggested that they might be the form in which these tissues utilized fat (see Chapter 5, Section A.2(b)). Following the demonstration that the plasma concentration of long-chain fatty acids increases in conditions such as starvation and that the half-life is extremely short (2–3 minutes), it was suggested that fatty acids could provide most of the fuel that was used for oxidation during starvation in man (Chapter 5). Furthermore, it was shown that adipose tissue released its stored triglyceride in the form of long-chain fatty acids which most tissues could oxidize. Therefore the position of ketone bodies in fat oxidation was overshadowed by the interest and research into the control of fatty acid mobilization and the physiological importance of the plasma fatty acid level. Indeed, in a review article published in 1968 Greville and Tubbs[12] commented, 'Clearly, it is not obvious in what ways ketogenesis in fasting is a good thing for the whole animal; should the liver be regarded as providing manna for the extrahepatic tissues or does it simply leave them to eat up its garbage?' However, in the last few years evidence has gradually accumulated to suggest that ketone bodies play an extremely important role in caloric homeostasis; they provide an important respiratory fuel for muscle and for brain and they function as part of a feedback regulatory loop which prevents excessive mobilization of fatty acids from adipose tissue.

It is possible to subdivide the conditions of ketosis (high ketone-body levels in the blood) into *physiological ketosis*, when the plasma concentration is about 2 mM, and *pathological ketosis* when the plasma concentration is as high as 20–30 mM.[13] Pathological ketosis is found in experimentally-induced diabetes (for example, in acute alloxan-diabetic animals), in some lactating cows (bovine ketosis) and in the clinical condition of severe diabetes mellitus. This discussion is restricted primarily to a consideration of physiological ketosis.

1. Biosynthesis of ketone bodies

Ketone bodies are formed by a specific biosynthetic pathway in the liver. Originally they were thought to be intermediates of fatty acid oxidation, but this was shown to be incorrect when it was discovered that the normal intermediates of fatty acid oxidation are CoA derivatives. Furthermore, the 3-hydroxybutyryl-CoA formed in the liver during the oxidation of fatty acids has the L configuration, whereas the 3-hydroxybutyrate found in blood has the D configuration.[14]

Ketone bodies are synthesized in the liver from acetyl-CoA via the hydroxymethylglutaryl-CoA (HMG CoA) pathway, which is sometimes known as the *Lynen cycle*.[15] This pathway is described in Figure 7.4. The first step is the formation of acetoacetyl-CoA from two molecules of acetyl-CoA catalysed by the enzyme acetoacetyl-CoA thiolase. The concentration of acetoacetyl-CoA is maintained at a very low level and it is probably bound to the enzyme HMG-CoA synthase.[12] This has the advantage of overcoming the unfavourable equilibrium of the acetoacetyl-CoA thiolase reaction. HMG-CoA synthase catalyses the conversion of acetoacetyl-CoA to HMG-CoA and this reaction is chemically analogous to the formation of

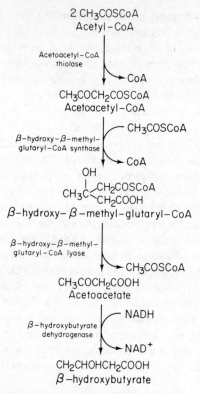

Figure 7.4. Pathway for the synthesis of ketone bodies in the liver (HMG-CoA cycle)

citrate by the condensation of oxaloacetate and acetyl-CoA. The HMG-CoA is a precursor of two pathways: first, it can be reduced by HMG-CoA reductase and NADPH to form mevalonic acid, which is an intermediate in the pathway for steroid biosynthesis; second, it can be cleaved by the enzyme HMG-CoA lyase to form acetoacetate and acetyl-CoA. Thus, the net reaction of the HMG-CoA pathway for ketone body formation is as follows:

$$2 \text{ acetyl-CoA} \rightarrow \text{acetoacetate} + 2\text{CoA}$$

A simpler mechanism for the formation of acetoacetate is that involving direct deacylation of acetoacetyl-CoA which was proposed by Stern and Miller in 1959[16]

$$\text{acetoacetyl-CoA} \rightarrow \text{acetoacetate} + \text{CoA}$$

It is now generally accepted that this is not involved to any large extent in the formation of ketone bodies. The activity of the deacylase in liver is less than 20% of the maximum rate of hepatic ketogenesis. Furthermore, the concentration of acetoacetyl-CoA in liver is very low, whereas the K_m of the deacylase for acetoacetyl-CoA is high.[5]

Hydroxybutyrate is formed from acetoacetate by reduction involving the enzyme D-3-hydroxybutyrate dehydrogenase

$$\text{acetoacetate} + \text{NADH} \leftrightarrows \text{D-3-hydroxybutyrate} + \text{NAD}^+$$

This enzyme, which is located on the inner membrane of rat-liver mitochondria, is very active and thus catalyses a reaction close to equilibrium. This property has been utilized in the investigation of the mechanism of ketosis (see Appendix 7.1).

2. Enzymatic pathway of ketone body utilization

Many tissues can oxidize ketone bodies, but liver is a notable exception. The utilization of acetoacetate by extrahepatic tissues involves the enzymes 3-oxoacid-CoA transferase and acetoacyl-CoA thiolase.

$$\text{acetoacetate} + \text{succinyl-CoA} \xrightleftharpoons{\text{3-oxoacid transferase}} \text{acetoacetyl-CoA} + \text{succinate}$$

$$\text{acetoacetyl-CoA} + \text{CoA} \xrightleftharpoons{\text{acetoacetyl-CoA thiolase}} 2\,\text{acetyl-CoA}$$

The equilibrium of the transferase reaction is towards the left (in favour of acetoacetate) but the equilibrium of the thiolase is towards the right (in favour of the formation of acetyl-CoA). Thus the linking of these two reactions overcomes the unfavourable equilibrium position of the former reaction. 3-hydroxybutyrate is metabolized by conversion to acetoacetate catalysed by the enzyme 3-hydroxybutyrate dehydrogenase. The activities of these enzymes in several tissues are presented in Table 7.2.

Table 7.2A. Relative activities in rat tissues of enzymes involved in ketone body utilization

| Tissue | Relative activities based on kidney = 100 | | |
	3-hydroxybutyrate dehydrogenase	3-oxoacid-CoA transferase	Acetoacetyl-CoA thiolase
Kidney	100	100	100
Heart	65	100	62
Adrenal glands	64	22	216
Brain	36	9	14
Lung	—	6	4
Spleen	2	5	10
Muscle (hind limb)	14	3	4
Liver	780	<0.5	140

The specific activities in the rat kidney are 1·5, 19·8 and 17·0 μmol/min/g fresh weight at 25 °C for hydroxybutyrate dehydrogenase, 3-oxoacid-CoA transferase and acetoacetyl-CoA thiolase, respectively.[23]

Table 7.2B. Activities of enzymes involved in ketone body utilization in different mammalian species[23]

Species	Enzyme activities (μmol/min/g fresh weight at 25 °C)					
	Kidney		Heart		Brain	
	3-oxoacid-CoA transferase	Acetoacetyl-CoA thiolase	3-oxoacid-CoA transferase	Acetoacetyl-CoA thiolase	3-oxoacid-CoA transferase	Acetoacetyl-CoA thiolase
Mouse	30·9	20·7	29·8	27·5	4·3	2·0
Gerbil (*Meriones lybicus*)	47·5	20·9	44·0	19·0	1·5	1·4
Golden hamster	16·7	16·3	29·1	6·6	0·7	0·4
Rat	25·5	14·4	24·8	8·9	2·1	2·1
Guinea pig	5·2	9·1	14·0	3·1	0·3	1·5
Sheep	35·4	13·2	2·7	1·3	0·2	0·4

There is some evidence to suggest that these enzymes catalyse reactions that are close to equilibrium. Although mass-action ratio data are not available, the maximum enzyme activities exceed the known rates of utilization of ketone bodies by heart and kidney, Furthermore, certain tissues (such as heart and kidney) are capable of *forming* ketone bodies if they are supplied with a high concentration of a precursor of acetyl-CoA (such as butyrate), despite the absence of the enzymes of the HMG-CoA cycle. The simplest hypothesis, which will explain this extrahepatic ketogenesis, is that the raised intracellular concentration of acetyl-CoA gives rise to acetoacetate via the reactions catalysed by acetoacetyl-CoA thiolase and 3-oxoacid-CoA transferase.[17]

E. PHYSIOLOGICAL IMPORTANCE OF KETONE BODIES

The concept of the glucose/fatty acid cycle emphasizes the importance of the plasma fatty acids in providing an alternative substrate to glucose for the provision of energy in tissues such as muscle. Since muscle can oxidize fatty acids, the obvious question is, why should fatty acids be converted to ketone bodies and provide yet another oxidative substrate? The answer to this problem lies in the toxicity of high concentrations of fatty acids in the blood and in the fact that they cannot be utilized to any large extent by brain.

1. Ketone bodies and long-chain fatty acids: complementary alternative substrates to glucose in muscle

The plasma concentrations of glucose, long-chain fatty acids and ketone bodies in rats and in human subjects during starvation are presented in Table 7.3. Starvation causes a 20–30% decrease in the plasma level of glucose, and increases in levels of fatty acids and ketone bodies of about 5-fold and 20-fold respectively. Since long-chain fatty acids are only slightly soluble in an aqueous medium, they are transported in the blood complexed with the plasma protein, albumin. At physiological pH and at physiological levels of fatty acid (1–2 mM) more than 99.9% of the fatty acid is probably complexed with albumin.[18] Under normal conditions, albumin is retained within the capillaries and thus it is found only in very low concentrations in the interstitial fluids (Figure 7.5). The concentration of long-chain fatty acid that will be present in the interstitial fluid will be less than 0·1% of the total concentration in the plasma—that is, about 0·001 mM. In resting muscle, when the vascular supply is reduced (vasoconstriction), the diffusion distance between the capillary and the muscle fibre may be considerable and, since the concentration of fatty acids is very low, the time taken for diffusion across the interstitial space may limit their utilization. On the other hand, ketone bodies are soluble in an aqueous medium and are free in the plasma

Table 7.3. Concentrations of glucose, long-chain fatty acids, ketone bodies, insulin and growth hormone during starvation in man and rat

Animal	Substrate or hormone	Fed	Concentrations in plasma (or serum) (mmol/l) Days of starvation							
			1	2	3	4	5	6	7	8
Man	Glucose	5.5	4.7	4.1	3.8	3.6	3.6	3.5	3.6	3.5
	Long-chain fatty acids	0.30	0.42	0.82	1.04	1.15	1.27	1.18	1.19	1.88
	Ketone bodies	<0.01	0.03	0.55	2.15	2.89	3.64	3.98	4.53	5.34
	Insulin*	>100	15.2	9.2	8.0	7.7	8.6	7.7	7.7	8.3
	Growth hormone†	—	1.9	3.1	5.8	3.7	8.8	6.0	2.5	3.4
				Concentrations in blood (mmol/l)						
Rat	Glucose	6.34	—	4.76	4.36	4.28				
	Long-chain fatty acids	0.66	—	1.31	—	—				
	Ketone bodies	0.22	—	2.81	3.03	3.35				
	Insulin*	28.7	—	4.2	—	—				

The concentrations in man represent the average of six normal subjects undergoing a prolonged voluntary fast. Day 1 represents an overnight fast and 2 to 8 represent each succeeding day of the fast. The information is taken from reference 37. The concentrations in the rat represent the average of a large number of rats. Two days represents the removal of food for 48 hours.[22,29]

* μ units/ml.   † ng/ml.

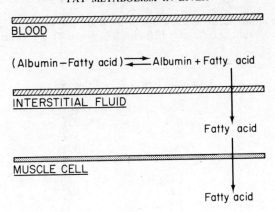

Figure 7.5

so that their concentration in the interstitial fluid will be about the same as in the plasma (2–3 mM during starvation). The concentration of glucose in the interstitial fluid will be about 4–5 mM. Consequently, ketone bodies will provide a fuel that will compete more effectively with glucose than will long-chain fatty acids. Indeed, in the case of heart muscle it has been observed that ketone bodies are oxidized in preference to fatty acids.[19,20] However, the diffusion distance for fatty acids is considerably reduced during mechanical activity when vasodilation occurs. Therefore the rate of fatty acid utilization will increase during exercise and the ability of this substrate to compete with glucose will be improved.

2. The utilization of ketone bodies by the brain

The work of Cahill, Owen and colleagues has established that in prolonged starvation in humans, ketone bodies can largely replace glucose as the important fuel of respiration for the brain (see also Chapter 6). Two lines of evidence support this conclusion. The most direct studies were performed on obese patients undergoing a 5–6 week period of therapeutic starvation.[21] The cerebral vessels of three such patients were catheterized and measurements were taken of arteriovenous differences in glucose, ketone bodies, fatty acids, lactate, pyruvate, oxygen and carbon dioxide. The rate of glucose oxidation by the brain could be calculated from these studies as about 24 g per day (cf. 120 g in the fed state) and that of ketone bodies as 37 g per day. This compares with an overnight fast, after which glucose oxidation accounts for more than 90% of the energy requirement of the brain (Table 7.4). An indirect estimate of glucose utilization by the brain during starvation can be obtained from the uptake of precursors of glucose by the liver and kidney (see Chapter 6, Section A.2(b)(i)). This estimate suggests that a maximum of about 33 g of glucose is available per day for the brain during

Table 7.4. The approximate fuel reserves of the body and the daily fuel consumption by different tissues during fasting for 12 hours, 8 days and 40 days in normal man under basal conditions[38]

	Overnight fast	8-day fast	40-day fast
	Body stores at end of period of fasting (kcal)		
Fat	100,000	88,000	42,000
Carbohydrate	680	380	380
Protein	25,000	23,000	18,500
Total	125,680	111,380	60,380
	Daily loss (last day of fasting period) (kcal)		
Fat	1,200	1,400	1,350
Carbohydrate	200	0	0
Protein	300	200	75
Total	1,700	1,600	1,425
	Fuel consumption (kcal)		
Brain: Glucose	400	100–150	50–75
Ketone	50	300–350	375–400
Carcass	1,250	1,150	975
Total	1,700	1,600	1,425

this prolonged fast, a figure which agrees reasonably well with the utilization rate of 24 g per day calculated from the arteriovenous difference. It can be concluded from this work that glucose utilization by the brain is reduced during prolonged starvation to approximately 25% of the requirement in the post-absorptive state (Table 7.4) and that ketone bodies are the major fuel for brain under these conditions.

Research into the utilization of ketone bodies by rat brain supports the conclusions reached from the studies with humans. The utilization of glucose and ketone bodies by rat brain has been measured *in situ* by catheterization techniques and it has been shown that in starvation (or following infusion of ketone bodies into a fed rat) the rate of ketone body utilization by the brain could account for about 20% of the oxygen uptake. In the fed rat the infusion of ketone bodies to a level of about 2 mM is sufficient to increase their utilization to a rate similar to that observed after 48 hours of starvation.[22] Complementary investigations into the activities of the enzymes that utilize ketone bodies (3-hydroxybutyrate dehydrogenase, 3-oxoacid-CoA transferase and acetoacetyl-CoA thiolase) have been carried out in brain. In both rat and human brain these enzymes are present at sufficiently high activities to account for the observed rates of ketone body utilization *in vivo*[23] (Table 7.5).

The work on rats has so far indicated that ketone body utilization can account for about 20% of the fuel requirement by the brain after 48 hours,

Table 7.5A. Activities of enzymes involved in ketone body utilization in brain from rats and humans[39]

Enzyme	Activities (μmol/min/g fresh weight at 25 °C)	
	Human brain (cortex)	Rat brain (whole)
3-hydroxybutyrate dehydrogenase	0·31	0·57
3-oxoacid-CoA transferase	1·63	2·53
Acetoacetyl-CoA thiolase	1·88	2·40
Approximate rate of ketone body utilization by brain *in situ* (μmol/min/g)	0·20	0·20

The rate of ketone body utilization by rat and human brain *in situ* is calculated from the arteriovenous difference and the rate of blood flow through the brain.[21,22]

Table 7.5B. Total activities of enzymes of the ketone body utilization pathway in brain, heart and kidney of suckling and adult rats

Enzyme	Tissue activities (μmol/min)					
	Suckling rats			Adult rats		
	Brain	Heart	Kidney	Brain	Heart	Kidney
3-hydroxybutyrate dehydrogenase	2·0	0·03	0·4	0·82	0·63	2·4
3-oxoacid-CoA transferase	7·2	0·9	3·0	3·7	11·5	32
Acetoacetyl-CoA thiolase	5·4	0·5	3·6	3·7	3·4	27

The total activity was calculated by multiplying the mean activity per gram fresh weight by the average weight of organ. Suckling rats were 20–24-day-old animals. Adults weighed 150–200 g.[24]

Table 7.5C. Activities of 3-hydroxybutyrate dehydrogenase and 3-oxoacid-CoA transferase in brain during postnatal development of the rat

Time after birth (days)	Enzyme activities (μmol/min/g fresh weight)	
	3-oxoacid-CoA transferase	3-hydroxybutyrate dehydrogenase
4	1·5	0·4
8	2·5	0·6
12	3·5	1·0
16	4·2	1·4
20	6·0	1·8
24	5·8	1·9
28	6·2	1·7
36	3·8	1·4
Adult	2·5	0·5

The activity of acetoacetyl-CoA thiolase remained fairly constant through this period at 4 μmol/min/g: the activity in the adult is about 2·3 μmol/min/g.[24]

or even after 96 hours, of starvation.[22] During prolonged starvation in obese humans, ketone body utilization can account for 75% of this fuel requirement. The reason for this species variation has not been explained. In rats the activities of the ketone-body-utilizing enzymes are not increased during starvation. Therefore the increased utilization is probably due to the elevation of the plasma levels of ketone bodies. Such experiments cannot be performed on human brain, so that it is not known if the increase in ketone body level is responsible for the increased utilization.

Another possible role for ketone bodies in the brain is the provision of precursor for fatty acid synthesis in the neonatal animal. Thus in the brain of the very young rat, the activities of the ketone-body-utilizing enzymes are higher than in the brain of an adult (Table 7.5). Indeed, from a comparison of the enzyme activities in various tissues in the neonatal rat, it can be suggested that the brain is the major organ for ketone body utilization at this stage of development.[24] Results of measurements of arteriovenous differences in the brain of the neonatal rat indicate that ketone body uptake is 3–4-fold greater than in the adult rat at the same plasma ketone body concentration.[22] This uptake occurs despite the fact that the plasma glucose and fatty acid levels are elevated. Thus it is unlikely that ketone bodies are being used only for energy production. Hence it is suggested that they may provide the precursor for the lipid synthesis, which is necessary at this stage of development for the myelination process. Perhaps long-chain fatty acids cannot be used because of a permeability barrier in the brain.

An important biochemical question still remains. How does the oxidation of ketone bodies by the brain cause inhibition of glucose utilization? The mechanism may be similar to that in muscle (Chapter 3, Section D.5) in that ketone body oxidation could elevate the levels of acetyl-CoA and citrate and cause inhibition of pyruvate dehydrogenase and phosphofructokinase. However, regulation of glycolysis by changes in the content of citrate may not be as straightforward in brain as it is in muscle. Thus, citrate plays an important role in the transfer of acetyl units across the mitochondrial membrane for the generation of acetyl-choline.[25] The only attempt to study this problem, so far, has been made with cerebral cortex slices of the guinea-pig.[26] In these experiments ketone bodies depressed glucose oxidation (about 20%) but did not inhibit glucose utilization (that is, glucose was converted to lactate instead of being oxidized). The depression of glucose utilization by ketone bodies, as well as the inability of brain to function totally on ketone bodies, remain problems of some biochemical and physiological importance.

3. Antilipolytic action of ketone bodies

Ketone bodies inhibit glucose utilization by isolated muscle and other tissue preparations. In vivo, high plasma levels of ketone bodies are always associated with conditions in which peripheral utilization of glucose is depressed. The glucose/fatty acid cycle (Chapter 5, Section C.1) which was originally based on such observations, predicts that the administration of ketone bodies to an animal should cause hyperglycaemia and a reduction in the rate of utilization of glucose. Somewhat surprisingly, experimental elevation of the ketone body level in a number of species results in hypoglycaemia. Madison and his colleagues[27] were first to demonstrate that in dogs the plasma concentrations of glucose and long-chain fatty acids were decreased by the infusion of ketone bodies. Moreover, the concentration of insulin in the pancreatic vein was increased. These observations suggested that high plasma levels of ketone bodies stimulate insulin release from the pancreas and that the resultant elevation in insulin level decreases lipolysis in adipose tissue. In some species (notably man) no appreciable changes in insulin levels are observed after administration of ketone bodies but nevertheless the plasma levels of fatty acids and glucose are depressed. These results may be explained by an inhibition of lipolysis in adipose tissue caused by ketone bodies. High concentrations of ketone bodies certainly decreased adrenaline-stimulated lipolysis *in vitro* in rat epididymal fat pads whereas malate, for example, has no effect.[28] However, the mechanism by which ketone bodies modify lipolysis is as yet unknown.

Experiments have been performed with rats in order to discover the means by which ketone bodies can influence fatty acid mobilization in this species. Sodium acetoacetate was infused into the inferior vena cava in fed, starved and streptozotocin-diabetic rats. (Rats are made diabetic by injection of streptozotocin which is thought to damage the β-cells of the pancreas more specifically than alloxan.) The results of this investigation[29] are shown in Table 7.6. In fed rats, the administration of ketone bodies lowered the plasma

Table 7.6. Effect of acetoacetate infusion on blood levels of glucose, long-chain fatty acids and insulin in the rat

Condition of rat	Time after acetoacetate infusion (min)	Glucose (mM)	Fatty acids (mM)	Insulin (μ units/ml)
Fed	0	6·2	0·82	20
	10	5·5*	0·73	50*
	30	5·2*	0·65*	29
Starved (48 hours)	0	4·0	1·2	6·4
	10	4·2	0·8*	18·5*
	30	3·6	0·8*	18·5*
Streptozotocin-diabetic rats maintained on insulin	0	3·3	0·8	47
	10	3·8	0·6*	43
	30	3·6	0·6*	33

The total concentration of ketone bodies in the blood during the experiment was 6–10 mM.[29]

* Indicates that the difference between the experimental and control (i.e. zero time) is statistically significant. Infusion of a similar concentration of NaCl has no statistically-significant effects.

glucose level by approximately 18 %, but there was no detectable change in the glucose levels in starved or diabetic rats. In all three conditions ketone bodies reduced the plasma level of fatty acids and, in the fed and starved animals (but not the diabetic), the level of insulin was raised. This work demonstrates that, although in all three conditions an elevation in the ketone body level causes a reduction in that of the fatty acids, the explanation for this effect may be different in the different physiological conditions. Thus, in the fed and starved rats the results could be explained by a stimulation of insulin release, whilst in the diabetic rats direct inhibition of lipolysis could be the answer.

Knowledge of the antilipolytic effect of ketone bodies makes possible a better understanding of the interrelationships between fat and carbohydrate metabolism in the whole animal. The plasma ketone body level is elevated whenever fatty acids are mobilized from adipose tissue. However, if the plasma fatty acid level is elevated to an excessive degree, the resultant elevation in ketone body level would inhibit fatty acid mobilization. This represents a feedback regulatory mechanism that will prevent *excessive* increases in the plasma fatty acid level, which is important since high concentrations of fatty acids are toxic.[30] This feedback mechanism incorporates at least two specific loops: a direct inhibition of lipolysis in adipose tissue and an indirect inhibition via stimulation of insulin release from the pancreas. Previously, the only mechanism for inhibition of fatty acid mobilization proposed for the cycle was via the increase in plasma glucose (and insulin) level that occurred in response to the inhibition of glycolysis by fatty acid oxidation. This is a very indirect mechanism of control. The plasma level of ketone bodies provides a more direct indicator of the fatty acid level and, since the process of converting fatty acids into ketone bodies in the liver results in amplification of changes in plasma fatty acid level (see above and Table 7.3), ketone bodies provide an ideal feedback regulator for lipolysis.[31] These antilipolytic effects of ketone bodies, together with the effects of ketone bodies on the glucose utilization by the brain, extend the original control mechanisms described in the glucose/fatty acid cycle (see Figure 7.6).

4. The role of the liver in fatty acid metabolism

Liver has the capacity to take up a large proportion of the fatty acids that are released by the adipose tissue (see Section C.1). These fatty acids can either be esterified (and secreted into the blood as VLDL) or oxidized to form ketone bodies. The liver has control over both of these pathways. The ketone bodies are released into the blood and can be oxidized by muscle, kidney and brain in which they provide an important alternative fuel to glucose during starvation (see above). Fatty acids can also be oxidized by muscle and they act as an alternative fuel to glucose (see Chapter 5). However,

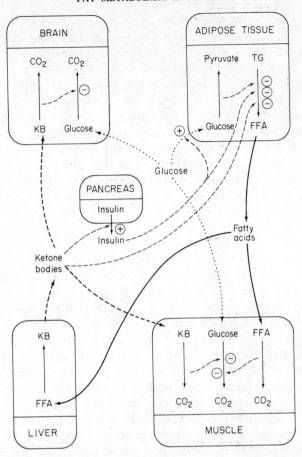

Figure 7.6. Extension of the glucose/fatty acid cycle. The regulatory cycle has been extended to include particularly the effect of ketone bodies on the brain and the direct and indirect antilipolytic actions of ketone bodies. Fatty acids are released from adipose tissue into the blood. The raised concentration of fatty acids in the blood increases the rate of fatty acid oxidation by muscle and liver. The increased oxidation in muscle reduces the rate of glucose utilization and oxidation. The oxidation of fatty acids in the liver leads to the production and release of ketone bodies into the blood. The increased concentration of ketone bodies in the blood increases the rate of their oxidation by the muscle and this further inhibits glucose utilization and oxidation in this tissue. The rate of ketone body utilization by the brain is increased and this leads to a reduction in glucose utilization by this tissue. The elevated concentration of ketone bodies in the blood stimulates the secretion of insulin by the pancreas; the increased concentration of insulin will inhibit lipolysis in adipose tissue. The increased concentration of ketone bodies in the blood inhibits lipolysis in the adipose tissue directly. These latter two effects on lipolysis provide a feedback mechanism so that the increase in concentration of fatty acids in the blood is not excessive. This figure should be compared with Figure 5.13

it is possible that during starvation ketone bodies provide the major oxidizable fat fuel for extrahepatic tissues. This implies that, at the levels of ketone bodies and fatty acids which occur in the blood during starvation, ketone bodies are the preferred fuel for muscle and kidney. (They are *known* to be the preferred fuel for brain; see above.) Some evidence in support of this idea has been obtained in the case of heart muscle. The presence of acetoacetate in the perfusion medium of rat heart reduces fatty acid oxidation by 75%.[19] In the dog heart *in situ*, catheterization studies have shown that the myocardial extraction of fatty acid is reduced when the blood level of acetoacetate is raised by infusion.[20] This should not imply that fatty acid oxidation *per se* is unimportant in starvation, it is merely restricted to one tissue, namely the liver. Ketone bodies, which are formed from the hepatic oxidation of fatty acids, are released by the liver for utilization by the other tissues. What does this obligatory 'predigestion' of the fatty acids by the liver mean in physiological terms? It means that the liver is endowed with the capacity to regulate fat metabolism in the whole animal. The liver can either increase the rate of general oxidation of plasma fatty acids by converting them to ketone bodies, or inhibit their general oxidation by esterification and the secretion of VLDL. Implicit in such a proposal is the suggestion that long-chain fatty acids are merely a means for transporting fat from the depot stores of the adipose tissue, via the blood, to the organ that will decide its eventual fate. The liver is, of course, ideally situated, both anatomically and physiologically, to decide the fate of fatty acids: the control mechanisms within the liver are continually assessing the level of blood glucose in the portal vein, the extent of the glycogen stores and the balance between glycolysis and gluconeogenesis. Moreover, this proposed role of the liver would provide an explanation for the fact that a large number of hormones stimulate the mobilization of fatty acids from adipose tissue (see page 224). Steinberg has commented upon the indiscriminative and unselective response of the lipolytic system in adipose tissue. However, this type of response is predictable if the liver is primarily responsible for the control of fatty acid oxidation. Thus, it *may* be necessary to oxidize fat in many different physiological situations in which different hormones will stimulate lipolysis. In all such conditions fatty acids must be made available in order for their fate to be decided in the liver. Therefore, adipose tissue must be responsive to a large number of different hormones. Finally, this hypothesis is consistent with the species variation in the proportion of the total body fat stored in the adipose tissue and in the liver: if the amount of fat stored in the liver is large, the adipose tissue stores are small and vice versa. The division of labour that has arisen in higher animals, in which the fat stores are dispersed throughout the body, demands a link between the liver and its fat store (the adipose tissue). This link is provided by the long-chain fatty acids (see Figure 7.7).

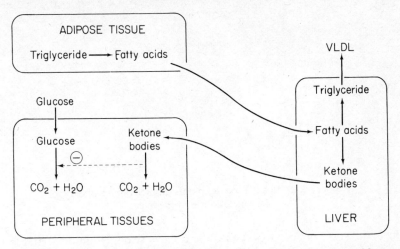

Figure 7.7. Diagram to illustrate the role of the liver in 'predigestion' of fatty acids to form ketone bodies.

F. REGULATION OF KETONE BODY FORMATION IN THE LIVER

The pathway for ketone body formation in liver, the HMG-CoA cycle, contains the enzymes acetoacetyl-CoA thiolase, HMG-CoA synthase and HMG-CoA lyase (see Figure 7.4). The maximum activities of these enzymes have been measured in liver and HMG-CoA synthase has the lowest activity. Therefore this enzyme may catalyse a non-equilibrium reaction and its activity might be modified by specific regulators. At present, little is known of the properties of this enzyme and consequently there are no theories of direct regulation of the HMG-CoA cycle apart from its regulation by substrate (that is, acetyl-CoA) concentration.

The close association of the elevated plasma fatty acid levels with ketosis has suggested that the rate of ketone body formation in the liver is regulated by the plasma fatty acid level. There is no doubt that the precursor for ketone body formation under conditions of prolonged ketosis (as in starvation) is plasma fatty acid. It has been demonstrated[32] that the liver may play some direct role in the regulation of ketone body formation (see Section C). The possible enzymatic sites at which the liver may exert this control (apart from the HMG-CoA cycle) are fatty acid esterification, fatty acid oxidation and the entry of acetyl-CoA into the TCA cycle (see Figure 7.8). The possible mechanisms for control of esterification and oxidation are discussed in Section C and the regulation of the activity of citrate synthase is discussed below. Indeed, investigations into the cause of ketosis at an enzymatic level have largely been devoted to the study of control of this enzyme. Thus, during

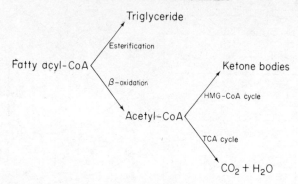

Figure 7.8. Possible control points (branch points) of fatty
acid metabolism in the liver

ketosis the entry of acetyl-CoA into the cycle is strongly inhibited and fatty
acid oxidation is arrested at the level of acetyl-CoA. The concentration of
acetyl-CoA is elevated and its metabolism is directed towards the HMG-CoA
cycle and the production of ketone bodies.

The evidence that the TCA cycle is inhibited under these conditions
arises from two types of investigation. First, oxygen uptake by the liver
can be accounted for primarily by two metabolic pathways, namely β-
oxidation of fatty acids to acetyl-CoA (and hence ketone bodies) and oxidation of acetyl-CoA through the TCA cycle. The stoichiometry of the pathway
from fatty acids to ketone bodies is well established and therefore the oxygen
consumed in the formation of ketone bodies can be calculated: one mole of
palmitate oxidized completely to acetoacetate requires 7 moles of oxygen,
whereas only 5 moles are required for formation of 3-hydroxybutyrate (one
mole of acetoacetate is equivalent to 1·75 moles of oxygen and one mole of
hydroxybutyrate is equivalent to 1·25 moles oxygen). The rates of acetoacetate and 3-hydroxybutyrate formation by the liver and the total oxygen
uptake can be measured experimentally. Using the theoretical oxygen-
requirement data, it is possible to calculate the oxygen that is required for the
ketone body formation and, by difference, the 'non-ketone oxygen' which is
used by the TCA cycle. Such calculations show that the 'non-ketone oxygen'
uptake is depressed by 80% during maximal rates of ketogenesis.[33] Second,
the release of $^{14}CO_2$ from ^{14}C-acetate, which provides some indication of the
activity of the TCA cycle, is severely depressed in liver slices and in the
perfused liver under conditions of ketosis.

1. Evidence that citrate synthase is a regulatory enzyme for the TCA cycle in liver

One problem in the application of the general approach to regulation is
the difficulty in identifying the regulatory enzymes in the TCA cycle. By

analogy with muscle, possible candidates are citrate synthase and isocitrate dehydrogenase (see Chapter 3, Section E.1). Although mass-action ratio data for both these reactions could be calculated, the interpretation of such data is complicated by the fact that all the participants of the reactions occur in both the mitochondrial and cytoplasmic compartments, whereas the TCA cycle operates only in the mitochondria. The maximum activity of citrate synthase in liver is low in relation to other enzymes of the cycle, and this is probably the best evidence for non-equilibrium character of this reaction. There are two types of isocitrate dehydrogenase in liver, an NAD^+-linked enzyme and an $NADP^+$-linked enzyme. At one time it was considered that only the NAD^+-linked enzyme was involved in the catabolic activity of the TCA cycle, but recent work in muscle has implicated both of these enzymes. The theories that have been proposed to explain the inhibition of the TCA cycle in liver during ketosis assume that citrate synthase is the enzyme that is inhibited. If it is assumed that this enzyme catalyses a non-equilibrium reaction, the increase in content of pathway substrate (acetyl-CoA), when flux through the cycle is depressed, indicates a regulatory enzyme according to the restricted definition of Chapter 1 (Section C.2). It must be emphasized that in this definition the substrate refers to acetyl-CoA and therefore one possible regulator is the alternative substrate for the enzyme, oxaloacetate.

(a) Theory of control of citrate synthase by availability of oxaloacetate

$$\begin{array}{ccc} \text{Acetyl-CoA} & & \text{Citrate} \\ + & \xrightarrow{\text{citrate synthase}} & + \\ \text{Oxaloacetate} & & \text{CoA} \end{array}$$

The important role of oxaloacetate in cellular respiration was known before the concept of the TCA cycle was developed. Indeed, it was suggested as early as 1937 that the large accumulation of ketone bodies observed in diabetes might be due to a deficiency of oxaloacetate.[13] It was readily demonstrated that homogenates of liver or isolated liver mitochondria produced ketone bodies when oxaloacetate was omitted from the incubation medium. However, neither the ketosis of human diabetics nor that of the alloxan-diabetic rat could be ameliorated by administration of oxaloacetate or any of its precursors (such as aspartate). A resurgence of interest in the role of oxaloacetate in the regulation of ketone body production resulted from the precise measurement of the content of oxaloacetate in freeze-clamped livers carried out by Wieland and his coworkers.[33] The content of oxaloacetate was found to be depressed in livers taken from alloxan-diabetic or starved rats, or from rats that had been fed a high-fat diet (see Table 7.7). Furthermore, when the mitochondrial concentration of oxaloacetate was calculated, it was found to be below the K_m of citrate synthase (that is, it could function as a regulator of this enzyme). Although there is general

Table 7.7. The contents of malate and oxaloacetate in normal and ketotic liver of the rat and cow[33,40]

Animal	Condition	Hepatic contents (μmol/g fresh weight liver)	
		Malate	Oxaloacetate
Rat	Control	294	5·9
	Alloxan-diabetic	444	2·2
	Fat-fed	555	0·47
Rat	Control	1,238	15·2
	Anti-insulin sera	1,690	11·2
Cow	Non-lactating	510	2·25
	Normal lactating	530	1·95
	Ketotic	530	0·65

agreement on the validity of these findings, Wieland and his coworkers have attempted to explain this decrease in oxaloacetate content according to changes in the redox state of the pyridine nucleotides, and this interpretation is disputed.

(i) *Control of oxaloacetate concentration via changes in redox state.* In ketotic conditions, the hepatic content of oxaloacetate is decreased but the content of malate, which is in equilibrium with oxaloacetate via the malate dehydrogenase reaction, is increased (Table 7.7). There are similar changes in the contents of other redox couples (such as pyruvate/lactate and dihydroxyacetone phosphate/glycerol phosphate)

$$malate + NAD^+ \leftrightharpoons oxaloacetate + NADH$$

$$lactate + NAD^+ \leftrightharpoons pyruvate + NADH$$

$$glycerol\ phosphate + NAD^+ \leftrightharpoons dihydroxyacetone\ phosphate + NADH$$

If these enzymes have access to the same pool of pyridine nucleotides in the cell, a change in the $NAD^+/NADH$ concentration ratio will produce changes in the same direction in all three redox pairs. Increased fatty acid oxidation in the liver results in a more reduced state of all these redox couples suggesting that the $[NAD^+]/[NADH]$ ratio has been decreased. Wieland and colleagues proposed that the decreased oxaloacetate concentration in the livers of ketotic animals was due to this change in redox state.

Lactate and glycerol phosphate dehydrogenases are found exclusively in the cytoplasmic compartment of the liver cell, whereas malate dehydrogenase occurs in both the cytoplasmic and the mitochondrial compartments. Therefore it is possible that the changes in the redox state are confined to the cytoplasm. Since citrate synthase is present within the mitochondria, it is the change in oxaloacetate *in this compartment* which is important for the control of the activity of this enzyme. The inner mitochondrial membrane is impermeable to oxaloacetate, therefore the near-equilibria catalysed by malate dehydrogenase on each side of the mitochondrial membrane may be different (see Figure 7.9). Indeed, the elegant work of Williamson, Lund and

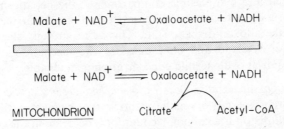

CYTOPLASM

Malate + NAD$^+$ ⇌ Oxaloacetate + NADH

Malate + NAD$^+$ ⇌ Oxaloacetate + NADH

MITOCHONDRION   Citrate   Acetyl–CoA

Figure 7.9

Krebs[34] has confirmed that such a difference exists. (See Appendix 7.1 for a discussion of the techniques for measuring cytoplasmic and mitochondrial [NAD$^+$]/[NADH] ratios.) The [NAD$^+$]/[NADH] ratios in the mitochondrial and cytoplasmic compartments were shown to be completely different. Moreover the cytoplasmic ratio decreased under ketotic conditions, whereas the mitochondrial ratio remained fairly constant (see Table 7.8).

Table 7.8. The calculated cytoplasmic [NAD$^+$]/[NADH] and [NADP$^+$]/[NADPH] ratios and the mitochondrial [NAD$^+$]/[NADH] ratios in livers from fed, starved and alloxan-diabetic rats

	[NAD$^+$]/[NADH]		
Condition of animal	Cytoplasmic	Mitochondrial	[NADP$^+$]/[NADPH]
Fed	725	7·8	0·012
Starved (48 hours)	528	5·6	0·002
Alloxan-diabetic	208	9·6	—
Sucrose-casein diet for 5 days	1,270	5·1	0·009
Low-carbohydrate diet for 5 days	443	4·0	0·002

The ratios are calculated from the formula, [NAD$^+$]/[NADH] (or [NADP$^+$]/[NADPH]) = [oxidized substrate]/[reduced substrate] × 1/K. The cytoplasmic and mitochondrial [NAD$^+$]/[NADH] ratios are calculated for the lactate dehydrogenase system and the 3-hydroxybutyrate system, respectively.[34] The cytoplasmic [NADP$^+$]/[NADPH] ratio is calculated from the NADP-linked malate dehydrogenase system (pyruvate + NADPH + CO$_2$ → malate + NADP).[36]

Knowledge of the mitochondrial ratio of [NAD$^+$]/[NADH] permits the calculation of the intramitochondrial concentration of oxaloacetate from the following equation

$$[\text{oxaloacetate}] = [\text{malate}] \times K_{MDH} \times \left(\frac{[\text{NAD}^+]}{[\text{NADH}]}\right)_{\text{mitochondria}}$$

Applying the assumption that malate is equally distributed between the mitochondrial and cytoplasmic compartments, the hepatic mitochondrial concentration of oxaloacetate increases from 0·11 μM in the fed state to 0·14 μM in the alloxan-diabetic state. This work strongly suggests that the hypothesis of Wieland and colleagues for the mechanism of control of the mitochondrial oxaloacetate concentration is untenable.

(ii) Control of oxaloacetate concentration via changes in gluconeogenic enzyme activities. Krebs and coworkers have shown that changes in the redox state within the mitochondria cannot account for a decrease in the concentration of oxaloacetate in this compartment. Nevertheless, they accept that a decreased mitochondrial concentration of oxaloacetate can explain the decreased activity of citrate synthase during ketogenesis. An alternative reason for the fall in oxaloacetate concentration is proposed. Conditions which cause high rates of ketone body production by the liver (for example, alloxan diabetes and bovine ketosis) are associated with an exceptionally high demand for glucose and it has been found that the maximum activities of a number of gluconeogenic enzymes increase under such conditions.[17] In the livers of alloxan-diabetic rats the activity of phosphoenolpyruvate carboxykinase is increased about two-fold whereas that of pyruvate carboxylase is hardly changed (Table 7.9). Therefore, the steady-state concentration of

Table 7.9. Activities of pyruvate carboxylase and phosphoenolpyruvate carboxykinase in normal and ketotic rat and cow liver[13,40]

Animal	Condition	Enzyme activities (μmol/min/g fresh weight liver)	
		Pyruvate carboxylase	Phosphoenol-pyruvate carboxykinase
Rat	Normal diet	1·18	0·48
	Starved (24 hours)	1·21	0·62
	Low-carbohydrate diet	0·94	0·74
	Alloxan-diabetic	1·26	0·92
Cow	Non-lactating	1·24	1·30
	Normal lactating	0·76	0·99
	Ketotic (lactating)	1·34	1·05

oxaloacetate should be decreased (see Figure 7.10). (The steady-state concentration of any intermediate depends upon the capacities of the reaction producing the intermediate and that removing it—see Table 4.4.

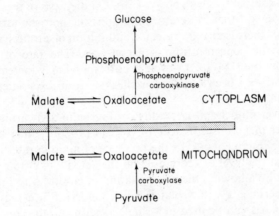

Figure 7.10. Role of pyruvate carboxylase and phosphoenolpyruvate carboxykinase in regulation of the concentration of oxaloacetate.

The limitation of this explanation for the change in mitochondrial oxaloacetate concentration is that it only applies in *severe* ketotic conditions (such as in alloxan diabetes). For this reason Krebs[13] has distinguished 'pathological ketosis', in which the ketone body level in the blood is very high, from 'physiological ketosis' in which the ketone body level in the blood is approximately 2 mM (as in starvation). In conditions of 'physiological ketosis' there is no change in the activities of pyruvate carboxylase or phosphoenolpyruvate carboxykinase (Table 7.9) and the above explanation for the decreased oxaloacetate concentration is untenable. Furthermore, it has also been shown that the activities of the two enzymes are unchanged in livers of cows suffering from bovine ketosis (see Table 7.9).

An important difference between these two theories for the control of the oxaloacetate concentration is that in Wieland's theory the total concentration of malate and oxaloacetate in the liver should either remain constant or increase, whereas in Krebs' theory the total concentration should be decreased. The hepatic contents of malate and oxaloacetate in various conditions are presented in Table 7.7. In alloxan diabetes and in animals that have been fed a high-fat diet the total content of oxaloacetate and malate in the livers is increased, whereas in bovine ketosis there is a decreased content of oxaloacetate but no detectable change in the content of malate.

(b) *Theory of control of citrate synthase by ATP*

If hepatic citrate synthase is a regulatory enzyme, its properties may provide the basis for a theory of control of the TCA cycle in liver. This enzyme is inhibited *in vitro* by ATP and to a lesser extent by ADP and AMP: the inhibition is competitive with acetyl-CoA. On the basis of these properties it has been proposed that in ketotic conditions the mitochondrial concentration of ATP is increased and this causes inhibition of citrate synthase and an elevation in the concentration of acetyl-CoA. The rate of ketone body production by the HMG-CoA cycle is correspondingly increased. Evidence for this theory has been obtained exclusively from experiments with liver mitochondria.[35]

Isolated liver mitochondria readily oxidize palmitoyl-carnitine to acetyl-CoA. Further metabolism of acetyl-CoA can produce either ketone bodies or TCA cycle intermediates. In the presence of fluorocitrate the TCA cycle is inhibited at the level of aconitase and the activity of citrate synthase can be measured by following the accumulation of citrate. A technical problem arises in experiments with isolated mitochondria. Since only a relatively few mitochondria can be used in a single experiment, the concentrations of citrate or ketone bodies that accumulate are too small to detect by conventional enzymatic analysis. This problem was elegantly overcome by relating the oxygen uptake and the amount of substrate (palmitoyl-carnitine) utilized in any one experiment to the eventual product of oxidation. The oxygen uptake by the mitochondria varies according to the amount of substrate utilized and according to the actual end-product of β-oxidation (acetoacetate, 3-hydroxybutyrate or citrate): the ratio of oxygen uptake to palmitoyl-carnitine utilized varies only with the product of β-oxidation (see Table 7.10). Using this technique it proved possible to detect whether mito-

Table 7.10. Stoichiometry of palmitoyl-carnitine oxidation by rat liver mitochondria[35]

Reaction	End product	Atoms oxygen/ moles palmitoyl-carnitine
A. Palmitoyl-carnitine + $7O_2 \rightarrow$ 4 acetoacetate	Acetoacetate	14
B. Palmitoyl-carnitine + $5O_2 \rightarrow$ 4 3-hydroxybutyrate	3-hydroxy-butyrate	10
C. Palmitoyl-carnitine + malate + $11O_2 \rightarrow$ 8 citrate	Citrate	22

chondria were producing citrate (that is, an active citrate synthase) or ketone bodies (that is, an active HMG-CoA cycle). The results of such experiments demonstrated that if conditions were selected such that the mitochondria produced sufficient ATP, ketone bodies were always the end-products of β-oxidation, but when the ATP concentration was experimentally reduced (for example, by addition of an uncoupling agent to the mitochondria), citrate was formed. These experiments provide good evidence that, in isolated mitochondria, citrate synthase could be regulated by the ATP concentration.

Measurement of the total ATP content of normal and ketotic livers provides another means for testing the theory. In the ketotic state the total hepatic content of ATP is *decreased* by about 15 % (Table 7.11). Therefore, if

Table 7.11. Effects of starvation and alloxan-diabetes on the contents of adenine nucleotides in rat liver*

Condition of rat	Hepatic content (μmol/g fresh weight)				
	ATP	ADP	AMP	ATP/ADP	ATP/AMP
Fed	2·45	0·760	0·130	3·2	18·8
Starved (24 hours)	1·78	0·778	0·155	2·2	11·7
Starved (48 hours)	1·86	0·825	0·184	2·3	10·4
Alloxan-diabetic	2·33	0·889	0·230	2·6	10·1

* The livers were freeze-clamped *in situ*.[41]

citrate synthase is inhibited by ATP in the liver under ketonic conditions, it is necessary to assume that the mitochondrial ATP concentration increases while that of the cytoplasmic compartment decreases. Furthermore one must assume that the ATP concentration in the mitochondria is so small in comparison with that in the cytoplasm that only the ATP concentration in the cytoplasmic compartment contributes significantly to the total cellular ATP content.

Satisfactory interpretation of all three hypotheses for the regulation of citrate synthase activity requires information concerning the distribution of metabolites between the mitochondrial and cytoplasmic compartments in the intact liver cell. At present, there are no methods available for such an experimental investigation, a fact which emphasizes a major limitation in modern biochemical technology, and which will restrict the development of knowledge in the field of metabolic biochemistry until it can be resolved.

APPENDIX TO CHAPTER 7

APPENDIX 7.1. THE $[NAD^+]/[NADH]$ RATIOS IN THE CYTOPLASMIC AND MITOCHONDRIAL COMPARTMENTS OF THE LIVER CELL

(a) Measurement of $[NAD^+]/[NADH]$ ratios

Lactate dehydrogenase, which is located solely in the cytoplasmic compartment in the liver cell, catalyses the following reaction

$$\text{lactate} + NAD^+ \leftrightarrows \text{pyruvate} + NADH + H^+$$

Since the enzyme is highly active in liver, it is assumed to catalyse a reaction close to equilibrium. Therefore the following equation should be approximately valid:

$$K_{LDH} = \frac{[\text{pyruvate}] \times [NADH]}{[\text{lactate}] \times [NAD^+]}$$

where K_{LDH} is the apparent equilibrium constant for the lactate dehydrogenase reaction at pH 0.

Therefore

$$\frac{[NAD^+]}{[NADH]} = \frac{[\text{pyruvate}]}{[\text{lactate}]} \times \frac{1}{K_{LDH}}$$

Since the contents of pyruvate and lactate can be measured in freeze-clamped liver and since the value for K_{LDH} can be measured in vitro (see Chapter 1, Appendix 1.1), the $[NAD^+]/[NADH]$ ratio in the cytoplasmic compartment of the liver cell can be calculated. This value is 725 in the liver of a well-fed rat and is decreased to values of 528 and 208 by starvation and alloxan-diabetes, respectively.[34]

The enzymes, 3-hydroxybutyrate dehydrogenase and glutamate dehydrogenase, are both located solely in the mitochondrial compartment of the liver cell where they catalyse the following reactions:

$$\text{3-hydroxybutyrate} + NAD^+ \leftrightarrows \text{acetoacetate} + NADH + H^+$$

$$\text{glutamate} + NAD^+ \leftrightarrows \text{oxoglutarate} + NADH + H^+ + NH_3$$

Since both enzymes are very active in liver, it is assumed that they catalyse reactions which are close to equilibrium. Therefore the following equations should be approximately valid

$$K_{HBD} = \frac{[\text{acetoacetate}] \times [\text{NADH}]}{[\text{3-hydroxybutyrate}] \times [\text{NAD}^+]} \qquad (7.1)$$

Therefore $\qquad \dfrac{[\text{NAD}^+]}{[\text{NADH}]} = \dfrac{[\text{acetoacetate}]}{[\text{3-hydroxybutyrate}]} \times \dfrac{1}{K_{HBD}}$

where K_{HBD} is the apparent equilibrium constant for this reaction at pH 0.

$$K_{GDH} = \frac{[\text{oxoglutarate}] \times [\text{NADH}] \times [\text{NH}_3]}{[\text{glutamate}] \times [\text{NAD}^+]}. \qquad (7.2)$$

Therefore $\qquad \dfrac{[\text{NAD}^+]}{[\text{NADH}]} = \dfrac{[\text{oxoglutarate}] \times [\text{NH}_3]}{[\text{glutamate}]} \times \dfrac{1}{K_{GDH}}$

where K_{GDH} is the apparent equilibrium constant for the reaction at pH 0*.

Since the contents of the redox couples and ammonia can be measured in freeze-clamped liver and since the equilibrium constants for the above reactions can be measured *in vitro*, the mitochondrial $[\text{NAD}^+]/[\text{NADH}]$ ratios can be calculated. For the 3-hydroxybutyrate dehydrogenase reaction the mitochondrial $[\text{NAD}^+]/[\text{NADH}]$ ratios were 7·8, 5·6 and 9·6 for livers from fed, starved and alloxan-diabetic rats, respectively. For the glutamate dehydrogenase reaction the corresponding values were 7·3, 4·7 and 10·8. Thus the two systems give rise to similar values for the mitochondrial $[\text{NAD}^+]/[\text{NADH}]$ ratios under various conditions.

(b) *The importance of the difference between mitochondrial and cytoplasmic redox states*

Measurements of the *total* contents of NAD^+ and NADH in liver tissue (or isolated compartments) do not provide valid information about the concentration of the pyridine nucleotides which are available to various dehydrogenase enzymes. Although the elegant work of Williamson, Lund and Krebs[34] enables the *concentration ratio* of $[\text{NAD}^+]/[\text{NADH}]$ to be measured in the two important compartments of the liver cell (mitochondria and cytoplasm), the *actual concentrations* of NAD^+ and NADH in these compartments are unknown. However, the results of this investigation have emphasized the restriction that is placed upon many, if not all, theories of control by the lack of information on such compartmentation. Despite the fact that the absolute concentrations of NAD^+ and NADH cannot be measured, it has been established that the mitochondrial and cytoplasmic compartments differ markedly in their redox state. Why should this difference arise? The cytoplasmic glyceraldehyde-3-phosphate dehydrogenase catalyses a reaction

---

* The values of the equilibrium constants used in the calculations of the $[\text{NAD}^+]/[\text{NADH}]$ ratios refer to pH 7·0, I 0·25 and 38 °C.

which, in liver, is probably close to equilibrium. Therefore the flux through this reaction depends upon the ratio of the concentrations of reactants and products.

$$NAD^+ + P_i + \text{glyceraldehyde-3-phosphate} \rightleftharpoons$$

$$NADH + 1:3\text{-diphosphoglycerate}$$

The rate of the reaction in the direction of glycolysis depends in part upon the concentration of glyceraldehyde-3-phosphate. This compound is in equilibrium with dihydroxyacetone phosphate via the action of triose phosphate isomerase and both triose phosphates are in equilibrium with fructose diphosphate via the action of aldolase. Since these equilibria are in favour of dihydroxyacetone phosphate (22/1) and fructose diphosphate (10/1) respectively, the concentration of glyceraldehyde-3-phosphate should be extremely low and this has been confirmed by the measurement of its content in liver. The low concentration of glyceraldehyde-3-phosphate will limit the flux through this reaction in the direction of glycolysis unless the [NAD$^+$]/[NADH] ratio is high.

However, in the mitochondria the [NAD$^+$]/[NADH] system must be maintained at a much more reduced level (about 10) in order to provide sufficient reducing power to 'drive' electrons along the electron-transport chain to generate ATP. If the ratio [NAD$^+$]/[NADH] in the mitochondria was as high as 10^3, reversal of oxidative phosphorylation would undoubtedly occur from the flavoprotein and cytochrome-c levels with consequent hydrolysis of ATP.

Thus, in order to maintain a satisfactory rate of glycolysis in the cytoplasm and a satisfactory rate of electron transport in the mitochondria, a large difference between the [NAD$^+$]/[NADH] ratios in the two compartments is required. This explains why the mitochondrial membrane is impermeable to pyridine nucleotides and why transportation of hydrogen across the mitochondrial membrane requires metabolite shuttles such as the glycerol-1-phosphate cycle (see Chapter 3, Section A.2). Moreover, these shuttles must be non-equilibrium processes if equilibration of the two redox pools on either side of the mitochondrial membrane is to be avoided.

Since the [NAD$^+$]/[NADH] ratio is very large in the cytoplasmic compartment, the ability of this system to cause reductions is limited. The reactions of glyceraldehyde-3-phosphate dehydrogenase and glycerol phosphate dehydrogenase, which are specific for NAD$^+$, can be used reductively in the biosynthesis of glucose and glycerol phosphate (for triglyceride formation). However, in the biosynthesis of fatty acids the C$=$O group has to be reduced to a CH$_2$ group and probably the NAD$^+$-NADH system in the cytoplasm of the liver cell is too oxidized to cause such a reduction. Consequently, fatty acid synthesis utilizes the NADP$^+$-NADPH system, which is maintained in a more reduced state. Recent work has shown that in the liver cell the $[NADP^+]/[NADPH]$ ratio is approximately 0.01 (Table 7.8). Therefore this system is five orders of magnitude more reduced than the $[NAD^+]/[NADH]$ system in the cytoplasm. This emphasizes the need for the two very similar pyridine nucleotide redox systems (NAD^+-NADH and $NADP^+$-NADPH) in living organisms.[36]

REFERENCES FOR CHAPTER 7

1. Vague, J. & Fenasse, R. (1965). In *Handbook of Physiology, Section 5, Adipose Tissue*, p. 25. Ed. A. E. Renold & G. F. Cahill. Washington, D.C.: American Physiological Society.
2. Robinson, D. S. (1970). In *Comprehensive Biochemistry*, **18**, 51. Ed. M. Florkin & E. H. Stotz. Amsterdam: Elsevier.
3. Mayes, P. A. (1970). In *Adipose Tissue*, p. 186. Ed. B. Jeanrenaud & D. Hepp. New York: Academic Press.
4. Williamson, D. H. (1973). In *Methods of Enzymatic Analysis*, 2nd edition (in press). Ed. H.-U. Bergmeyer. London: Academic Press.
5. Williamson, D. H. & Hems, R. (1970). In *Essays in Cell Metabolism*, p. 257. Ed. W. Bartley, H. L. Kornberg & J. R. Quayle. London: Wiley
6. Fritz, I. B. (1963). *Adv. Lipid Res.* **1**, 286.
7. Bode, C. & Klingenberg, M. (1964). *Biochem. Z.* **341**, 271.
8. Bunyan, P. J. & Greenbaum, A. L. (1965). *Biochem. J.* **96**, 432.
9. Shepherd, D., Yates, D. W. & Garland, P. B. (1966). *Biochem. J.* **98**, 3C.
10. Jaksch, R. von (1883). *Z. Physiol. Chem.* **7**, 487.
11. Minkowski, O. (1884). *Arch. Expt. Path. Pharmak.* **18**, 35.
12. Greville, G. D. & Tubbs, P. K. (1968). *Essays in Biochemistry*, **4**, 155. Ed. P. N. Campbell & G. D. Greville. London: Academic Press.
13. Krebs, H. A. (1966). *Adv. Enz. Reg.* **4**, 339.
14. Lehninger, A. L. & Greville, G. D. (1953). *Biochim. biophys. Acta*, **12**, 188.
15. Jaenicke, L. & Lynen, F. (1960). In *The Enzymes*, **3** (Part B), p. 3. Ed. P. D. Boyer, H. Lardy & K. Myrbäck. New York: Academic Press.
16. Stern, J. R. & Miller, G. E. (1959). *Biochim. biophys. Acta*, **35**, 576.
17. Krebs, H. A. (1969). In *Current Topics in Cellular Regulation*, **1**, 45. Ed. B. L. Horecker & E. W. Stadtman. New York: Academic Press.
18. Goodman, D. S. (1958). *J. Amer. Chem. Soc.* **80**, 3892.
19. Olson, R. E. (1962). *Nature, Lond.* **195**, 597.
20. Bassenge, E., Wendt, V. E., Schollmeyer, P., Blümchem, G., Gudbjärnason, S. & Bing, R. J. (1965). *Amer. J. Physiol.* **208**, 162.
21. Owen, O. E., Morgan, A. P., Kemp, H. G., Sullivan, J. M., Herrara, M. G. & Cahill, G. F. (1967). *J. clin. Invest.* **46**, 1589.
22. Hawkins, R. A., Williamson, D. H. & Krebs, H. A. (1971). *Biochem. J.* **122**, 13.
23. Williamson, D. H., Bates, M. W., Page, M. A. & Krebs, H. A. (1971). *Biochem. J.* **121**, 41.
24. Page, M. A., Krebs, H. A. & Williamson, D. H. (1971). *Biochem. J.* **121**, 49.
25. Srere, P. A. (1965). *Nature, Lond.* **205**, 766.
26. Rolleston, F. S. & Newsholme, E. A. (1967). *Biochem. J.* **104**, 519.
27. Madison, L. L., Mebane, D., Unger, R. H. & Lochner, A. (1964). *J. clin. Invest.* **43**, 408.
28. Björntorp, P. (1966). *J. Lipid Res.* **7**, 621.

29. Hawkins, R. A., Alberti, K.G.M.M., Houghton, C. R. S., Williamson, D. H. & Krebs, H. A. (1971). *Biochem. J.* **125**, 541.
30. Kerr, J. W., Pirrie, R., MacAulay, I. & Bronte-Stewart, B. (1965). *Lancet*, **1**, 1296.
31. Krebs, H. A., Williamson, D. H., Bates, M. W., Page, M. A. & Hawkins, R. A. (1971). *Adv. Enz. Reg.* **9**, 387.
32. Williamson, D. H., Veloso, D., Ellington, E. V. & Krebs, H. A. (1969). *Biochem. J.* **114**, 575.
33. Wieland, O. (1968). *Adv. Metabolic Disorders*, **3**, 1.
34. Williamson, D. H., Lund, P. & Krebs, H. A. (1967). *Biochem. J.* **103**, 514.
35. Garland, P. B. (1968). In *Metabolic Roles of Citrate*, p. 41. Ed. T. W. Goodwin. New York: Academic Press.
36. Krebs, H. A. & Veech, R. L. (1970). In *Pyridine Nucleotide-Dependent Dehydrogenases*, p. 413. Ed. H. Sund. Berlin: Springer-Verlag.
37. Cahill, G. F., Herrera, M. G., Morgan, A. P., Soeldner, J. S., Steinke, J., Levy, P. L., Reichard, G. A. & Kipnis, D. M. (1966). *J. clin. Invest.* **45**, 1751.
38. Cahill, G. F. & Owen, O. E. (1968). In *Carbohydrate Metabolism and its Disorders*, **1**, 497. Ed. F. Dickens, P. J. Randle & W. J. Whelan. London: Academic Press.
39. Page, M. A. & Williamson, D. H. (1971). *Lancet*, **2**, 66.
40. Baird, G. D., Hibbit, K. G., Hunter, G. D., Lund, P., Stubbs, M. & Krebs, H. A. (1968). *Biochem. J.* **107**, 683.
41. Start, C. & Newsholme, E. A. (1968). *Biochem. J.* **102**, 942.

INDEX OF METABOLIC EFFECTS
OF HORMONES

A. INSULIN

1. Effects on muscle

(a) In vitro

(i) Glucose transport. Insulin increases the transport of glucose across the muscle cell membrane. This is a specific stimulation of the membrane transport process (Chapter 3, Section C.2), the mechanism of which is not known.

(ii) Glycolysis. Insulin increases the rate of glycolysis in muscle. The resultant increase in flux through the hexokinase and phosphofructokinase reactions is likely to be caused solely by an increase in the concentrations of their substrates. Insulin, in the isolated rat heart perfused with a concentration of 5 mM glucose, increases the intracellular concentration of glucose and the contents of glucose-6-phosphate, fructose-6-phosphate and fructose diphosphate.[1] Thus, the stimulation of glucose transport raises the intracellular concentration of glucose and consequently stimulates hexokinase. The increased hexokinase activity raises the concentrations of glucose-6-phosphate and fructose-6-phosphate which relieves the ATP inhibition of phosphofructokinase and increases the activity of this enzyme[1] (Chapter 3, Section D.2). This theory proposes that glycolysis is increased primarily by the increase in the concentration of intracellular glucose. If intracellular glucose concentration could be measured precisely, it might be possible to ascertain, from a consideration of the properties of hexokinase *in vitro*, if this increase was sufficient to account for the observed stimulation of hexokinase activity. Unfortunately it is not possible to measure the precise concentration of intracellular glucose (see Chapter 3, Section C.2). Cori and coworkers proposed long ago that insulin stimulates hexokinase activity directly (see Chapter 3, Section C.2). There is, of course, no direct evidence to support such an effect, but the fact that, of the four known isoenzymes of hexokinase in mammalian tissues, type II predominates in the insulin-sensitive tissues,[2] has renewed interest in this possibility.

(iii) UDPG-glucosyltransferase. Insulin stimulates markedly the conversion of glucose to glycogen in muscle (Chapter 4, Section E.1). The activity of the regulatory enzyme for glycogen synthesis, UDPG-glucosyltransferase, is increased by insulin: the less active D form is converted into the more active I

form (Chapter 4, Section E.3). This conversion is achieved as a result of a decrease in the activity of protein kinase. However, in muscle, this is not brought about by a reduction in the cyclic AMP content. Two forms of protein kinase exist in equilibrium in the cell, one form is active in the absence of cyclic AMP (the C form) and the other requires cyclic AMP for activity (the RC form) (Chapter 4, Section E.5(b)). The effect of insulin may be to move the equilibrium in favour of the RC form so that the activity of protein kinase is reduced, despite the fact that the concentration of cyclic AMP in the cell is unchanged (Chapter 4, Section E.5(b)). It is not known how insulin could modify the equilibrium of the two forms of protein kinase.

(*iv*) *Protein synthesis.* Insulin increases the rate of protein synthesis in muscle tissue both *in vivo* and *in vitro*. The subject of the hormonal control of protein synthesis has not been discussed in this book since, if it were to be covered adequately, another volume would be required. In brief, insulin stimulates at least two processes in protein synthesis in muscle: the transport of amino acids across the cell membrane and the conversion of t-RNA-bound amino acids into protein (the process of translation which occurs at the ribosomal level). Most of the current research effort is concentrated upon an understanding of the effect of insulin on the translational process but there are a number of different theories which attempt to explain this effect. Several excellent reviews have been written on this subject of hormones and the control of protein synthesis.[3,4,5,6,7,8] One of the major difficulties in understanding the action of hormones on protein synthesis is that many of the enzymatic reactions at the ribosomal level have not yet been elucidated. Therefore it is not yet possible to define potential regulatory sites for the pathway of protein synthesis and this makes it exceedingly difficult to propose satisfactory theories of control according to the approach outlined in Chapter 1 (Section C).

The effects of insulin on protein synthesis and on carbohydrate metabolism are known to be independent—that is, the stimulation of protein synthesis by insulin is not dependent upon an effect on carbohydrate metabolism, and vice versa. Thus, in the absence of glucose in the incubation medium or in the presence of phloridzin (a potent inhibitor of glucose uptake by muscle), insulin stimulation of protein synthesis can be demonstrated[9] and, conversely, insulin increases glucose transport and glycolysis in the presence of inhibitors of protein synthesis (such as puromycin).[10]

(*v*) *RNA synthesis.* Insulin increases the rate of RNA synthesis in muscle. This is undoubtedly related to the effect of insulin on protein synthesis (see references 4, 6 and 8).

(*b*) *In vivo*

The *in vitro* effects of insulin on carbohydrate metabolism and on protein synthesis outlined above can also be demonstrated *in vivo*. Thus, both protein synthesis and glucose utilization by muscle are markedly reduced in alloxan-diabetic animals. Nevertheless, it is possible to speculate that the effect of insulin in stimulation of membrane transport of glucose is of little physio-logical importance under most conditions. Thus, the sensitivity to insulin of the glucose uptake process in muscle is much less than the lipolytic process in adipose tissue.[11] Consequently, *in vivo* it is possible that changes in the circulating level of insulin may influence glucose utilization in muscle not directly, but indirectly, via changes in the plasma fatty acid concentration. A decrease in plasma insulin level will increase the rate of fatty acid mobiliza-tion from adipose tissue (see below) so that the plasma fatty acid level is elevated and this in turn inhibits glucose uptake by muscle. An increase in plasma insulin level will lower the plasma fatty acid level and increase glucose utilization (see Chapter 3, Section D.5 and Chapter 5, Sections B.3 and B.4(b)(ii)). Possibly these indirect effects represent the mechanism by which insulin normally controls the rate of glucose uptake and only when excessive carbohydrate has been ingested is the level of insulin raised sufficiently to exert a direct effect on glucose uptake by the muscle.

In any discussion of the hormonal control of carbohydrate metabolism by muscle, the effects of hormones on fatty acid mobilization from adipose tissue must be considered, since these hormones *indirectly* modify carbo-hydrate metabolism in the muscle (see Chapter 5, Sections B.3, B.4 and C).

2. Effects on adipose tissue

(*i*) *Glucose transport and glycolysis.* Insulin increases the transport of glucose into the adipose tissue cell and increases the rate of glycolysis. The stimula-tion of glycolysis may be caused solely by the increase in the rate of transport of glucose into the cell and the resultant increase in the concentration of intracellular glucose (Chapter 5, Section A.1(b)(iii)). There is some evidence that insulin can modify the concentration of hexokinase in adipose tissue. The activity of this enzyme is decreased in starvation and alloxan diabetes and increased upon re-feeding or following insulin administration.[12]

(*ii*) *Esterification.* Insulin increases the rate of esterification in adipose tissue and this is particularly important in the control of fatty acid mobilization. The increased entry of glucose and the consequent stimulation of glycolysis may be responsible for an increase in the content of glycerol-1-phosphate which in turn may be the direct cause of the increase in esterification. How-ever, insulin might exert a more direct effect on one of the enzymes involved in the esterification process (see Chapter 5, Section B.3).

(*iii*) *Lipogenesis.* Insulin increases the rate of triglyceride synthesis from either glucose or acetate. The pathway from acetyl-CoA to long-chain acyl-CoA, like the glycolytic pathway, is stimulated by insulin. However, the mechanism by which insulin modifies the rate of this pathway is unknown.

Since acetyl-CoA carboxylase is considered to be the regulatory enzyme in this pathway and since it is activated by citrate, it is possible that insulin may increase the *cytoplasmic* concentration of citrate. However, insulin has no effect upon the *total* citrate content in isolated adipose tissue (see Chapter 5, Section A.1(b)(iv)). Recently, pyruvate dehydrogenase from adipose tissue has been found to exist in two forms, inactive (phosphorylated) and active (dephosphorylated), which are interconvertible via phosphokinase and phosphatase reactions. Insulin increases the proportion of the dephosphorylated (i.e. active) form in the tissue and this action may be important in the stimulation of the conversion of glucose and glycolytic residues into fat (Chapter 5, Section A.1(b)(iv)). However, this effect cannot explain how the hormone stimulates the conversion of acetate into fat.

(*iv*) *Pentose phosphate pathway.* The pentose phosphate pathway in adipose tissue is responsible for the generation of at least part of the reducing power (NADPH) necessary for fatty acid synthesis. Insulin increases the rate of the pentose phosphate pathway. The evidence indicates that this pathway is regulated by the availability of $NADP^+$, which implies that the insulin effect is due to a stimulation of fatty acid synthesis and a consequent increase in the concentration of $NADP^+$ (see Chapter 5, Section A.1(b)(ii)).

(*v*) *Lipolysis.* Insulin decreases the rate of release of fatty acids and glycerol from adipose tissue. This effect may be explained by a decrease in the concentration of cyclic AMP and a consequent decrease in the activity of triglyceride lipase (see Chapter 5, Section B.4(b)(ii)). It is not known how insulin lowers the cyclic AMP concentration. The antilipolytic action of insulin on adipose tissue is observed at lower concentrations than are required to stimulate glucose uptake by muscle.[12] This fact re-emphasizes the speculative possibility that under most normal conditions the physiological action of insulin in lowering the blood sugar level may be related to its ability to lower the plasma fatty acid (and ketone body) level rather than its ability to influence glucose uptake by muscle.

(*vi*) *Lipoprotein lipase.* Insulin increases the lipoprotein lipase activity in adipose tissue and consequently facilitates the uptake of plasma triglyceride. The increase in activity may be caused by a stimulation of the synthesis of this enzyme rather than an increase in specific catalytic activity and it is possible that the decrease in concentration of cyclic AMP plays some part in this postulated change in rate of enzyme synthesis.[13]

(*vii*) *Protein synthesis.* Insulin increases protein synthesis in adipose tissue, but this has not been studied to any large extent in this tissue.

3. Effects on liver

The liver differs from both adipose tissue and muscle in an important respect. The transport of glucose across the liver cell membrane is an equilibrium process and is thus not modified by insulin. Nonetheless, insulin is able to modify the rates of release and uptake of glucose by the liver both *in vivo* and *in vitro*.[14,15]

(*i*) *Glucokinase activity.* The role of glucokinase in the regulation of uptake and *release* of glucose by the liver has been discussed in Chapter 6 (Section B.1). The amount of glucokinase in this tissue appears to be regulated by the plasma levels of glucose and insulin: it has been suggested that insulin causes a specific increase in the synthesis of this enzyme in liver. There is no doubt that the activity of this enzyme increases in the liver under conditions when the plasma insulin level is high (as in carbohydrate feeding) and it decreases when the plasma insulin level is low (as in starvation and alloxan diabetes). The activity of glucose-6-phosphatase also changes but in the opposite direction to that of glucokinase. Insulin may be responsible for both of these changes (see Chapter 6, Section B.1). Since these changes in enzyme activity are the result of modifications in the amount of enzyme-protein, there is a time lag of several hours before these effects are observed. These changes in enzyme activity may be responsible, in part, for the effects of insulin on glucose uptake and release by the liver.

(*ii*) *Glycogen synthesis.* Insulin increases the rate of glycogen synthesis in liver by stimulating the synthesis of UDPG-glucosyltransferase as well as by causing the conversion of some of the D form of the enzyme into the I form.[16] Insulin may lower the concentration of cyclic AMP in the liver (Chapter 6, Section C.10(c)) and this could be responsible for the conversion of D form into the I form via an inhibition of protein kinase. The effects of insulin upon both UDPG-glucosyltransferase and glucokinase may be important in causing increased glucose uptake by the liver.

(*iii*) *Gluconeogenesis.* Insulin decreases the rate of gluconeogenesis in the liver. The reduced concentration of cyclic AMP may be responsible for this effect, although the mechanism by which cyclic AMP modifies gluconeogenesis is not known (see Chapter 6, Section C.10(c)). Insulin may also modify the rate of gluconeogenesis by reducing the availability of the precursors, amino acids and glycerol, in the plasma (see Chapter 6, Sections C.9 and C.11).

(*iv*) *Fatty acid and triglyceride synthesis.* Insulin increases the rate of fatty acid synthesis and triglyceride formation (esterification) in liver. Unfortunately, little is known about the regulation of these pathways in the liver (see Chapter 7, Section C.1).

(v) *Protein and RNA synthesis.* Insulin increases protein and RNA synthesis in the liver.[3,5,8]

4. Brain and kidney cortex

Despite the fact that insulin probably has no direct effect upon carbohydrate metabolism in brain or in kidney cortex, it does modify the metabolism in both tissues *indirectly* by changing the plasma concentrations of ketone bodies (see Chapter 6, Sections A.2(b)(i) and C.6; Chapter 7, Section E.2).

5. Other tissues

Insulin may modify the metabolism of other tissues but since these have not been discussed in this book they have been omitted from this index.

B. GROWTH HORMONE

There are several good reviews describing the metabolic and physiological effects of growth hormone (see particularly references 17, 18, 19).

1. Effects on adipose tissue

Growth hormone stimulates the mobilization of fatty acids from adipose tissue and hence causes an increase in the plasma fatty acid and ketone body levels. This effect is only observed in the presence of glucocorticoids. The stimulation may be explained by an increase in the concentration of adenyl cyclase in the cell, so that the concentration of cyclic AMP is elevated and the activity of the triglyceride lipase is increased (see Chapter 5, Section B.4(b)(i)). This effect of growth hormone may explain, at least in part, the long-established antagonism between the secretions of the anterior pituitary (particularly growth hormone and ACTH) and the secretions of the β-cells in the pancreas (insulin).[17]

2. Effects on muscle

The effects of growth hormone on muscle *in vitro* that have been described to date[8] are probably physiologically unimportant. However, its effects *in vivo* are of fundamental importance. First, growth hormone acts by increasing the mobilization of fatty acids from adipose tissue. The plasma concentrations of fatty acids and ketone bodies are increased and these inhibit glucose utilization by muscle and antagonize the action of insulin (Chapter 3, Section D.5). This is the basis of the glucose/fatty acid cycle (Chapter 5, Section C). Second, growth hormone, as its name implies, stimulates RNA and protein synthesis in muscle and other tissues.[3,5,8] In terms of rational metabolic effects of hormones, growth hormone may appear to be somewhat enigmatic. It is responsible, in part, for fatty acid mobilization from adipose tissue during starvation (that is, when there is no growth, or even negative growth), yet it also plays an important role in stimulation of RNA and protein synthesis and the control of growth. This apparent paradox only reflects our inability to understand fully the complex interplay of metabolic factors involved in the process of growth. Although an oversimplification, a possible explanation for this metabolic paradox has been proposed by Rabinowitz and Zierler.[21,22] They suggest that the period after a meal may be divided into at least three stages: immediate post-prandial, delayed post-prandial and remote post-absorptive.

In the immediate post-prandial stage, insulin is the dominant hormone so that storage of available fuels obtained from the diet takes place. In the delayed post-prandial stage, both insulin and growth hormone are present in the blood. This results in some fatty acid oxidation and spares carbohydrate and amino acids for biosynthetic reactions necessary for growth, which occurs at this stage. In the remote post-absorptive stage growth hormone is dominant and fatty acids are oxidized in preference to glucose, in order to conserve this fuel. This is the beginning of the starvation period. In other words, the metabolic effects of growth hormone may be divided into two classes, insulin-like and contra-insulin. The insulin-like or growth-promoting effects of growth hormone are obtained only in the presence of insulin. The contra-insulin effect (fatty acid mobilization) is obtained in the absence of insulin.[22]

3. Effects on other tissues

Growth hormone probably has a stimulatory effect on protein and RNA synthesis in most tissues, although its effects on these processes in tissues other than muscle and liver have not been studied in detail. Growth hormone can indirectly modify the metabolism of the liver by increasing the plasma concentration of fatty acids, so that the rates of triglyceride and ketone body formation increase (Chapter 7, Sections C.1 and C.2). An increase in the plasma level of ketone bodies stimulates gluconeogenesis in the kidney cortex (Chapter 6, Section C.6) and inhibits glucose utilization in brain (Chapter 7, Section E.2).

C. ADRENALINE AND GLUCAGON

Both these hormones activate the enzyme adenyl cyclase in a variety of tissues and therefore increase the concentration of cyclic AMP. At physiological concentrations of the hormones adrenaline should affect muscle and adipose tissue and glucagon should affect liver and adipose tissue.[23]

In muscle the biochemical and physiological effects of adrenaline are to activate phosphorylase and stimulate glycogen breakdown, so that glycolytic intermediates are provided for the energy that will be necessary in the 'fight or flight' muscular activity. A detailed discussion of the evidence and the physiological importance of the mechanism by which adrenaline controls phosphorylase is presented in Chapter 4 (Section D.3). In muscles which possess endogenous triglyceride (usually red muscles), an elevation in the cyclic AMP content may activate the triglyceride lipase and provide fatty acyl-CoA, as a fuel for respiration, in addition to glycolytic intermediates obtained from glycogen. In adipose tissue, the triglyceride lipase is stimulated by the rise in cyclic AMP level, fatty acids are mobilized, and the plasma fatty acid level is increased. This is important in conditions of stress, since both the endogenous fuels (glycogen and triglyceride in the muscles) and the exogenous fuels (fatty acids and glucose in the blood) are mobilized. The hormonal control of fatty acid mobilization during stress is discussed in detail in Chapter 5 (Section B.4(a)).

In terms of the molecular action of hormones, the mechanisms by which glucagon and adrenaline activate adenyl cyclase are important, since they must represent very early biochemical events in the actions of these hormones. At present, it seems likely that the hormone initially binds to an acceptor molecule on the surface of the cell membrane and this somehow modifies the catalytic activity of adenyl cyclase. This elevates the intracellular concentration of cyclic AMP which functions as a 'secondary messenger' *inside* the cell.[24]

Glucagon stimulates triglyceride lipase activity in adipose tissue and this results in fatty acid mobilization. This effect of glucagon may be of physiological importance in starvation (see Chapter 5, Section B.4(b)(iii)). In liver, glucagon raises the intracellular concentration of cyclic AMP and this stimulates glycogenolysis and gluconeogenesis (see Chapter 6, Sections A.2(a) and C.10, C.11). Glucagon also increases the entry of amino acids into liver, which is possibly important in the control of gluconeogenesis (Chapter 6, Section C.9). However, it is not known if this effect of glucagon is dependent upon changes in the cyclic AMP concentration in the liver cell.

REFERENCES FOR HORMONE INDEX

1. Newsholme, E. A. & Randle, P. J. (1964). *Biochem. J.* **93**, 641.
2. Katzen, H. M. & Schimke, R. T. (1965). *Proc. Nat. Acad. Sci. U.S.A.* **54**, 1218.
3. Korner, A. (1962). In *Protein Metabolism*, p. 2. Ed. F. Gross. Berlin: Springer-Verlag.
4. Wool, I. G. (1965). In *Mechanisms of Hormone Action*, p. 98. Ed. P. Karlson. New York: Academic Press.
5. Korner, A. (1965). *Rec. Prog. Horm. Res.* **21**, 205.
6. Wool, I. G., Stirewalt, W. S., Kurihara, K., Low, R. B., Bailey, P. & Oyer, D. (1968). *Rec. Prog. Horm. Res.* **24**, 139.
7. Tata, J. R. (1966). *Prog. Nucleic Acid Res. molec. Biol.* **5**, 191.
8. Manchester, K. L. (1968). In *The Biological Basis of Medicine*, **2**, 221. Ed. E. E. Bittar & N. Bittar. London: Academic Press.
9. Manchester, K. L. & Young, F. G. (1961). *Vitamins & Hormones*, **19**, 95.

10. Ebaue-Bonis, D., Chambaut, A. M., Volfin, P. & Clausser, H. (1963). *Nature, Lond.* **199**, 1183.
11. Zierler, K. L. & Rabinowitz, D. (1963). *Medicine*, **42**, 385.
12. Katzen, H. M. (1967). *Adv. Enz. Reg.* **5**, 335.
13. Wing, D. R. & Robinson, D. S. (1968). *Biochem. J.* **109**, 841.
14. Steele, R. (1966). *Ergebnisse der Physiol.* **57**, 91.
15. Randle, P. J. (1964). In *The Hormones*, **4**, 481. Ed. G. Pincus, K. V. Thimann & E. B. Astwood. New York: Academic Press.
16. Steiner, D. F. & King, J. (1964). *J. biol. Chem.* **239**, 1292.
17. Ketterer, B., Randle, P. J. & Young, F. G. (1957). *Ergebnisse der Physiol.* **49**, 127.
18. Daughaday, W. H. & Kipnis, D. M. (1966). *Rec. Prog. Horm. Res.* **22**, 49.
19. Tata, J. R. (1970). In *Biochemical Actions of Hormones,* **1**, 89. Ed. G. Litwack. New York: Academic Press.
20. McGarry, E. E. & Beck, J. C. (1972). In *Human Growth Hormone*, p. 25. Ed. A. Stuart Mason. William Heinemann Medical Books Ltd.
21. Rabinowitz, D. & Zierler, K. L. (1963). *Nature, Lond.* **199**, 913.
22. Rabinowitz, D., Merimee, T. J. & Burgess, J. A. (1966). *Diabetes*, **15**, 905.
23. Exton, J. H., Mallette, L. E., Jefferson, L. S., Wong, E. H. A., Friedmann, N., Miller, T. B. & Park, C. R. (1970). *Rec. Prog. Horm. Res.* **26**, 411.
24. Sutherland, E. W., Øye, I. & Butcher, R. W. (1965). *Rec. Prog. Horm. Res.* **21**, 623.

INDEX